Marinella Astuto

Editor

Basics

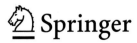 Springer

Marinella Astuto, MD
Department of Anesthesia and Intensive Care
Pediatric Anesthesia and Intensive Care Section
Catania University Hospital
Catania, Italy

Library of Congress Control Number: 2008936497

ISBN 978-88-470-0654-6 Springer Milan Berlin Heidelberg New York
e-ISBN 978-88-470-0655-3

Springer is a part of Springer Science+Business Media
springer.com
© Springer-Verlag Italia 2009

Cover design: Simona Colombo, Milan, Italy
Typesetting: Graphostudio, Milan, Italy
Printing and binding: Grafiche Porpora, Segrate (MI), Italy

Printed in Italy
Springer-Verlag Italia S.r.l. – Via Decembrio 28 – I-20137 Milan

*To my father, who would have been the first
and most interested reader of this book,
and to Maria, my teacher, both of anesthesia and of life*

Foreword

In March 2006 I took up my new position as Chairman of the Department of Anesthesia and Intensive Care and Director of the School at the University of Catania, a position that represents an ideal continuity with 30 years of professional teaching at the bed-side involving several hundred students and anesthesiologists in training at Trieste Medical School.

In Catania the excellent working group of anesthesiologists established a cooperative program with the prestigious Children's Hospital of McGill University in Montreal, Canada.

Giuliana Rizzo, MD, during 2 years of fellowship in Montreal was interested in taking part actively in a dynamic process of development in clinical anesthesia, intensive care and pain management in neonates and children. The excellent background of Giuliana Rizzo gained at the University of Catania in this field favored her appointment to the staff of the Children's Hospital with autonomy and decision making ability in routine procedures and also in the management of difficult and life-threatening critical care conditions.

In September 2007 a special task force coordinated by Marinella Astuto, MD, as clinical leader of the Catania team in pediatric anesthesia, in collaboration with the Montreal group directed by Prof. Ronald Gottsman, organized a 3-day masterclass in pediatric anesthesia, intensive care and pain in which 45 experts from several regions of Italy participated.

During 2008 the two groups worked actively to finalize the 19 chapters which are collected in the present volume. My hope is that residents and practicing anesthesiologists find the contents of this book a useful guide to good clinical practice.

Catania, 27 September 2008   *Prof. Antonino Gullo*
Director, Department and School of Anesthesia
and Intensive Care, Catania School of Medicine, Catania, Italy
Council World Federation Societies of Intensive
and Critical Care Medicine (WFSICCM)

Preface

The success of the fellowship program developed by the School of Medicine of Catania in collaboration with McGill University of Montreal led to the organization of the first masterclass in anesthesia, intensive care and pain in neonates and children, held in September 2007 in Catania with a selected group of participants.

An additional remarkable outcome of this cooperation is the present book published by Springer-Verlag Italia and based on the content of the masterclass including formal lectures, interactive sessions, case presentation, and problem solving.

It is my opinion that anyone who anesthetizes infants and children, who takes care of children in the ICU or who manages pain in children must understand the differences in physiology and clinical pharmacology that exist between children and adults. For many years it has been considered that infants and children are small adults, but in the majority of situations this is no true. The anesthesiologist who fails to understand these differences will have a hard time when facing unexpected events, and the result could be dangerous for the patient.

My goal was to produce a book that provides a basic approach to anesthesia, perioperative medicine, intensive care and pain management in pediatric patients (from the neonate to the child). To reach this goal, I convinced a group of pediatricians, experts on infectious diseases, and anesthesiologists to contribute with their talent to pass on their expertise to all allied professionals interested in the field.

I thank Prof. Gullo for his enthusiasm and strong support for an exciting and successful initiative. Finally, I am grateful to the residents; I have learned as much from them as they have heard from me. Their curiosity and their interest in improving their knowledge and professional skill shows to all that the mission to achieve excellence may be possible.

Catania, 27 September 2008   *Marinella Astuto, MD*

Table of Contents

List of Contributors XIII

List of Abbreviations XVII

Part I: Highlights

1   **Anatomy and Physiology in Neonates and Children**   3
    M. Astuto, A.L. Paratore, A. Gullo

2   **Strategy to Manage Pediatric Patients: the Family and the Child**   11
    G. Rosano, M. Antoci, M. Astuto

3   **Off-Label Drugs in Pediatric Perioperative Medicine**   19
    M. Astuto, M. Antoci, A. Gullo

Part II: Guidelines and Standardization of Procedures

4   **The Pediatric Difficult Airway**   31
    T. Valois

5   **Central Venous Cannulation Techniques**   49
    N. Disma, M. Astuto

6   **Prevention of Bloodstream Infections**   61
    H.K.F. van Saene, K. Thorburn, A.J. Petros

Part III: Perioperative Medicine, Intensive Care, Pain

7   **Preoperative Evaluation**   71
    I. Salvo, A. Camporesi

8 Anesthesia Induction 85
M. Astuto, D. Lauretta

**9 Monitoring the Level of Anesthesia and Sedation in Children:
An Overview** 101
N. Disma, A.J. Davidson, M. Astuto

10 Locoregional Anesthesia in Children 113
M. Astuto

11 Perioperative Fluid Management 135
D.E. Withington

12 Adrenal Insufficiency in Pediatric Critical Illness 151
G. Rizzo, K. Menon

13 Perioperative Care in Pediatric Cardiac Surgery 161
J. Lavoie

14 Acute Pain Service: Clinical Assessment and Standard of Care 173
J. Desparmet

15 Anesthesia Outside the Operating Room 185
T. Valois

16 Tracheotomy in Children 197
G. Rizzo, P. Murabito, F. Rubulotta, C. Cutuli, M. Sorbello, M. Astuto

17 Infection Control in Neonates and Children 215
R.E. Sarginson, H.K.F. van Saene, A. Gullo

18 Pediatric Palliative Care in the Intensive Care Unit 231
S. Liben

**19 Chronic Pain Management: Organization,
Techniques and Guidelines** 241
J. Desparmet

Subject Index 255

List of Contributors

Manuela Antoci
Department of Anesthesia and Intensive Care, Postgraduate School of Anesthesia
and Intensive Care, Catania University Hospital, Catania, Italy

Marinella Astuto
Department of Anesthesia and Intensive Care, Pediatric Anesthesia and Intensive
Care Section, Catania University Hospital, Catania, Italy

Anna Camporesi
Department of Pediatric Anesthesia and Intensive Care, "V. Buzzi" Hospital,
Milan, Italy

Carmela Cutuli
Department of Anesthesia and Intensive Care, Postgraduate School of Anesthesia
and Intensive Care, Catania University Hospital, Catania, Italy

Andrew J. Davidson
Department of Anesthesia and Pain Management, Royal Children's Hospital,
Melbourne, Australia

Joëlle Desparmet
Acute and Chronic Pain Service (Pediatric), Montreal Children's Hospital,
Montreal, Canada

Nicola Disma
Department of Anesthesia, Pediatric and Neonatal Intensive Care, "G. Gaslini"
Children's Hospital, Genoa, Italy

Antonino Gullo
Department of Anesthesia and Intensive Care, Postgraduate School of Anesthesia
and Intensive Care, Catania University Hospital, Catania, Italy

Daniela Lauretta
Department of Anesthesia and Intensive Care, Postgraduate School of Anesthesia and Intensive Care, Catania University Hospital, Catania, Italy

Josée Lavoie
"McGill" University, Pediatric Cardiac Anesthesia, Montreal Children's Hospital "McGill" University Health Center, Montreal, Canada

Stephen Liben
Palliative Care Program, Montreal Children's Hospital, Montreal, Canada

Kusum Menon
Children's Hospital of Eastern Ontario, University of Ottawa, Ottawa, Canada

Paolo Murabito
Department of Anesthesia and Intensive Care, Postgraduate School of Anesthesia and Intensive Care, Catania University Hospital, Catania, Italy

Anna L. Paratore
Department of Anesthesia and Intensive Care, Postgraduate School of Anesthesia and Intensive Care, Catania University Hospital, Catania, Italy

Andy J. Petros
Paediatric Intensive Care Unit, "Great Ormond Street" Children's Hospital - PICU, London, U.K.

Giuliana Rizzo
Department of Anesthesia and Intensive Care, Pediatric Anesthesia and Intensive Care Section, Catania University Hospital, Catania, Italy;
Department of Anesthesia and Palliative Care, Montreal Children's Hospital, "McGill" University, Montreal, Canada

Giuseppe Rosano
Department of Anesthesia and Intensive Care, Pediatric Anesthesia and Intensive Care Section, Catania University Hospital, Catania, Italy

Francesca Rubulotta
Department of Anesthesia and Intensive Care, Postgraduate School of Anesthesia and Intensive Care, Catania University Hospital, Catania, Italy

Ida Salvo
Department of Pediatric Anesthesia and Intensive Care, "V. Buzzi" Hospital, Milan, Italy

Richard E. Sarginson
Paediatric Intensive Care Unit, Royal Liverpool Children's NHS Trust Alder Hey
Hospital, Liverpool, U.K.

Massimiliano Sorbello
Department of Anesthesia and Intensive Care, Postgraduate School of Anesthesia
and Intensive Care, Catania University Hospital, Catania, Italy

Kentigern Thorburn
Department of Paediatric Intensive Care, Royal Liverpool Children's Hospital,
Alder Hey, Liverpool, U.K.

Teresa Valois
Department of Anesthesia, Montreal Children's Hospital, Montreal, Canada

Hendrick K.F. van Saene
Department of Medical Microbiology/Infection Control, Royal Liverpool
Children's NHS Trust Alder Hey Hospital, Liverpool, U.K.

Davinia E. Withington
Department of Anesthesia, Montreal Children's Hospital, Montreal, Canada

List of Abbreviations

AAI	A-line ARX Index
AAP	American Academy of Pediatrics
AAP	American Association of Pediatrics
ACE	Angiotensin-converting Enzyme
ACTH	Adrenocorticotropin Hormone
ADH	Antidiuretic Hormone
AGNB	Anaerobic Gram-negative Bacteria
AHC	Adrenal Hypoplasia Congenita
ALD	Adrenoleukodystrophy
AOP	Apnea of Prematurity
APS	Acute Pain Service
APS	Anesthesia Patient Safety Foundation
ASA	American Society of Anesthesiologists
ASA-PS	American Society of Anesthesiologists Physical Status
ASD	Atrial Septal Defect
ATP	Adenosine-5'-triphosphate
ATPase	Adenosine-5'-triphosphatase
BHR	Bronchial Hyperresponsiveness
BIS	Bispectral Index
BMI	Body Mass Index
BSI	Bloodstream Infections
BUN	Blood Urea Nitrogen
CBG	Corticosteroid-binding Globulin
CDC	Center for Disease Control and Prevention
CHD	Congenital Heart Disease
CHEOPS	Children's Hospital of Eastern Ontario Pain Scale
CI	Confidence Interval
CNS	Central Nervous System
CNS	Coagulase-negative Staphylococcus
CPAP	Continuous Positive Airway Pressure
CPB	Cardiopulmonary Bypass
CPNB	Continuous Peripheral Nerve Block
CRH	Corticotropin-releasing Hormone

CRPS	Complex Regional Pain Syndromes
CSF	Cerebrospinal Fluid
CSI	Cerebral State Index
CVC	Central Venous Catheter
CVP	Central Venous Pressure
DMD	Duchenne's Muscular Dystrophy
Doppler US	Doppler ultrasound
DPA	Difficult Pediatric Airway
ECMO	Extracorporeal Membrane Oxygenation
EEG	Electroencephalography
EMLA	Eutectic Misture of Local Anesthetics
ETT	Endotracheal Tube
ENT	Endonasal Tube
ESBL	Extended-spectrum Beta-lactamase
FDA	Food and Drug Administration
FEV1	Forced Expiratory Volume in one second
FLACC	Face, Legs, Activity, Cry, Consolability scale
FRC	Functional Residual Capacity
FVC	Forced Vital Capacity
GABA	γ-aminobutyric Acid
HIV	Human Immunodeficiency Virus
HPA	Hypothalamic-pituitary-adrenal axis
IASP	International Association for the Study of Pain
ICU	Intensive Care Unit
IJV	Internal Jugular Vein
INR	International Normalized Ratio
JCAHO	Joint Commission on Accreditation of Healthcare Organizations
LMA	Laryngeal Mask Airway
LOR	Loss of Resistance
LST	Life-sustaining Treatment
MAC	Minimum Alveolar Concentrations
MAP	Mitogen-activated Protein
MEAC	Minimum Effective Analgesic Concentration
MH	Malignant Hyperthermia
MRA	Magnetic Resonance Angiography
MRSA	Methicillin-resistant Staphylococcus Aureus
NICE	National Institute for Clinical Excellence
NIRS	Near Infrared Spectroscopy
NIS	Near Infrared Spectroscopy
NMDA	Receptor blocker N-methyl-D-aspartic Acid
NSAIDs	Nonsteroidal Antiinflammatory Drugs
OAA/S Scale	Observer's Assessment of Alertness/Sedation Scale
OR	Odds Ratio
OR	Operating Room
OSAS	Obstructive Sleep Apnea Syndrome

PACU	Postanesthesia Care Unit
PAP	Pulmonary Artery Pressure
PCA	Patient-controlled Analgesia
PEEP	Positive End-Expiratory Pressure
PICC	Peripherally Inserted Central Catheter
PICU	Pediatric Intensive Care Unit
PIP	Pediatric Investigation Plan
PPMs	Potential Pathogenic Microorganisms
PT	Prothrombin Time
PTT	Partial Thromboplastin Time
PTT	Pediatric Tracheotomy Teams
PVC	Polyvinyl Chloride
RAP	Recurrent Abdominal Pain
RCTs	Randomized Controlled Trials
RR	Relative Risk
RRS	Rapid Response Systems
RSD	Reflex Sympathetic Dystrophy
SDD	Selective Digestive Decontamination
SIRS	Systemic Inflammatory Response Syndrome
SIT	Simultaneous Interview Technique
SOAPME	Suction, Oxygen, Airway equipment, Pharmaceutical (medications), Monitors, Equipment (special)
SSRI	Selective Serotonin Reuptake Inhibitors
SVC	Superior Vena Cava
TCD	Transcranial Doppler Ultrasonographic
TD	Transcranial Doppler
TEE	Transesophageal Echocardiography
TENS	Transcutaneous Electrical Stimulation
TRAMS	Tracheostomy Review and Management Service
UMSS	University of Michigan Sedation Scale
URTI	Upper Respiratory Tract Infections
US	Direct Ultrasonographic Visualization
VAD	Ventricular Assist Devices
VAS	Visual Analogue Scales
VRE	Vancomycin-resistant Enterococcus
WDP	Widespread Diffuse Pain
WHO	World Health Organization

Part I
Highlights

Chapter 1

Anatomy and Physiology in Neonates and Children

Marinella Astuto, Anna L. Paratore, Antonino Gullo

Introduction

Pediatric anesthesia involves patients ranging from preterm infants to teenagers, and these groups require different anesthetic equipment and techniques. Successful and safe anesthetic management in pediatric patients depends on an appreciation and clear understanding of the physiological, anatomic, pharmacological and psychological differences among the pediatric age groups and between pediatric and adult patients. Changes in the airways, cardiovascular system, renal function, central and autonomic nervous system, gastrointestinal system and thermoregulation that take place during development make anesthetic management different and extremely challenging. Pediatric anesthesia management requires an understanding and knowledge of the differences and characteristics unique to the child and infant. Infants and children have unique anatomic, physiological, pharmacological, and psychological issues relating to perioperative management [1].

Pediatric Airways

We briefly discuss the functional characteristics of the developing airway, the impact of mechanical ventilation on airway function, and the clinical assessment of airway function in neonates and children [2].

The differences in anatomy of the pediatric airway are related to the prominence and size of the occipital bone, relative macroglossia, the narrowness of the nasal passages, and anterior and cephalic larynx (at C3-C4 vertebral level), and the larger, longer and omega-shaped epiglottis. The cricoid cartilage (subglottis) is the narrowest point of the airway in children under 5 years of age. So, 1 mm of edema will have a proportionately greater effect in children because of their smaller tracheal diameter. Also, due to the shorter length of the trachea endobronchial intubation and accidental extubation with head movement are more common.

M. Astuto (ed), *Basics*, Anesthesia, Intensive Care and Pain in Neonates and Children.
ISBN 978-88-470-0654-6 © Springer-Verlag Italia 2009

Due to the large occiput, a small pillow placed under the occiput will flex the head on the neck instead of extending it for the sniffing position. Thus it is preferable to place a pad under the neck and shoulders, with a large ring under the occiput to stabilize the head to help achieve the optimum head position for laryngoscopy.

Regarding the physiology of the respiratory system, the respiratory rate in children is three times that in adults, alveolar ventilation is high (double that in adults), and the functional residual capacity (FRC) is minor [3]. Oxygen consumption in the neonate is almost twice the adult value (newborn 4–6 ml/kg per minute, adult 2 ml/kg per minute). This is seen as increased minute ventilation (200 ml/kg per minute) in the newborn as compared to 100 ml/kg per minute at puberty. As tidal volume remains constant at 7 ml/kg through life, an increase in ventilation occurs by an increase in respiratory rate, which is approximately 30 per minute at birth progressively falling to adult values by adolescence. In young infants the FRC during complete relaxation (central apnea, general anesthesia, use of muscle relaxants) decreases to 10–15% of total lung capacity. This low FRC is caused by low closing capacity and results in atelectasias, ventilation/perfusion imbalance, and hemoglobin desaturation.

The small diameter of the airways results in high resistance. Infant airways are highly compliant and poorly supported by the surrounding structures. The chest wall is also highly compliant, so that the ribs provide little support to the lungs. Therefore negative intrathoracic pressure is poorly maintained so breathing work is approximately three times that in the adult.

Another difference concerns the composition of the respiratory muscles: type I muscle fibers which are fatigue-resistant and able to perform repeated exercise are deficient in the newborn and infant. Adult fiber configuration is reached only by approximately 2 years of age. So any factor increasing the work of breathing contributes to early fatigue of the respiratory muscles [4]. The fatigue can lead to apnea or carbon dioxide retention and respiratory failure.

Prematurely born infants, especially those with a history of apnea, are at risk (20 to 40%) of developing postoperative apnea. Apnea occurs mostly during the first 12 hours of the postoperative period, especially in the presence of certain risk factors which include postconceptual age <60 weeks, prematurity, anemia, and continuing apnea. Finally, the central coordination of breathing function is completed only after 3–5 months of extrauterine life. Neither the hypoxic nor the hypercapnic ventilatory drive is well developed in neonates and infants.

Immature respiratory control combined with an increased susceptibility to fatigue of the respiratory muscles may be responsible for the increased risk of postoperative apnea especially in preterm infants with a gestational age less than 46 weeks. For all these reasons respiratory reserve and apnea tolerance are strongly reduced and hypoxia may suddenly appear and quickly worsen.

Cardiovascular System

Cardiovascular physiology differs between neonates, infants, children, and adolescents because of continuing development and maturation of the cardiovascular system [5]. Many changes occur in the cardiovascular system at birth, and with growth and development [6]. Table 1.1 shows the principal differences between the immature and mature myocardium. Thus, there are differences between the human infant up to approximately 6 months of age and the adult in the cellular elements of the cardiac myocytes, in the adrenergic receptors, in the intracellular receptors, in the interaction of contractile proteins, and in calcium cycling and regulation. Moreover in neonates, the diastolic and systolic myocardial velocities of the left ventricle are significantly lower than in children. The decreased myocardial tissue values of neonates might reflect the immaturity of the neonatal myocardium. As a consequence of this immaturity, myocardial sequelae of longstanding congenital heart disease are hypertrophy of the cardiac chambers, increase in wall thickness (hypertrophy of cardiac myocytes and non-contractile elements), reduction in wall stress and ventricular function (particularly diastolic function), and finally reduction in myocardial function.

Table 1.2 shows the principal differences in hemodynamic parameters between the immature and adult heart. Cardiac output is strongly related to heart rate [7]. Contractility, catecholamine response and compliance are lower, the Starling response is limited, and ventricular interdependence is greater in the

Table 1.1 Immature versus adult myocardium

Newborn	Adult
Few contractile elements	Many contractile elements
Fewer mitochondrial rows along contractile elements	Mitochondria form rows along contractile elements
Reduced sarcoplasmic reticulum	Abundant sarcoplasmic reticulum
Poorly formed T-tubules	Well-formed T-tubules
Lower myofibrillar ATPase activity	Normal myofibrillar ATPase activity
More potential for glycolytic ATP generation	Oxidative metabolism
Decreased developed tension	Normal developed tension
Decreased output with increasing preload	Able to maintain output with increase in preload
Ca^{2+} for excitation–contraction coupling trans-sarcolemmal	Ca^{2+} for excitation–contraction coupling sarcoplasmic reticulum

Table 1.2 Differences between the immature and adult heart

	Neonate	Adult
Cardiac output	Rate-dependent	Increased by stroke volume/heart rate
Contractility	Reduced	Normal
Starling response	Limited	Normal
Catecholamine response	Reduced	Normal
Compliance	Reduced	Normal
Afterload mismatch	Susceptible	Resistant
Ventricular interdependence	Increased	Normal

neonate. In particular, cardiac output at birth is 200 ml/kg per minute and progressively decreases to 100 ml/kg per minute by adolescence. Resting stroke volume remains fairly constant at about 1 ml/kg per minute, the increased cardiac output in younger patients being maintained by an increase in the heart rate (which progressively decreases throughout childhood).

Renal Function

Glomerular filtration and tubular function are reduced at birth because of the immaturity of the kidneys, but reach adult values by 2 years of age by which time complete maturation of renal function has occurred [8]. Premature neonates often possess multiple renal defects, including decreased creatinine clearance, impaired sodium retention, glucose excretion, bicarbonate reabsorption and poor diluting and concentrating abilities [9]. Thus, meticulous attention to fluid administration and balance is essential [10]. Perioperative fluid management includes maintenance fluid requirements and replacement of fluid deficit and losses.

Fluid deficits are calculated and replaced based on duration of fasting, presence of associated conditions (for example, fever, vomiting, diarrhea, sweating) and the presence of particular disease states or surgical problems likely to affect fluid status (for example, bowel obstruction or peritonitis). Intraoperative losses are subdivided into third space loss and blood loss. Third space losses may be estimated from the extent of surgery (the magnitude of this loss is usually highest in infants undergoing intraabdominal procedures and least in those undergoing superficial surgery, with range of 1–10 ml/kg per hour) and the clinical response to appropriate fluid replacement (i.e. sustained and adequate blood pressure and heart rate, adequate perfusion, and a urine output of 1–2 ml/kg per hour). The anesthesiologist should also have a preoperative plan regarding replacement of blood loss based on the patient's preoperative condition, preoperative hematocrit, and the nature of the surgery.

Central and Autonomic Nervous Systems

Although the nervous system is anatomically complete at birth, myelination continues and functionally it remains immature [11, 12]. Myelination of the nervous system is rapid during the first 2 years of life and is complete by 7 years of age.

Lack of myelin, small size of the nerve fibers and short distance between successive nodes of Ranvier favor penetration of local anesthetics and rapid onset of nerve blockade even with the use of diluted solutions. Following differentiation at birth, the spinal cord ends at the intervetebral level L3, reaching the adult level of L1 to L2 at the age of 8 years. Due to this lower termination, lower intervertebral approaches to epidural and subarachnoid spaces are recommended to avoid any neurological damage. The anesthesiologist should aim to attenuate the stress response as well as to prevent the perception of pain by administering sufficient analgesia [13]. Neonates respond to noxious stimuli with facial grimaces and cardiovascular and metabolic stress responses, suggesting perception of pain. Moreover, in neonates sympathetic and parasympathetic functions do exist, with a predominance of the parasympathetic response system, but do not mature until later in infancy.

Gastrointestinal System

At birth the functional maturity of the liver is incomplete but, as the infant grows, hepatic blood flow increases and the enzyme systems develop and are induced. So the ability to metabolize drugs increases rapidly [14, 15].

In neonates conjugation reactions are often impaired, resulting in jaundice and a decrease in degradation reaction leading to long drug half-lives. In neonates and infants, lower esophageal sphincter tone is decreased, and also the ability to coordinate swallowing with respiration is not fully matured until 4–5 months of age. These two factors lead to an increase in the incidence of gastroesophageal reflux.

Thermoregulation System

Infants are particularly vulnerable to hypothermia because of both a large body surface area to weight ratio and a limited ability to cope with cold stress [16].

Temperature derangements are frequently associated with anesthesia, and transient dysfunction in the thermoregulatory system may lead to potentially serious complications. During the perioperative period patients are at risk of developing thermoregulatory disturbances due to both anesthesia and surgery. It is important to minimize heat loss by various methods including the use of a warming mattress, blankets, warm intravenous fluids and blood, warming and humidifying anesthetic gases, overhead radiant heaters or incubators for transport, plastic wrap to decrease evaporative loss, warming of preparation solution, and increasing the operating room temperature [17, 18].

Conclusion

Pediatric anesthesia involves patients during the perioperative period and those in critical care of all ages ranging from preterm infants to teenagers. Differences in physiological characteristics make anesthetic management different and extremely challenging for the anesthesiologist. It is imperative to have a good knowledge of the anatomic and physiological differences among the pediatric age groups (neonates, infants, children, teenagers) and between pediatric and adult patients for the conduct of successful and safe anesthesia [1].

References

1. Breschan C, Likar R (2006) Anaesthetic management of surgery in term and preterm infants. Anaesthetist 55:1087–1098
2. Levy RJ, Helfaer MA (2000) Paediatric airway issues. Crit Care Clin 16:489–504
3. Stocks J (1999) Respiratory physiology during early life. Monaldi Arch Chest Dis 54:358–364
4. Fisher JT (1992) Airway smooth muscle contraction at birth: in vivo versus in vitro comparisons to the adult. Can J Physiol Pharmacol 70:590–596
5. Rychik J (2004) Fetal cardiovascular physiology. Pediatr Cardiol 25:201–209
6. Strafford MA (1996) Cardiovascular physiology. In: Motoyama EK, Davis PJ (eds) Smith's anesthesia for infants and children. Mosby, pp 69 –104
7. DiPietro JA, Bornstein MH, Hahn C-S et al (2007) Fetal heart rate and variability: stability and prediction to developmental outcomes in early childhood. Child Dev 78:1788–1798
8. Strazdins V, Watson AR, Harvey B (2004) Renal replacement therapy in children: European Guidelines. Pediatr Nephrol 19:199–207
9. Blackburn ST (1994) Renal function in the neonate. J Perinat Neonatal Nurs 8:37–57
10. Way C, Dhamrait R, Wade A, Walker I (2006) Perioperative fluid therapy in children: a survey of current prescribing practice. Br J Anaesth 97:371–379
11. Appenzeller O, Ogin G (1973) Myelinated fibres in the human paravertebral sympathetic chain; quantitative studies on white rami communicantes. J Neurol Neurosurg Psychiatry 36:777–785
12. Dietrich KN, Eskenazi B, Schantz S, Yolton K (2005) Principles and practices of neurodevelopmental assessment in children: lesson learned from the Centers for Children's Environmental Health and Disease Prevention Research. Environ Health Perspect 113:1437–1446
13. American Academy of Pediatrics. Committee on Fetus and Newborn. Committee on Drugs. Section on Anesthesiology. Section on Surgery. Canadian Paediatric Society. Fetus and Newborn Committee (2000) Prevention and management of pain and stress in the neonate. Pediatrics 105:454–461
14. Mahmood I (2006) Prediction of drug clearance in children from adults: a comparison of several allometrics methods. Br J Clin Pharmacol 61:545–557

15. Yao L, Horn PS, Heubi JE, Woollett LA (2007) The liver plays a key role in whole body sterol accretion of the neonatal Golden Syrian hamster. Biochim Biophys Acta 1771:550–557
16. Cross KW, Hey EN, Kennaird DL et al (1971) Lack of temperature control in infants with abnormalities of central nervous system. Arch Dis Child 46:437–443
17. Bissonnette B (1992) Temperature monitoring in paediatric anesthesia. Int Anesthesiol Clin 30:63–76
18. Insler SR, Sessler DI (2006) Perioperative thermoregulation and temperature monitoring. Anesthesiol Clin 24:823–837

Chapter 2

Strategy to Manage Pediatric Patients: the Family and the Child

Giuseppe Rosano, Manuela Antoci, Marinella Astuto

Introduction

An important responsibility of physicians who care for children is the elimination of anxiety and suffering whenever possible, especially during the preoperative period. It is known that preoperative anxiety in children is associated with adverse postoperative outcomes (i.e. increased incidence of emergence delirium, increased pain) and so an adequate preparation programme should be applied routinely. The strategy to manage the pediatric patient should include the parents to avoid increasing the parents' anxiety and concomitantly the child's anxiety.

Good communication and parental involvement have been demonstrated to be of benefit to the child during hospitalization. Several studies and particularly a randomized controlled trial study by Kain et al. have demonstrated that a family-centered preoperative behavioral intervention not only reduces children's anxiety, but also reduces the incidence of postoperative delirium, shortens the time to discharge and reduces the consumption of analgesics [1].

The Importance of a Team Approach

The need for a collaborative, multidisciplinary approach to manage the pediatric patient has become apparent. The optimal application of various techniques depends on the cooperation between different members of the health-care team, including patients and their parents. So anesthesiologists, nurses and parents should actively collaborate in the management of the child.

Multidisciplinary discussions about the indications, urgency and timing of interventions requiring anesthesia may be of benefit, as well as placing difficult children first on the theatre list to minimize waiting periods and list delays. An early start also allows an early recovery and return home, if appropriate.

M. Astuto (ed), *Basics*, Anesthesia, Intensive Care and Pain in Neonates and Children.
ISBN 978-88-470-0654-6 © Springer-Verlag Italia 2009

Preparing the Child for Surgery

Fear and anxiety are common responses in children during hospitalization. Anxiety is normal in stressful situations and its effects are well known and are associated with significant distress in the parents and child before surgery. Preoperative anxiety is characterized by subjective feelings of tension, apprehension, nervousness and worry, and it is influenced by various factors such as: anticipation of pain, fear of separation from parents, loss of control, unfamiliar routines, hospital procedures, and surgical instruments.

Anxiety in children may lead to immediate negative postoperative responses such as nightmares, separation anxiety, eating disturbances and new-onset enuresis. Anxiety also may activate a stress response, resulting in catabolism, delayed wound healing and postoperative immune suppression [2]. Preoperative parental anxiety has also been demonstrated to result in increased anxiety in the child, which has implications not only at the time of surgery but also after surgery and hospitalization.

Preparing children for surgery is an appropriate strategy to prevent many behavioral and physiological manifestations of anxiety. The aims of preoperative preparation are a reduction in preoperative anxiety levels in children and parents, a reduction in negative postoperative behavior, improved parental satisfaction, facilitation of the consent process, and improvement in the profile of the anesthesiologist.

Considering the correlation between a child's anxiety and the parents' anxiety, both children and parents should receive appropriate information about what to expect and appropriate preparation about how to minimize distress. Preparation for anesthesia may include, besides queries regarding current medical conditions and history, perioperative information and preparation of the child and parents. In particular, there is a need for the preparation of parents so that they are in a position to contribute constructively to the hospital stay of their child [3].

The treatment approach for preoperative anxiety in children should be multimodal and meet the child's needs and nowadays several techniques are available such as psychological and behavioral intervention and a pharmacological strategy [4].

Priorities and Satisfaction in Pediatric Care

The level of patient and parent satisfaction is an important factor in the quality of the health care. Satisfaction with the health-care environment concerns not only clinical aspects but also the quality of communication between health-care staff and patients and the comfort offered by the centre, and also includes a subjective component related to the quality of the assistance provided [5]. Identification of parents' priorities (e.g. concerning the patient's preferences or desires) may be an important approach to measuring and improving the quality of health care [6].

The contact with the physician is of great importance. To reduce stress and to improve satisfaction, pediatric anesthesiologists must give full information about the anesthesia and the postoperative course to both patient and parents. Parents in fact want detailed information about the specific anesthetic techniques, the risks and personnel roles, so by giving adequate information preoperatively the anesthesiologist may reduce parental and the child's anxiety and increase their satisfaction. In particular, written information may improve parent knowledge and ensure satisfaction [7].

Another important strategy to reduce parental anxiety before surgery and improve the parents' level of satisfaction is to allow a parent to be present during induction of anesthesia. This issue has been a controversial topic for many years, but has become commonplace in several countries as a result of its potential benefits, which include reducing or avoiding the fear and anxiety in both the child and parents on their separation as the child is taken to the operating room, reducing the need for preoperative premedication, and improving the child's compliance during anesthesia induction. However, despite these benefits, there are also potential disadvantages of the presence of a parent which include possible adverse reactions of the parent as a result of anxiety which may result in prolonged anesthesia induction and may put additional stress on the anesthesiologist. So the final decision whether or not to allow a parent to be present at induction must be made on an individual basis following careful preoperative assessment. Furthermore, to maximize the benefit of having a parent present in the operating room and to reduce the possible negative consequences, the parents must be provided with adequate preoperative information and education [8].

Having confidence in the doctors and the behavior of the nurses and doctors have been shown to be determinants of satisfaction, although a short waiting time was one of the items given the highest priority score [6]. A long waiting period for an operation is stressful for family and child and is an emotionally charged issue for the parents. They feel that the waiting period should not exceed 3 months, and a waiting time perceived as excessively long causes frustration and therefore dissatisfaction [9].

In conclusion, the waiting time and communication with parents are the highest priorities for improving satisfaction and are the principal factors in providing care and treatment that meet with parents' needs, but careful planning and coordination of teaching efforts are necessary for parental preparation.

Preinduction Techniques

Preparing pediatric patients for their surgical experience is a complex process that may be facilitated by pharmacological and nonpharmacological techniques.

Several techniques are often utilized in the preoperative setting to decrease the anxiety level of pediatric patients and their parents, and include the administration of a sedative drug, parental presence during induction, and a variety of other nonpharmacological modalities. These techniques must be associated as indicated, for example, by evidence that parental presence during induction of anesthesia in a child undergoing general anesthesia enhances the effect of oral midazolam on emergence behavior [10].

Pharmacological Techniques

In some cases parental preparation alone is not enough, and the use of premedication is advisable. Premedication may help and should be acceptable and effective. Drugs (especially benzodiazepine) can be useful to calm the child and may therefore help achieve a good anesthesia induction. Children can be premedicated via the oral, intranasal or rectal route, and a further consideration is the unpleasant taste of some current formulations.

Although a variety of preinduction techniques exist, the most popular technique involves administering a sedative premedication, such as midazolam. Preoperative administration of midazolam, alone or combined with other pharmacological agents, is the most effective technique to reduce anxiety in the child and parents [11].

Nonpharmacological Techniques

Psychoeducational care has a beneficial effect on distress after surgery and if the various techniques are used correctly pharmacological premedication can be avoided. But these methods require specific staff preparation and they cannot be applied to all children and to all ages.

Nonpharmacological strategies to manage children's and parent's preoperative anxiety include the presence of one or two parents during induction of anesthesia, psychological preparation of the child and other techniques that include: distraction (toys, television, DVDs, video games, clowns), techniques involving the imagination (recalling pleasurable events, listening to stories) and conscious hypnosis [11].

In particular, it has been found that children are good hypnotic subjects and are highly responsive to suggestion, and such techniques effectively reduce procedural distress and anxiety during hospitalization [12]. Many experienced pediatric anesthesiologists use hypnotic language in their daily work, frequently without realizing they are doing so. Hypnosis in children has been defined as an alternative state of awareness where the focus of attention is on a particular idea or image with the specific purpose of achieving a particular goal. Suggestion is a verbal or nonverbal communication that results in an apparent spontaneous change in perception or behavior. For example, in the study by Fukumoto et al. in which the anesthesiologist suggested under hypnosis that the smell of the face mask could be magically changed into the child's favorite smell, children were found to have an innate ability to change their perception of smell to facilitate their anesthesia [13].

Some children will benefit from the presence of a parent during anesthesia induction, after adequate preoperative preparation, and sometimes the presence of others in the operating room, together with the parent, may reduce anxiety in children and parents and may smooth the anesthesiologist's work during induction of anesthesia. An example is the presence of a clown in the preoperative room, but some questions exist about their usefulness. Some studies, such as that by Vagnoli et al., highlight the benefit to the child of a clown's presence: those who had a clown present during induction were significantly less anxious than those who did not (the control group). At the same time, the majority of physicians and nurses considered that the operating room routine was disturbed because the clown delayed the procedures and interfered in the relationship between the medical personnel and the child [14].

Another possible technique is the introduction of small animals into wards to support hospitalized children. For children who are severely ill and hospitalized, and therefore cut off from their everyday lives, animals can be very important. Indeed, they can help children cope with separation from their family, chronic disease, pain, death and bereavement. A project has been started at the Meyer Children's Hospital with the introduction of pets into different wards. Parents and medical staff view this as a positive event, and have expressed satisfaction because of the participation of the hospitalized children [15].

It is clear that a comfortable environment in hospital is pleasant to both child and parents. Institutions vary in their practice but the final decision should be agreed between the anesthesiologist and the parents.

The Difficult Child

A few children violently resist interventions even after careful preparation, and represent a challenging group of patients who risk: *damage* to themselves, *disruption* and *delays* to the surgery lists, and *stress* to their family and staff. It is important that staff are aware of and recognize the difficult child. It is known that children who are combative at home or have resisted other therapeutic interventions are also likely to resist anesthesia [16].

It is possible to identify some of the factors that predispose to the development this problem. Such factors include:

- Neurological developmental disabilities
- Behavioral disorders
- Autism
- Mental health problems
- Personality problems
- History of combativeness
- Recent history of physical/psychological trauma.

Physical Restraint

Occasionally the anesthesiologist is confronted with a child who refuses anesthesia. In such a case physical restraint may be the only option, but its use requires clear indications, safe application, reassessment guidelines, and use only after consideration of alternative methods. Children and adolescents may need to be physically or chemically restrained for various procedures, because of disruptive behavior, or to prevent injury to themselves or others [17].

The Joint Commission on Accreditation of Healthcare Organizations categorizes the use of restraint as a special treatment procedure requiring special justification for its use. Situations that may require the short-term use of restraint of a child or adolescent include extreme, disruptive, self-injurious, or aggressive behavior as a result of drug intoxication, head injury, cerebrovascular hemorrhage, multiple trauma, or acute psychiatric disorder.

Restraints may be chemical of physical. Chemical restraints include the use of psychotropic drugs, sedatives or paralytic agents. Physical restraints include the use of cloth, leather, metal handcuffs or shackles, car seats or seat belts.

Management options may be discussed with the parents, whilst recruiting their help and the choice of strategy can be discussed by telephone or at the routine preoperative visit and should be documented. If parents believe that careful restraint is used in their child's best interest, they are likely to be supportive. Also nursing groups have developed clinical guidelines and a protocol for procedural restraints.

Conclusion

The pediatric anesthesiologist has to deal with different types of child, pathologies and ages, and has to take care of the whole family. A family-centered intervention is mandatory to manage children and should be incorporated in all aspects of a child's medical experience.

References

1. Kain ZN, Caldwell-Andrews A, Mayes L et al (2007) Family-centered preparation for surgery improves perioperative outcomes in children: a randomized controlled trial. Anesthesiology 106:65–74
2. Kain ZN, Mayes LC, O'Connor TZ et al (1996) Preoperative anxiety in children. Predictors and outcomes. Arch Pediatr Adolesc Med 150:1238–1245
3. Shirley PJ, Thompson N, Kenward M, Johnston G (1998) Parental anxiety before elective surgery in children. Anaesthesia 53:956–959
4. Kain ZN, Caldwell-Andrews AA (2005) Preoperative psychological preparation of the child for surgery: an update. Anesthesiol Clin North Am 23:597–614
5. Iacobucci T, Federico B, Pintus C, De Francisci G (2005) Evaluation of satisfaction level by parents and children following paediatric anaesthesia. Paediatr Anaesth 15:314–320
6. Ammentorp J, Mainz J, Sabroe S (2006) Determinants of priorities and satisfaction in pedi-

atric care. Pediatr Nurs 333:340-348

7. Spencer C, Franck LS (2005) Giving parents written information about children's anesthesia: are setting and timing important. Paediatr Anaesth 15:547–553

8. Astuto M, Rosano G, Rizzo G et al (2006) Preoperative parental information and parents' presence at induction of anaesthesia. Minerva Anestesiol 72:461–465

9. Miller GG (2003) Waiting for an operation: parents' perspectives. Can J Surg 47:179–181

10. Arai YC, Ito H, Kandatsu N et al (2007) Parental presence during induction enhances the effect of oral midazolam on emergence behaviour of children undergoing general anaesthesia. Acta Anaesthesiol Scand 51:858–861

11. Bailey PD Jr, Bastien JL (2005) Preinduction techniques for paediatric anaesthesia. Curr Opin Anaesthesiol 18:265–269

12. Lucas-Polomeni MM (2004) Hypnosis: a new anaesthetic technique! Pediatr Anesth 14:975–976

13. Fukumoto M, Arima H, Ito S (2005) Distorted perception of smell by volatile agents facilitated inhalational induction of anaesthesia. Pediatr Anesth 15:98–101

14. Vagnoli L, Caprilli S, Robiglio A, Messeri A (2005) Clown doctors as a treatment for preoperative anxiety in children: a randomized, prospective study. Paediatrics 116:563–567

15. Caprilli S, Messeri A (2006) Animal-assisted activity at A. Meyer Children's Hospital: a pilot study. Evid Based Complement Alternat Med 3:379–383

16. American Academy of Pediatrics (1997) The use of physical restraint interventions for children and adolescents in the acute care setting. American Academy of Pediatrics Committee on Pediatric Emergency Medicine. Pediatrics 99:497–498

17. Christiansen E, Chambers N (2005) Induction of anesthesia in a combative child; management and issues. Paediatr Anaesth 15:421–425

Chapter 3

Off-Label Drugs in Pediatric Perioperative Medicine

Marinella Astuto, Manuela Antoci, Antonino Gullo

Introduction

The drug licensing system was introduced with the aim of ensuring that medicines are marketed only after having been examined for safety, efficacy and quality. So, before a drug is allowed on the market, a favorable balance between beneficial and harmful effects has to be demonstrated. Often this has been established only in adults and once a drug is approved, it may be prescribed by a physician for any population or disease state desired. Many drugs pass through the licensing process without being evaluated in children. The product license often contains statements such as "not recommended for use in children" or "no evidence for use in children." This usually reflects an absence of data in children rather than a specific reason for the drug not to be used.

The term "off-label" has been applied to describe the use of these drugs in either populations or disease states not listed as indicated in the package insert. "Off-label" drug use refers to the use of drugs outside the terms of the product license in terms of dose, patient age, route of administration, indications and contraindications. Licensed drugs are often prescribed outside the terms of the product license (off-label) in relation to age, indications, dose frequency, route of administration, or formulation. The use of a drug in children is considered "unlicensed" when the drug has not received market authorization for such use [1], but the term "unlicensed" does not imply disapproval or that the practice is improper. It only implies that pharmaceutical companies have not performed clinical trials and therefore evidence of tolerability and efficacy is not available to satisfy licensing authorities [1].

"On-label" drug use refers to the use of a drug according to the product license.

Unlicensed and off-label drug use in children is widespread and there is insufficient information about safety and efficacy for such use [2].

M. Astuto (ed), *Basics*, Anesthesia, Intensive Care and Pain in Neonates and Children.
ISBN 978-88-470-0654-6 © Springer-Verlag Italia 2009

Drug Regulation

In the US the Food and Drug Administration (FDA) has responsibility for the licensing process for all drugs. Under current law, when the FDA reviews an application for a new drug, it holds the drug to both safety and efficacy requirements before granting a license. Prescribing FDA-approved drugs for off-label uses often is necessary for optimal patient care. The FDA never has had authority to regulate the practice of medicine; physicians may use legally marketed drugs or devices in any way that they believe, in their professional judgment, will best serve their patients [3, 4].

The European Regulation on medicines for pediatric use came into force on 26 January 2007. It encourages the development of medicines for pediatric age groups and improves the availability of information on the use of medicines in children. For the first time, companies will be required to study medicines in the pediatric population and develop age-appropriate formulations. The Regulation establishes a European pediatric clinical trials network and a pediatric study program for off-patent medicines. A Paediatric Committee, based at the European Medicines Agency, will be responsible for agreeing the pediatric investigation plan (PIP) with companies. This will describe the clinical trials and other measures necessary to investigate a particular medicine in the pediatric population [5]. Several concerns exists in Europe and the US about the use of unlicensed and off-label drugs in children, but there is little information on the extent to which these types of treatments are used.

The FDA has provided financial incentives for the development and marketing of medicines for children. But compelling and motivating companies to undertake pediatric clinical trials is not the whole answer to the issue. There is a need to identify and address factors that make the conduct of pediatric clinical trials difficult. The factors include those related to difficulty in recruitment, obtaining ethical clearance, and having sensitive and trained investigators.

There are too many variations in clinical circumstances and too much time delay in regulations to allow governments to impede the physician's ability to practice in a way that is medically appropriate [5]. For a product to have the most effective potential benefits, law and regulation should and must follow, not precede, science.

Pediatric Labeling

Off-label use of approved drugs is very common in all areas of medicine and it is quite common in children, as most drugs are developed only on the basis of trials in adults. Licensed drugs are often prescribed outside the terms of the product license (off-label) in relation to age, indications, dose frequency, route of administration, or formulation.

Almost all medicines are licensed for use in adults but only one-third are licensed for use in children. This situation primarily results from lack of data because there are fewer clinical trials undertaken in children. Moreover, data from studies in adults cannot be extrapolated to predict the pharmacokinetics, toxicity and therapeutic effects of a medicine in children. Drug metabolism, clearance and distribution alter throughout childhood because of maturing hepatic and renal functions, particularly in neonates and infants. So, separate clinical trials in children are necessary to assess appropriate dosage regimens in order to achieve the desired therapeutic effect whilst avoiding toxicity [6].

For several years, children have been excluded from clinical trials carried out during the process of market authorization as society and law makers have thought it prudent not to expose children to molecules whose safety and efficacy has not been established. This has resulted in drugs being marketed without pediatric safety and efficacy data.

The pharmaceutical industry has been less enthusiastic in conducting clinical trials in children as they are costlier and logistically more challenging to undertake [6]. There are several other reasons why pharmaceutical companies are reluctant to study medicines in children: the market for the sale of medicines for use in children is much smaller than that for adults; it is unrealistic for the pharmaceutical industry to carry out large randomized clinical trials in children to meet the registration requirement since the investment is not financially attractive; and there are ethical and technical difficulties to performing clinical trials in children. Moreover, nonavailability of pediatric formulations is a common reason for unlicensed drug use. Young children require liquid preparations and dispersible tablets, and for many molecules, such preparations are not available.

Defining the optimal dose, the dose range for a given patient population, and the dose adjustments required as a result of physiological, pathological or iatrogenic interventions, remains one of the most challenging tasks in drug development and clinical care.

Literature reviews of articles on off-label and unlicensed drug use in children have confirmed a widespread attitude to prescribing medicines to children outside their product license both in hospital and in the community [7, 8]. Over 67% of children admitted to wards in five European hospitals received drugs prescribed in an unlicensed or off-label manner. This suggests the need for immediate action for a more rational use of drugs in the pediatric population, to avoid exposing children and infants to risks, but also to avoid depriving them of potentially effective and sometimes life-saving therapies [8, 9].

In a study of unlicensed and off-label drug use on five pediatric wards in European countries, 39% of 2,262 drug prescriptions given to children over a 4-week period were off-label [10].

Legal Issues and Implications for Safety

Physicians who treat children often prescribe drugs for off-label uses because little information is available from well-controlled studies on dosage, formulation, effectiveness, and safety in children.

When devices and drugs are used off-label the primary purpose is to benefit the individual patient.

When a drug is used outside the limits of its label, neither the company nor the authorities take any legal or ethical responsibility for the occurrence of an unexpected event. It may still be proper and lawful for a doctor to prescribe a drug off-label but the responsibility lies entirely with the prescriber. The decision to use the drug and its dose should be based on evidence and authoritative professional opinion, even though the licensing authorities may not have enough evidence about the drug's efficacy, safety and risk-benefit ratio, the label on the drug does not indicate a particular dose, the scientific information available from the medical literature is confusing at best, and there is hardly any single authoritative source of reference available. The doctor may fear being sued for malpractice for indulging in off-label drug use should an unexpected event occur. However, it needs to be emphasized that the doctor would be able to justify such use provided the decision is based on what is good medicine and what is best for the patient regardless of whether such use conforms to the labeling. If there is no high-quality evidence supporting off-label use of a particular medicine, and it is not suitable for exceptional use (justified by individual clinical circumstances) or research indications, its use is generally not recommended.

At the same time, it is not ethical for a doctor to withhold using a potentially useful drug from a patient, just because it would amount to off-label use. The American Academy of Pediatrics has also pointed out that failure to use a drug off-label where appropriate under the standard of care may also constitute malpractice. So, a doctor could be subject to a claim of malpractice if a patient is denied the best potential treatment just because it was unlicensed or off-label.

Pediatricians and other prescribers caring for children are faced with difficult choices and are forced into a situation of having to prescribe unlicensed or off-label drugs in order to ensure the most effective treatment regimen for children, because the benefit of using unlicensed or off-label drugs is more likely to outweigh the risk of using them [11]. The risk associated with unlicensed and off-label drug use appears to be greater than for prescribing in accordance with the product license [12, 13]. This risk may be higher in those children with more severe clinical conditions and with young age [14].

A Medline search relating to the period 1990 to 2006 by Cuzzolin et al. identified a total of 52 studies. From the authors' analysis of the literature, the extent of pediatric unlicensed/off-label use is higher in neonatal and pediatric intensive care units and oncology wards than in primary care. Moreover, among the nine studies reporting the contribution of an off-label/unlicensed drug use to the occurrence of adverse events, the percentage of unlicensed and/or off-label prescriptions involved in an adverse drug reaction ranged between 23% and 60% [15]. The incidence of adverse drug reactions associated with the unlicensed and/or off-label use of drugs is yet to be established. Neubert et al. found that in a pediatric isolation ward the incidence of adverse drug reactions caused by unlicensed or off-label drug use was not significantly more than that caused by licensed drug use [16].

The prescribing of medicine to children in an unlicensed manner and/or off-label may often be appropriate, and sometimes health professionals have no alternative but to use unlicensed and off-label medicines. However, children constitute a vulnerable group, since new drugs are released to the market without the benefit of even limited experience in them. So, drug safety monitoring, i.e. early detection of possible adverse effects of a drug, especially a newly introduced one, is crucial in this patient group.

Examples of Unlicensed and Off-Label Drugs

Off-label use is an international problem with comparable rates reported in European countries and North America [15, 16]. The extent of pediatric unlicensed/off-label use is higher in neonatal and intensive care units and oncology wards than in primary care. The drugs most commonly used in an off-label or unlicensed manner are usually established drugs for which there is a large amount of clinical information available [17].

Approximately half of the uses of anticancer chemotherapy drugs are for indications other than those referred to in the FDA-approved label. Some managed care organizations and private health insurance plans have declined to reimburse the cost of drugs used off-label to threat cancer on the grounds that these uses are "experimental" or "investigational" [18].

Moreover, many respiratory drugs are not available in formulations suitable for infants and toddlers [19, 20]. The phenomenon of off-label drug use also exists in pediatric cardiology [21]. The findings imply that the phenomenon of off-label and unlicensed use of drugs in children can be correlated with the deficiency of pediatric drug formulations on the global market and insufficient data from clinical studies which must be performed to confirm the efficacy and safety of drugs in the pediatric population [22]. Several literature reviews of articles on off-label and unlicensed drug use in children have been performed using Medline and Embase [11, 22–24] (Table 3.1).

Pandolfini et al. [34] analyzed prescriptions given to all children admitted to nine general pediatric hospital wards from December 1998 to February 1999, and found that the most common off-label categories were dosage/frequency (50% of prescriptions), and indication and lack of pediatric license (7% each). The majority of the prescriptions (60%, range between centers 44–71%) were off-label and concerned 89% of children receiving medications (80–96%). The main drug classes were antibacterials, antiasthmatics and analgesics, which represented 56% of off-label prescriptions.

Another review [21] included 30 studies during the period 1985–2004. In general, off-label/unlicensed prescription rates ranged from 11% to 80%, and higher rates were found in younger than in older patients and in the hospital setting than in the community setting. On pediatric hospital wards, off-label/unlicensed prescriptions ranged from 16% to 62%, and were most often for acetaminophen, cisapride, chloral hydrate, and salbutamol. In the neonatal wards,

Table 3.1 Selected studies estimating the use of drugs beyond license

Investigators	Year	Clinical setting	Country	No. of prescriptions	No. of patients	Unlicensed or off-label drug use (%)
Turner et al. [25]	1996	Pediatric intensive care unit	UK	862	166	31
Turner et al. [22]	1998	Two pediatric wards	UK	20,013	609	25
Conroy et al. [26]	1999	Neonatal intensive care unit	UK	455	70	64.6
Turner et al. [24]	1999	Five pediatric wards	–	4,455	936	48
Wilton et al. [27]	1999	Community	–	NA	24,337	12.6
't Jong et al. [28]	2000	Four pediatric wards	–	2,139	238	66
Conroy et al. [10]	2000	Five pediatric wards	Five European countries	2,262	624	46
Gravilov et al. [29]	2000	Pediatric ambulatory hospital ward	Israel	222	132	42
Chalumelau et al. [30]	2000	77 pediatricians	France	2,522	989	33
McIntyre et al. [31]	2000	Pediatric ambulatory	UK	33,457	1,175	10.8
Craig et al. [32]	2001	Pediatric unit	UK (Northern Ireland)	237	74	22.8
't Jong et al. [33]	2001	Pediatric ward + three pediatric intensive care units	The Netherlands	2,139	237	66
Pandolfini et al. [34]	2002	Nine pediatric wards	Italy	4,625	1,461	60
O'donnell et al. [35]	2002	Neonatal intensive care unit	Australia	1,442	97	58
't Jong et al. [36]	2002	Community	The Netherlands	17,453	6,141	28.9
Bucheler et al. [37]	2002	Records of health insurer	Germany	1.74 million	–	13.2
Carvalho et al. [38]	2003	Pediatric intensive care unit	Brazil	747	51	54.2
Schirm et al. [39]	2003	Community	The Netherlands	66,222	18,943	37.2
Neubert et al. [16]	2004	Pediatric isolation ward	Germany	740	178	22.7

rates ranged from 55% to 80% and the prescriptions often involved caffeine. In the community setting, rates ranged from 11% to 37% and the prescriptions were most commonly for salbutamol and amoxicillin. In children, all classes of drugs are involved.

Examples of the use of off-label drugs include diazepam rectal solution in children under 1 year of age (not licensed for age group), amiloride tablets in any children (formulation) and rectal injection of lorazepam in a child with an acute seizure (route). An example of unlicensed use is the preparation of a suspension from a tablet by the hospital pharmacy. The 20 most frequently prescribed off-label and unlicensed drugs are: furosemide, lincomycin i.v., digoxin, amoxicillin, propanolol, spironolactone, acetylsalicylic acid, captopril, amikacin, carvedilol, propofol, bupivacaine, fentanyl, clonidine, ondansetron, meperidine, bupivacaine, diazepam, hydromorphone, and gabapentin.

Conclusion

Off-label use of drugs remains a concern for anesthesiologists and physicians caring for children. To ensure that children are not exposed to unnecessary risks, controlled clinical trials are required to determine the most appropriate dose in children of different ages.

The new European guidance on the clinical investigation of medical products in children encourages pharmaceutical companies that wish to introduce new products to investigate these in children when clinically appropriate. Off-label prescribing remains acceptable if there is no suitable alternative and physicians are confident that they are using agents in accordance with the body of respected medical opinion.

Physicians undertake a risk/benefit analysis of proposed treatments, whether they are on-label or off-label, based on their assessment of the unique medical needs of individual patients. Fortunately, much information about off-label prescribing is now available in the medical literature, from professional associations and pharmaceutical sources, to help physicians make appropriate decisions. For the potential benefits of a product to be maximized, law and regulation should and must follow, not precede, science.

The problem of off-label and unlicensed drug prescribing in children is a European problem that requires European action [11].

References

1. Gazarian M, Kelly M, McPhee JR et al (2006) Off-label use of medicines: consensus recommendations for evaluating appropriateness. Med J Aust 185:544–548
2. Schirm E, Tobi H, de Jong-van den Berg LT (2003) Risk factors for unlicensed and off-label drug use in children outside the hospital. Pediatrics 111:291–295
3. Beck JM, Azari ED (1998) FDA, off-label use, and informed consent: debunking, myths and misconception. Food Drug Law J 53:71–104

4. Novak E, Allen PJ (2007) Prescribing medications in pediatrics: concerns regarding FDA approval and pharmacokinetics. Pediatr Nurs 33:64–70
5. Dunne J (2007) The European Regulation on medicines for paediatric use. Paediatric Respir Rev 8:177–183
6. Poetsch J (2006) Legal issues in the off-label use of drug medication in paediatrics. J Dtsch Dermatol Ges 4:421–426
7. Lifshitz M, Gavrilov V, Gorodischer R (2001) Off-label and unlicensed use of antidotes in paediatric patients. Eur J Clin Pharmacol 56:839–841
8. Conroy S, McIntyre J, Choonara I, Stephenson T (2000) Drugs trials in children: problems and the way forward. Br J Clin Pharmacol 49:93–97
9. Cuzzolin L, Zaccaron A, Fanos V (2003) Unlicensed and off-label uses of drugs in paediatrics: a review of the literature. Fundam Clin Pharmacol 17:125–131
10. Conroy S, Choonara I, Impicciatore P et al (2000) Survey on unlicensed and off-label drug use in paediatric wards in European countries. BMJ 320:79–82
11. Pandolfini C, Bonati M (2005) A literature review on off-label drug use in children. Eur J Pediatr 164:552–558
12. Caron S, Choonara I, Impicciatore P (2000) Survey on unlicensed and off-label drug use in paediatric wards in European countries. BMJ 320:79–82
13. Bennet WM (2004) Off-label use of approved drugs: therapeutic opportunity and challenges. J Am Soc Nephrol 15:830–831
14. Choonara I (2004) Unlicensed and off-label drug use in children: implications for safety. Expert Opin Drug Saf 3:81–83
15. Cuzzolin L, Atzei A, Fanos V (2006) Off-label and unlicensed prescribing for newborns and children in different settings: a review of the literature and a consideration about drug safety. Expert Opin Drug Saf 5:703–718
16. Neubert A, Dormann H, Weiss J et al (2004) The impact of unlicensed and off label drug use on adverse drug reactions in paediatric patients. Drug Saf 27:1059–1067
17. Dell'Aera M, Gasbarro AR, Padovano M (2007) Unlicensed and off-label use of medicines at a neonatology clinic in Italy. Pharm World Sci 29:361–367
18. American Society of Oncology (2006) Reimbursement for cancer treatment: coverage of off-label drug indications. J Clin Oncol 24:3206–3208
19. Shah SS, Hall M, Goodman DM et al (2007) Off-label drug use in hospitalized children. Arch Pediatr Adolesc Med 161:282–290
20. Jong GW, Eland IA, Sturkenboom MC et al (2004) Unlicensed and off-label prescription of respiratory drugs to children. Eur Respir J 23:310–313
21. Bajetic M, Jelisavcic M, Mitrovic J et al (2005) Off-label and unlicensed drugs use in paediatric cardiology. Eur J Clin Pharmacol 61:775–779
22. Turner S, Longworth A, Ninn AJ, Choonara I (1998) Unlicensed and off-label drug use in paediatric wards: prospective study. BMJ 316:343–345
23. Choonara I, Conroy S (2002) Unlicensed and off-label drug use in children: implications for safety. Drug Saf 25:1–5
24. Turner S, Nunn AJ, Fielding K, Choonara I (1999) Adverse drug reactions to unlicensed and off-label drugs on paediatric wards: a prospective study. Acta Paediatr 88:965–968
25. Turner S, Gill A, Nunn T et al (1996) Use of "off-label" and unlicensed drugs in paediatric intensive care unit. Lancet 347:549–550
26. Conroy S, McIntyre J, Choonara I (1999) Unlicensed and off label drug use in neonates. Arch Dis Child Fetal Neonatal Ed. 80:F142-4; discussion F144–145
27. Wilton LV, Pearce G, Mann RD (1999) The use of newly marketed drugs in children and adolescents prescribed in general practice. Pharmacoepidemiol Drug Saf 8 Suppl 1:S37–45
28. 't Jong GW, Vulto AG, de Hoog M et al (2000) Unapproved and off-label use of drugs in a children's hospital. N Engl J Med 343:1125
29. Gavrilov V, Lifshitz M, Levy J, Gorodischer R (2000) Unlicensed and off-label medication use in a general pediatrics ambulatory hospital unit in Israel. Isr Med Assoc J 2:595–597
30. Chalumeau M, Tréluyer JM, Salanave B et al (2000) Off label and unlicensed drug use among French office based paediatricians. Arch Dis Child 83:502–505

31. McIntyre J, Conroy S, Avery A et al (2000) Unlicensed and off label prescribing of drugs in general practice. Arch Dis Child 83:498–501

32. Craig JS, Henderson CR, Magee FA (2001) The extent of unlicensed and off-label drug use in the paediatric ward of a district general hospital in Northern Ireland. Ir Med J 94:237–240

33. 't Jong GW, Vulto AG, de Hoog M et al (2001) A survey of the use of off-label and unlicensed drugs in a Dutch children's hospital. Pediatrics 108:1089–1093

34. Pandolfini C, Impicciatore P, Provasi D et al; Italian Paediatric Off-label Collaborative Group (2002) Off-label use of drugs in Italy: a prospective, observational and multicentre study. Acta Paediatr 91:339–347

35. O'Donnell CP, Stone RJ, Morley CJ (2002) Unlicensed and off-label drug use in an Australian neonatal intensive care unit. Pediatrics 110:e52

36. 't Jong GW, van der Linden PD, Bakker EM (2002) Unlicensed and off-label drug use in a paediatric ward of a general hospital in the Netherlands. Eur J Clin Pharmacol 58:293–297. Epub 2002 Jun 15

37. Bücheler R, Schwab M, Mörike K et al (2002) Off label prescribing to children in primary care in Germany: retrospective cohort study. BMJ 324:1311–1312

38. Carvalho PR, Carvalho CG, Alievi PT et al (2003) Prescription of drugs not appropriate for children in a Pediatric Intensive Care Unit. J Pediatr (Rio J) 79:397–402

39. Schirm E, Tobi H, de Vries TW et al (2003) Lack of appropriate formulations of medicines for children in the community. Acta Paediatr 92:1486–1489

Part II
Guidelines and
Standardization of Procedures

Chapter 4
The Pediatric Difficult Airway

Teresa Valois

Introduction

It is a common adage in pediatric anesthesia practice that: "children are not small adults", and in airway management this is especially true. The anatomical and physiological characteristics of children, together with developmental changes, make a careful and thorough approach necessary to guarantee success.

In this chapter, we review the features of the normal pediatric airway and difficult airway, different approaches and techniques currently available, complications and areas of research for the future.

Early in the 1950s, with the increase in practice of endotracheal intubation for general anesthesia, the clinical features of the normal pediatric airway were described in detail by Eckenhoff [1], and some of these features have been confirmed and revised with the aid of current video technology and imaging [2–4].

Characteristics of the Pediatric Upper Airway

Anatomical

Tongue The tongue is larger in proportion of the rest of the oral cavity.

Epiglottis The epiglottis is omega shaped, narrow and inclined away from the axis of the trachea (slanted). Also, the angle between the glottic opening and epiglottis is more acute. Dalal et al. [5], using videobronchoscopy found a mean coronal angle of the superior aspect of the epiglottis of 62.8°, and a positive correlation between weight and height. According to these authors, it reaches the adult angle (approximately 90°) at around the age of 6 years. This difference in angle is attributed to the intimate attachment of the hyoid bone of the infant to the thyroid cartilage [1].

Larynx The superior portion of the larynx is located at the level of the third and fourth cervical vertebrae (C3–C4) at birth in a term baby, and reaches C5 by 5–6

M. Astuto (ed), *Basics*, Anesthesia, Intensive Care and Pain in Neonates and Children.
ISBN 978-88-470-0654-6 © Springer-Verlag Italia 2009

years of age, and its adult location (C7) by 13 years [1]. The cricoid ring is the narrowest point in the internal diameter of the larynx. The vocal folds are slanted anteriorly; this contributes to the difficulties in passing the endotracheal tube (ETT) during routine laryngoscopy and also during fiberoptic intubation.

Technical

Positioning In infants, due to the large occiput, extension of the cervical spine (neck extension) during laryngoscopy tends to flatten the airway (increasing the submandibular space), causing some degree of obstruction to visualization of the cords. Extension of the cervical spine should always be done gently, especially in children with Down's syndrome [6].

Laryngoscopy The shallow vallecula, especially in infants, makes it difficult to lift the epiglottis during laryngoscopy.

Physiological

The higher metabolic rate in children decreases the time for desaturation [7] and response to an obstruction. There is decreased functional residual capacity. At birth there are 25 million alveoli, and this number reaches 360 million by 8 years of age [8]. Respiratory muscles are rich in type II fibers (fast twitch, low oxidative) which increases the risk of fatigue. Adult fiber levels are reached by 2 years of age [8]. The trachea is short and narrow and angled posteriorly. Increased viscosity of mucus in the newborn may lead to rapid ETT obstruction. There is decreased total lung capacity and a faster respiratory rate.

The Difficult Airway

Definition

The current definition of a difficult airway, as stated by the American Society of Anesthesiologists Task Force on Management of the Difficult Airway [9], is a clinical situation in which a conventionally trained anesthesiologist experiences difficulty with face-mask ventilation of the upper airway, difficulty with tracheal intubation, or both [9]. Within this definition are included more specific descriptions, in terms of which step of the airway management is compromised:
- Difficult face-mask ventilation
- Difficult laryngoscopy: visualization
- Difficult tracheal intubation: multiple attempts
- Failed intubation: placement of an ETT [9].

Epidemiology

In non-obstetric adult surgical patients, the incidence of failed intubation is 1:2,303, whereas in the obstetric population it is as high as 1:300 [10]. Difficult intubation occurs at a rate between 1.5% and 13% [9]. In a recent meta-analysis by Shiga et al. [11] the incidence of unanticipated difficult intubation was 5.8% in an adult population. Conversely, the exact incidence of difficult airway is unknown in the pediatric population; it is thought to be rare [10]. The difficult intubation registry from The Children's Hospital of Philadelphia indicates an incidence of approximately 0.25% [12]; however, this may underestimate the real incidence given its retrospective nature. Akpek et al. [13] and Bevilacqua et al. [14], focusing on patients with cardiac disease, found a frequency of difficult intubation of 1.25% and 4.6%, respectively. In the latter study [14] it was also found that difficult intubation in infants (1 year old and younger) was 5.3 times greater than in children (more than 1 year old), and 2.26 times greater than in neonates (younger than 1 month). These findings suggest that age distribution may affect the incidence of difficult airway in children.

Classification

Various classifications have been suggested to facilitate the approach to the difficult pediatric airway, including anatomical, pathophysiological, and other classifications. Hall [15] has classified the difficult pediatric airway into four types (Fig. 4.1).

This classification might allow difficulties at induction to be anticipated and emphasizes the importance of looking for symptoms and signs in the history and on physical examination. In the first group, congenital abnormalities, the pathophysiological event to be considered is chronic obstruction which can be seen in laryngomalacia, glottic webs, vascular rings, hemangioma and hypoplastic mandible. In patients with congenital or acquired abnormalities, subjacent anatomic malformation makes visualization of the glottis difficult by direct laryngoscopy. This group includes those with trisomy 21, Pierre Robin syndrome, Treacher Collins syndrome or Goldenhar syndrome. Of these syndromes the most commonly found in daily practice is trisomy 21, in which there is anatomic as well as chronic obstruction.

In these patients the most important anesthetic considerations are the following:
- Atlantoaxial instability
- Approximately one-quarter of the children require an ETT one or two sizes smaller than predicted, although at least some of this may be due to the generally smaller size of these patients
- Postoperative stridor and respiratory complications are more common than in the general population
- Macroglossia and pharyngeal muscle hypotonia may lead to upper airway obstruction; patients must be observed closely in the postanesthetic care unit

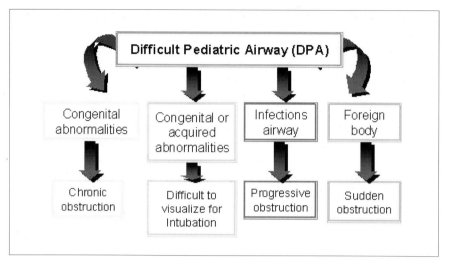

Fig. 4.1 Classification of the difficult pediatric airway

- Some patients also have some degree of pulmonary hypertension, due to either heart disease or chronic upper airway obstruction, or a combination of both. Subacute bacterial endocarditis prophylaxis may be required
- These patients are relatively difficult to sedate, particularly those requiring monitored anesthesia care, without causing hypoventilation [16]
- Airway infections are considered one of the thorny issues in pediatric anesthesia, due first to the progressive obstruction they entail, which is associated with an increased risk of airway complications perioperatively [17]. In this group we find those with epiglottitis, croup, and diphtheria, among others. Patients with a recognized difficult airway, in the elective setting, should not have upper respiratory tract infections at the time of surgery
- In the fourth group, sudden obstruction, as well as the location of the foreign body, is the main concern.

Another way of classifying the difficult pediatric airway in practical terms is: expected or recognized difficult pediatric airway and unanticipated difficult pediatric airway. The first includes mostly patients with known congenital malformations or craniofacial anomalies, which allows preparation and planning to instrument the airway. The latter entails recognizing and effectively overcoming unforeseen risks.

Diagnosis

During the preanesthetic interview, there are key questions that facilitate predicting the likelihood of difficult face-mask ventilation: previous history of anesthesia problems, snoring history (for more details on perioperative management of patients with obstructive sleep apnea, see Gross et al. [18]), apnea, daytime somnolence, stridor, hoarse voice, and sleeping position.

Physical examination will provide more information about intubation. There is scarce information regarding airway indexes validated in children. The Mallampati score is limited to age groups that cooperate to open their mouths, although it does not accurately predict a poor view of the glottis during laryngoscopy [19]. Three features are, however, highly suggestive of difficult laryngoscopy in children: the presence of micrognathia, limited mouth opening, and protruding teeth [10]. It has been suggested that an acceptable submandibular distance as measured from the middle of the inside of the mentum to the hyoid bone is 1.5 cm (approximately one finger breadth) in infants and changes proportionately with age to the adult distance of 3 cm (two finger breadths) [8].

The successful management of the difficult pediatric airway requires prompt diagnosis, a careful and detailed plan, and the participation of an expert airway team.

Equipment

Difficult Airway Cart

A difficult airway cart should always be present in the operating room when a patient with a difficult airway is being anesthetized. Table 4.1 show the contents of the difficult airway cart at the Montreal Children's Hospital. The contents may vary according to staff preferences and the techniques used in different institutions.

Face Mask

Face masks come in different sizes that should fit the nasal bridge [20], include the mouth, and not obstruct the eyes of the patient. Also they should provide a tight seal. Several sizes should be available. The appropriate size will have a minimum dead space, optimizing oxygenation.

Oral Airway

Oral airways (Guedel airways) also should be available in different sizes; the appropriate size for the patient can be determined from the angle of the mandible to the lips. An oral airway that is too small will worsen obstruction by splitting the tongue and pushing the base towards the posterior pharyngeal wall. An oral airway that is too large may push the tip of the epiglottis, causing obstruction and worsening the ventilation and even precipitating laryngospasm (see Fig. 4.2). Adequate anesthetic depth should be ensured before inserting an oral airway.

Table 4.1 Difficult airway cart contents in the Montreal Children's Hospital

Drawer	Equipment	Size/quantity[a]
First drawer	Magill forceps	Neonate, pediatric, adult
	Throat pack	Large x2, small x2
	Intubation stylets	6F, 10F, 14F
	Trachlight handle	x2
	Trachlight intubation stylet	Infant x2, pediatric x2, adult x2
	Oral airways	Each size x2
	Intubating stylet aluminum/plastic precut	
	Laryngoscope handles	Neonate, pediatric, adult
	Laryngoscope blades	
	Mac	1, 2, 3, 4
	Miller	00, 0, 1, 2, 3
	Robertshaw	0,1
	Philips	1x2
	Laryngoscope light bulbs	
	Laryngoscope batteries	Cx2, Nx2, 123
	Suture 4.0 silk, needle driver	
Second drawer	LMA airways	
	Classic	Sizes 1, 1.5, 2.5, 3, 4, 5
	ProSeal	Sizes 2, 3, 4
	Fastrach	
	Nasal airways	12F to 32F
	Lubricant and gauzes	2x2 inches
	Viewmax fiber optic blades	Pediatric, adult
Third drawer	Cricothyrotomy Melker emergency catheter set	Needle 6.0 mm ID, 18 G, 7 cm long, x2
	Jet-ventilator catheter	14 G x2, 16 G for babies x2
	Emergency transtracheal airway catheter	6F 5 cm x2; 6F 7.5 cm x2
	Easy Cap II CO_2 detector	
	Pedi-Cap CO_2 detector	
	CO_2 Microstream	

LMA, laryngeal mask airway

cont. →

continue **Table 4.1**

Fourth drawer	LMA precut	Sizes 1, 1.5, 2, 2.5, 3, 4
	Oral intubating bite blocks	x2
	Tongue depressors	
	Tongue forceps + needle driver	
	Forceps with rubber	
	Antifog kit	x4
	Lens cleaner	
	Silicone spray can for bronchoscope	
	Swivel adaptor	
	Malleable connector	
	Loss of resistance syringe	x2
	Syringes	3 cm^3, 5 cm^3, 10 cm^3, 20 cm^3, 60 cm^3
	Needles	22 G, 18 G
	Trach tie	x5
	Simms adapter for suction port	x2
	Tapes	
	Medications	
	Drixoral decongestant nasal pump	
	Lidocaine 2%	2-ml plastic container, x2
	Lidocaine 2% viscous	100-ml bottle
	Lidocaine 4% topical solution	50-ml bottle
	Lidocaine	aerosol spray and nozzle
	Lidocaine 2% jelly	Prepackage
	Lidocaine 1%	10-ml plastic container
	Xylocard cardiac	100 mg 20 mg/ml, x2
Fifth drawer	Endotracheal tubes cuffed and uncuffed	Every size, x2
	Microlaryngoscopy tubes	4.0 and 5.0 cuffed, x3
	Endoscope/fiberscope masks	1, 3, 5
	Extra membranes	

cont. →

continue **Table 4.1**

Sixth drawer	Jet ventilation catheters	6F, 8F, 10F, 14F, 18F
	Small green guidewire	
	Aerosol delivery kit	Neonate, pediatric, adult
	PEEP value administration set up	
	Light bulbs for light source	
	Extra O_2 tubing	x2
	Rubber pieces for bronchoscopes	
	Disposable endotracheal tube introducer	15F 70 cm, x2
Vertical drawer	Bronchoscopes	
	Olympus neonatal	
	Pentax neonatal	
	Pentax pediatric (battery operated or light source)	x2
	Endotracheal tube exchangers	ID >3 mm, >4 mm, >5 mm short, >5 mm long, >7 mm
	Fogarty catheter	3F
	Eschmann tracheal tube guide	x2
	Frova intubation introducer	ID >3 mm, >6 mm

[a]Quantity if more than one. *PEEP*, positive end-expiratory pressure

Supraglottic Devices

The use of the laryngeal mask airway has been reviewed by Ecoffey [21]. Currently, the most commonly used supraglottic device is the LMA Classic. Its applications in the difficult airway are multiple: rescue from difficult face-mask ventilation, conduit for intubation [22], and ventilation device, among others. As a rescue for difficult face-mask ventilation, it bypasses all potential obstacles and forms an airtight seal around the larynx, thereby making it a more effective supraglottic ventilating device than the face mask [23].

Flexible bronchoscopy through the laryngeal mask airway facilitates the intubation process, as the patient's ventilation is achieved more easily. Secondly, the rigidity of the laryngeal mask airway makes it a perfect conduit for the bronchoscope. Nonetheless, threading the ETT through the laryngeal mask airway without dislodging it is a challenging task, that to date has not been fully resolved in airways other than the LMA Fastrach, or intubating LMA airway (not available in sizes smaller than 3). Among the solutions proposed is the use of a longer ETT threaded in the proximal end with an ETT half a size smaller. The extra length allows the tube to be held while the laryngeal mask airway is removed. Caution should be exercised when trying to pass the tube through the glottic opening as this is not possible with direct visualization; repeated trauma will cause undesirable airway edema.

In some cases laryngeal mask airway removal is not possible without dislodging the ETT. In these cases keeping the laryngeal mask airway *in situ* should be considered, after thorough deliberation upon the length and location of the surgery, intraoperative airway protection and postoperative airway edema.

In the last decade multiple alternatives to the LMA Classic have become available in the market, and their advantages and disadvantages are presented in Table 4.2.

Endotracheal Tubes: Uncuffed vs. Cuffed

Historically much controversy existed and still exists as to whether the ideal ETT is cuffed or uncuffed. Current research has demonstrated various shortcomings in the design of pediatric ETTs, including among others the distance from cuff to tip, the design and material for the cuff, the length of the tube, and the length the markings. Present recommendations for resuscitation include using cuffed tubes in neonatal and pediatric patients [27]. Currently a new ETT with a high-volume/low-pressure polyurethane cuff is being studied [28, 29], but evidence to date is not sufficient to recommend one over another. It is the author's opinion that in patients who are expected to remain intubated in the postoperative period a cuffed tube is preferable. First, it allows the pressure in the cuff to be controlled intraoperatively (cuff pressure monitoring is highly recommended), and later it allows the leak around the tube to be progressively increased, making the ventilation and extubation process easier.

Table 4.2 Supraglottic devices

Device	Advantages	Disadvantages
LMA Classic	Easy insertion Low level of skill Can be used as a guide for intubation	Supraglottic device Small sizes designed by downsizing adult LMAs Low pressure seal [24] Age: 6 months to 1 year Increased risk of laryngospasm and dislodgement [25]
LMA ProSeal	Small sizes designed according to pediatric airway anatomy Small LMAs seat better, less risk of dislodgement Higher airway leak pressure [24] Decrease gastric insufflation [23]	Airway compression
Cuffed oropharyngeal airway	Positive pressure can be achieved up to a pressure of 30 cm H_2O [26]	Inflation pressure <50 cm H_2O (mucosal perfusion)

Anesthetic Management

The most important element of a successful management of a difficult pediatric airway is planning. This should take into account patient factors (age, current health status, etc), anesthesiologist factors (experience, familiarity with different techniques, personnel and equipment availability), and surgical factors (type, length, positioning and extent of surgery). The plan should include induction, as well as how the patient will be extubated, and where the patient will be monitored postoperatively and followed-up.

Once the approach has been decided it should be discussed with the members of the operating room team so that everybody is aware of how to respond to unexpected events.

The ideal induction plan [30]:
1. Maintains oxygenation and ventilation
2. Provides as smooth an induction as possible
3. Has back-up options in case the original plan fails
4. Can be safely aborted if the back-up plan fails
5. Involves airway experts and experienced personnel.

Familiarity with the patient's pathological features (hemifacial microsomia, obstructing mass, small mouth opening, etc) should guide the planning process.

Meticulous equipment preparation (age-appropriate face mask, oral and nasal airways, and laryngoscope blades) and careful positioning of the patient (the use of a shoulder roll may be necessary, or occiput elevation). External laryngeal manipulation may be necessary; clear instructions to the person assisting should be given.

Deciding on the induction technique in children, as opposed to the process in adults, requires balancing the advantages and disadvantages of inhalational versus intravenous induction.

Regardless of which induction technique is chosen, the patient should have an intravenous line in place before any attempt is undertaken to instrument the airway, and antisialagogues are highly recommended (atropine or glycopyrrolate). Induction should be smooth, careful and gradual. The priority is ventilating the patient. This can be achieved by having the appropriate face mask for the patient's size with a good seal, by using maneuvers such as chin lift and jaw thrust, and by using continuous positive airway pressure (CPAP), oral and nasopharyngeal airways, and two-person mask ventilation [31, 32]. In patients with soft-tissue masses in the sub- and retromandibular regions, jaw thrust can decrease airway patency [33].

Laryngospasm can be precipitated if anesthetic depth is inadequate. In the context of the difficult airway, it is a true emergency. It should be established whether the laryngospasm is incomplete (mainly supraglottic component; stridor and cords are partially open, end-tidal CO_2 still present) or complete (supraglottic and glottic component; cords closed, absence of end-tidal CO_2). Figure 4.2 lists different treatment options. For a more detailed description of the laryngospasm pressure point see Larson [34].

Table 4.3 Advantages and disadvantages of different induction techniques in difficult pediatric airway management

| | Induction technique | |
	Inhalational	Intravenous
Advantages	No need for sedation Allows preservation of spontaneous ventilation	
Disadvantages	Risk of apnea Laryngospasm Loss of the airway	Need for sedation (N_2O) More difficult Laryngospasm Loss of the airway
Agents	Sevoflurane, halothane	Propofol, ketamine, dexmedetomidine

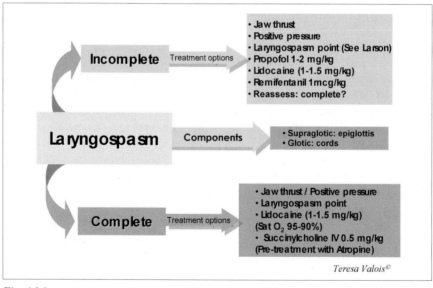

Fig. 4.2 Laryngospasm

As a rescue device for ventilation, the laryngeal mask airway has gained popularity due to: ease of insertion, low level of skill needed for successful placement, and usefulness as a guide for intubation [22, 35]. Although valuable, it is a supraglottic device and poses the risk of aspiration.

Techniques: Inhalational vs. Total Intravenous Anesthesia

Sevoflurane

This inhalational agent possesses two key advantages in the management of the difficult pediatric airway [36]: it allows spontaneous ventilation and quick reversal of anesthetic effects.

Remifentanil

This ultrashort-acting opioid is very useful in the context of the difficult airway due to its ultrashort half-life and easy titration, and the fact that it allows preservation of spontaneous ventilation. However, in children it should be used with caution as a bolus due to its bradycardic effect.

Remifentanil can be used with propofol as separate infusions or mixed in one syringe. Independent infusion enables independent titration of the drugs [23]. Ansermino et al. showed that a dose of 0.05 µg/kg per minute allows spontaneous ventilation in more than 90% of patients [37].

Dexmedetomidine

Multiple reports [38–42] of the use of this new α2 agonist for fiberoptic intubation have been recently published. Among its advantages is that it provides sedation allowing spontaneous ventilation. However, severe bradycardia has been reported after bolus administration [43–46]. Intubation has to be performed with meticulous technique to limit the number of attempts so that trauma and airway edema are minimized [32]. Muscle relaxants have the advantages of reducing the risk of laryngospasm and patient movement, but they render the patient apneic and may worsen airway obstruction due to the decrease in muscle tone.

Multiple techniques have been described to approach the difficult pediatric airway (Table 4.4); every practitioner should choose two or three alternative techniques to direct laryngoscopy. These should be practiced in normal airways to facilitate recognition of anatomical structures. Regular practice will ensure good technical skill for when it is needed.

Extubation and Follow-up

Patients should be extubated when fully awake, with protective airway reflexes intact. For patients undergoing surgery involving the airway, or prolonged surgery with the associated risks (spinal fusion), admission to the intensive care unit should be considered. Patients should be observed in the postanesthetic care

Table 4.4 Suggested approaches for different airway pathologies

Pathology	Difficulties	Suggested technique
Cervical neck instability/cervical spine fusion	Inability to extend the neck	Nasal fiberoptic intubation. Light wand
Mid-facial hypoplasia (Treacher Collins syndrome, Crouzon disease)	Difficult mask ventilation (inability to fit the mask) but not necessarily difficult laryngoscopy [32]. Treacher Collins syndrome (mandibular hypoplasia): difficult laryngoscopy	Awake fiberoptic intubation (oral or nasal). Preserve spontaneous ventilation
Micrognathia	Decreased space for laryngoscopy and manipulation. ENT should be aware of case and prepared for tracheotomy. After induction may be difficult to ventilate, due to decreased tone (base of the tongue)	Preserve spontaneous ventilation. Fiberoptic intubation. Intubating LMA. Fiberoptic intubation through LMA
Small mouth opening	Possible difficult mask ventilation. LMA not suggested	Nasal fiberoptic intubation (awake). Blind nasal intubation
Airway trauma	Difficulty to visualize due to bleeding	Direct laryngoscopy or tracheotomy
Airway masses	Difficult to visualize due to mass effect and risk of rupture. Direct vision techniques preferred to blind techniques. Careful and gentle technique is mandatory to avoid rupture or spillage	Direct laryngoscopy. Fiberoptic intubation
Hurler or Hunter syndrome	Distortion of facial features and macroglossia [32] (snoring history): face mask and direct laryngoscopy are difficult. Airway becomes worse with age	Preserve spontaneous ventilation. Fiberoptic intubation through LMA. Awake fiberoptic intubation
Pierre Robin syndrome	Micrognathia, difficult direct laryngoscopy. Airway improves with age. May be associated with cleft lip and/or palate	Preserve spontaneous ventilation. Fiberoptic intubation
Goldenhar syndrome	Hemifacial hypoplasia: difficult face mask and direct laryngoscopy. Airway difficulty worsens with age	Preserve spontaneous ventilation. Fiberoptic intubation. Fiberoptic intubation through LMA

ENT, endonasal tube

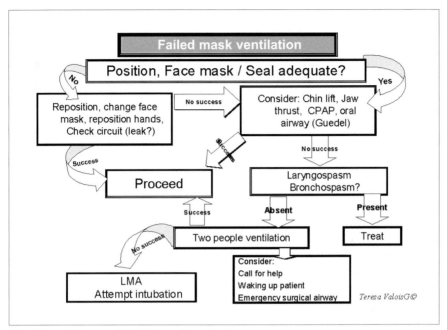

Fig. 4.3 Decision tree for failed mask ventilation

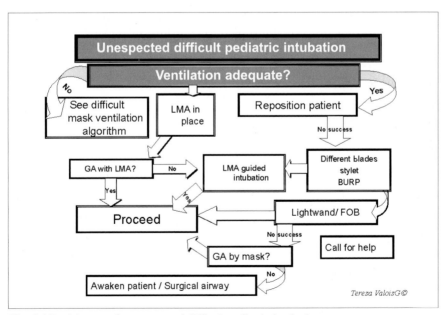

Fig. 4.4 Decision tree for unexpected difficult pediatric intubation

unit or in the intensive care unit for complications such as croup, bleeding, tracheal or esophageal perforation, pneumothorax, trauma (lip, tongue, teeth, larynx), aspiration or postobstructive pulmonary edema.

Prior to discharge parents should be given a detailed explanation and informative letter describing what was used to instrument their airway and a clear description of the maneuvers done. It is of outmost importance to classify difficulties in ventilating, intubating or both.

The following are points to consider in extubating pediatric patients with a difficult airway:

- Plan for reintubation in case of failure to extubate
- Airway cart available
- Anesthesiologist(s) in place
- May be necessary to extubate the patient in the operating room
- ENT in place
- ETT exchanger could be left in place in cooperative patients after extubation to enable quick reintubation in in the event of sudden deterioration. The ETT exchanger is less bulky and irritating than a bougie.

Future Directions

Definitions of a difficult airway specific to the pediatric population are needed, as extrapolations from adult definitions are not always applicable. Also, prospective studies concerning the incidence of difficult face-mask ventilation, intubation and laryngoscopy, and the associated risk factors would help current and future practitioners to successfully approach the difficult pediatric airway.

References

1. Eckenhoff JE (1951) Some anatomic considerations of the infant larynx influencing endotracheal anesthesia. Anesthesiology 12:401–410
2. Litman RS, Weissend EE, Shibata D et al (2003) Developmental changes of laryngeal dimensions in unparalyzed, sedated children. Anesthesiology 98:41–45
3. Litman RS, Wake N, Chan LM et al (2005) Effect of lateral positioning on upper airway size and morphology in sedated children. Anesthesiology 103:484–488
4. Litman RS, Weissend EE, Shrier DA et al (2002) Morphologic changes in the upper airway of children during awakening from propofol administration. Anesthesiology 96:607–611
5. Dalal PG, Feng A, Molter D et al (2007) Morphologic changes in the pediatric epiglottis: an age-based comparison in normal children using video-bronchoscopy (abstract P45). Society for Pediatric Anesthesia. Pediatric Anesthesiology (2007 Winter Meeting), Phoenix
6. Reber A (2004) The pediatric upper airway: anaesthetic aspects and conclusions. Curr Opin Anaesthesiol 17:217–221
7. Farmery AD, Roe PG (1996) A model to describe the rate of oxyhaemoglobin desaturation during apnoea. Br J Anaesth 76:284–291
8. Wheeler M (1998) Management strategies for the difficult pediatric airway. Anesthesiol Clin North America 16:743–761

9. American Society of Anesthesiologists Task Force on Management of the Difficult Airway (2003) Practice guidelines for management of the difficult airway: an updated report by the American Society of Anesthesiologists Task Force on Management of the Difficult Airway. Anesthesiology 98:1269–1277

10. Frei FJ, Ummenhofer W (1996) Difficult intubation in paediatrics. Paediatr Anaesth 6:251–263

11. Shiga T, Wajima Z, Inoue T et al (2005) Predicting difficult intubation in apparently normal patients: a meta-analysis of bedside screening test performance. Anesthesiology 103:429–437

12. Tong DC, Litman RS (2007) The Children's Hospital of Philadelphia Difficult Intubation Registry (abstract P43). Society for Pediatric Anesthesia. Pediatric Anesthesiology (2007 Winter Meeting), Phoenix

13. Akpek EA, Mutlu H, Kayhan Z (2004) Difficult intubation in pediatric cardiac anesthesia. J Cardiothorac Vasc Anesth 18:610–612

14. Bevilacqua S, Nicolini A, Del Sarto P (1996) Difficult intubation in paediatric cardiac surgery. Significance of age. Association with Down's syndrome. Minerva Anestesiol 62:259–264

15. Hall SC (2001) The difficult pediatric airway – recognition evaluation, and management. Can J Anesth 48:R1–R5

16. Baum VC, O'Flaherty JE (2006) Anesthesia for genetic, metabolic & dysmorphic syndromes of childhood, 2nd edn. Lippincott Williams and Wilkins, Philadelphia

17. Tait AR, Malviya S (2005) Anesthesia for the child with an upper respiratory tract infection: still a dilemma? Anesth Analg 100:59–65

18. Gross JB, Bachenberg KL, Benumof JL et al (2006) Practice guidelines for the perioperative management of patients with obstructive sleep apnea: a report by the American Society of Anesthesiologists Task Force on Perioperative Management of patients with obstructive sleep apnea. Anesthesiology 104:1081–1093

19. Gregory GA, Riazi J (1998) Classification and assessment of the difficult pediatric airway. Anesthesiol Clin North America 16:729–741

20. Constant I (2003) Choosing an endotracheal intubation set in paediatric anaesthesia (in French). Ann Fr Anesth Reanim 22:890–895

21. Ecoffey C (2003) Laryngeal mask airway in paediatrics: when? How? (in French). Ann Fr Anesth Reanim 22:648–652

22. Selim M, Mowafi H, Al-Ghamdi A et al (1999) Intubation via LMA in pediatric patients with difficult airways. Can J Anaesth 46:891–893

23. Goldmann K (2006) Recent developments in airway management of the paediatric patient. Curr Opin Anaesthesiol 19:278–284

24. Goldmann K, Roettger C, Wulf H (2006) The size 1(1/2) ProSeal laryngeal mask airway in infants: a randomized, crossover investigation with the Classic laryngeal mask airway. Anesth Analg 102:405–410

25. Bordet F, Allaouchiche B, Lansiaux S et al (2002) Risk factors for airway complications during general anaesthesia in paediatric patients. Paediatr Anaesth 12:762–769

26. Polaner DM (2006) Supraglottic devices in pediatrics. Proceedings of the Fifth International Symposium on the Pediatric Airway, Pittsburgh, PA, 8–11 June 2006

27. American Academy of Pediatrics/American College of Emergency Physicians (2007) APLS course manual (4th edn). American Academy of Pediatrics, Elk Grove Village, IL

28. Dullenkopf A, Gerber AC, Weiss M (2005) Fit and seal characteristics of a new paediatric tracheal tube with high volume-low pressure polyurethane cuff. Acta Anaesthesiol Scand 49:232–237

29. Weiss M, Dullenkopf A, Bottcher S et al (2006) Clinical evaluation of cuff and tube tip position in a newly designed paediatric preformed oral cuffed tracheal tube. Br J Anaesth 97:695–700

30. Marraro GA (2001) Airway management. In: Bissonnette B, Dalens BJ (eds) Pediatric anesthesia: principles and practice. McGraw-Hill, New York, p 778

31. von Ungern-Sternberg BS, Erb TO, Reber A et al (2005) Opening the upper airway – airway maneuvers in pediatric anesthesia. Paediatr Anaesth 15:181–189

32. Wheeler M (2000) The difficult pediatric airway. In: Hagberg CA (ed) Handbook of difficult airway management, 1st edn. Churchill Livingstone, London, pp 257–300

33. von Ungern-Sternberg BS, Erb TO, Frei FJ (2005) Jaw thrust can deteriorate upper airway patency. Acta Anaesthesiol Scand 49:583–585

34. Larson CP Jr (1998) Laryngospasm – the best treatment. Anesthesiology 89:1293–1294

35. Nussbaum E, Zagnoev M (2001) Pediatric fiberoptic bronchoscopy with a laryngeal mask airway. Chest 120:614–616

36. Kandasamy R, Sivalingam P (2000) Use of sevoflurane in difficult airways. Acta Anaesthesiol Scand 44:627–629

37. Ansermino JM, Brooks P, Rosen D et al (2005) Spontaneous ventilation with remifentanil in children. Paediatr Anaesth 15:115–121

38. Abdelmalak B, Makary L, Hoban J et al (2007) Dexmedetomidine as sole sedative for awake intubation in management of the critical airway. J Clin Anesth 19:370–373

39. Bergese SD, Khabiri B, Roberts WD et al (2007) Dexmedetomidine for conscious sedation in difficult awake fiberoptic intubation cases. J Clin Anesth 19:141–144

40. Scher CS, Gitlin MC (2003) Dexmedetomidine and low-dose ketamine provide adequate sedation for awake fibreoptic intubation. Can J Anaesth 50:607–610

41. Shimabukuro A, Satoh K (2007) Airway management with dexmedetomidine for difficult airway (in Japanese). Masui 56:681–684

42. Siobal MS, Kallet RH, Kivett VA et al (2006) Use of dexmedetomidine to facilitate extubation in surgical intensive-care-unit patients who failed previous weaning attempts following prolonged mechanical ventilation: a pilot study. Respir Care 51:492–496

43. Finkel JC, Quezado ZM (2007) Hypothermia-induced bradycardia in a neonate receiving dexmedetomidine. J Clin Anesth 19:290–292

44. Hammer GB, Drover DR, Cao H et al (2008) The effects of dexmedetomidine on cardiac electrophysiology in children. Anesth Analg 106:79–83

45. Berkenbosch JW, Tobias JD (2003) Development of bradycardia during sedation with dexmedetomidine in an infant concurrently receiving digoxin. Pediatr Crit Care Med 4:203–205

46. Tobias JD (2007) Dexmedetomidine: applications in pediatric critical care and pediatric anesthesiology. Pediatr Crit Care Med 8:115–131

Chapter 5

Central Venous Cannulation Techniques

Nicola Disma, Marinella Astuto

Introduction

Central venous cannulation (CVC) is a commonly performed procedure in anesthesia and intensive care. It facilitates optimal anesthetic and perioperative management particularly the management of high-risk patients and the long-term management of those with chronic underlying diseases. To insert a central venous line means to place a catheter within the thoracic cavity, with the tip terminating in the joint between the right atrium and the superior vena cava (SVC). CVC is important in infants and children because of the need to establish and maintain a vascular access.

The principal reasons that a CVC is requested are:
- Central venous pressure (CVP) measurement
- Monitoring of mixed venous and bulb oxygen saturation
- Insertion of pacing wires or pulmonary artery catheters
- CVP waveform analysis
- Delivery of drugs to the central circulation
- Administration of high-concentration parenteral alimentation
- Rapid infusion of large volumes of fluids or blood products
- Replacement of circulating volume
- Administration of chemotherapy
- If peripheral access is difficult and for frequent blood sampling
- Administration of vasoconstrictor inotropes
- Hemodialysis or hemofiltration
- Plasmapheresis.

Above all long-term central venous access devices are used in the treatment of pediatric oncology patients offering considerable advantages for both patients and the treatment team. They may be classified as: short-term, long-term, and single or multiple lumen. Sizes vary from less than 1F to 14F.

M. Astuto (ed), *Basics*, Anesthesia, Intensive Care and Pain in Neonates and Children.
ISBN 978-88-470-0654-6 © Springer-Verlag Italia 2009

Insertion Techniques

Providing a long enough catheter is used, any peripheral vessel can be used to access a central vein. Deep veins available for CVC placement are: the internal jugular vein (IJV), the femoral vein, and the subclavian vein. The central circulation can be accessed via peripheral veins such as the external jugular, antecubital and saphenous veins (such a device is referred to as a peripherally inserted central catheter, PICC).

The three percutaneous techniques commonly used are:
1. The Seldinger technique
2. The through-the-needle technique
3. The combined technique.

In the *Seldinger technique* a needle mounted on a syringe is used to search percutaneously the desired vessel. The syringe is removed from the needle when the aspired blood flows freely. The needle is removed after a guidewire has been passed. The skin is dilated with the set dilator to allow the catheter to be inserted over the wire. The guidewire is removed gently after the catheter is introduced in the proper position.

In the *through-the-needle technique* a needle is used large enough to accommodate a catheter. Once a vessel is cannulated, the catheter is advanced into the vessel and then the introducing needle is removed. This technique is especially useful in premature infants for placing small catheters into a vessel and advancing them to the central circulation.

In the *combined technique* the same guidewire approach is used. A peel-away sheath is introduced over the wire into the vessel and the wire is removed. A catheter of smaller diameter than the peel-away sheath is introduced into the vessel, and after the catheter is positioned as desired, the sheath is pulled and peeled, leaving the catheter in place. Because this technique allows the use of vessel dilators and the sheath offers little resistance to the advancement of a floppy catheter, it is useful for the placement of soft, large-diameter catheters.

Technique and Anatomical Landmarks

The IJV is frequently chosen for a CVC. In particular, the right IJV is most frequently cannulated because it is larger and straighter than that on the left side. Moreover, it is more convenient for right-handed practitioners and avoids the possibility of injury to the thoracic duct. Four different approaches have been described: central, low, anterior and posterior. The central approach is commonly used.

First, the table is tilted head down to increase the diameter of the vein and to prevent air embolism. A small pillow can be placed under the shoulders to extend the patient's neck and the head is turned slightly away from the site of puncture. The needle is inserted at the apex of the triangle formed by the two heads of the sternomastoid muscle and the clavicle, just lateral to the carotid artery. It is directed caudally towards the ipsilateral nipple at an angle of 30–40° to the skin. The subclavian vein is believed to be held open by surrounding tissue, even in severe circulatory collapse. The right subclavian vein is preferred because this approach avoids damage to the thoracic duct. In children the use of a pillow under the shoulders can be avoided during subclavian vein cannulation, and a more physiological position is preferred. The head can be turned away from the site of insertion, even though tilting the head toward the catheterization side has been demonstrated to be the best method for facilitating placement in the subclavian vein cannulation (SVC) and reducing the likelihood of malpositioning of the catheter. In the infraclavicular approach the needle is inserted just below the lower border of the clavicle at the border of the medial and middle thirds. The needle is kept in the horizontal plane and advanced medially and posteriorly to the clavicle, aiming for the sternal notch. The needle should not pass further than the sternal head of the clavicle.

The femoral vein may be cannulated with a low risk of serious short-term complications. The large diameter of the femoral vein allows infusion and removal of large volumes of fluid, and because of this it is commonly used in the pediatric intensive care unit for placement of short-term hemofiltration catheters. The patient is positioned supine in the frog-leg position. The pulsation of the femoral artery is palpated caudally to the inguinal ligament. Then needle is inserted medial to the pulsation, aiming medially towards the head at an angle of 20–30° to the skin.

A summary of the techniques described above is presented in Table 5.1.

Table 5.1 Sites of insertion and summary of techniques

Site of insertion	Technique
Internal jugular vein	1 Apex of the triangle
	2 Level of the cricoid
	3 Angle of 30° to the coronal plane
	4 Needle caudal and parallel to the sagittal plane or slightly down toward the ipsilateral nipple
Subclavian vein	1 Introduce needle at the junction of the middle and the medial thirds of the clavicle
	2 Direct it toward the suprasternal notch
	3 Syringe parallel to the frontal plane, lying in the pectoral shoulder groove
	4 After free flow rotate the needle 90° to facilitate passage of the guidewire
Femoral vein	1 Frog-leg position
	2 Medial to the femoral pulse
	3 1–2 cm below the inguinal ligament
	4 Advancing cephalad at an angle of 45°

Complications of Central Venous Catheterization

Mechanical, cardiopulmonary, infectious and thromboembolic complications can occur. Infections are the most serious and frequent catheter-related complication and for this reason are described fully below. The other complications are only mentioned briefly.

Mechanical
- Migration and malpositioning
- Occlusion (clotting)
  - Thrombus formation
  - Fat deposition
  - Chemical occlusion
  - Tip laying against the vessel wall
  - Kinking
- Fractures
- Curling inside the heart
- Dislodgement

Cardiopulmonary
- Pneumothorax and hydrothorax
- Hemothorax
- Hemorrhage
- Arrhythmia
- Arterial puncture
- Hematoma
- Embolism
- Right atrial thrombus
- Endocarditis
- Cardiac tamponade
- Thoracic duct damage

Infectious
- Local infection
- Bacteremia, sepsis

Thromboembolic
- Vessel thrombosis
- Venous air embolism
- Catheter/guidewire embolism

Infections

The American Academy of Pediatrics (AAP) recently developed the *Guidelines for the Prevention of Intravascular Catheter-related Infections* [1]. The guidelines aim to provide practical indications for surveillance and control of catheter-related infections in hospital, outpatient, and home health-care. Guidelines are really important because a long-term catheter puts patients at risk of local and systemic infectious complications, including local site infection, catheter-related blood-stream infections (BSI), septic thrombophlebitis, endocarditis, and other metastatic infections (lung abscess, brain abscess, osteomyelitis, and endophthalmitis). The incidence of catheter-related BSI varies considerably by type of catheter, frequency of catheter manipulation, and patient-related factors (underlying disease and acuity of illness), and the incidence of infection is often higher in the ICU setting than in the less-acute inpatient or ambulatory setting.

The rate of all catheter-related infections (including local infections and systemic infections) is difficult to determine. Although catheter-related BSI is the best indicator because it is the most serious catheter-related infection, the rate of catheter-related BSI depends on how it is defined. Health-care professionals should recognize the difference between surveillance definitions and clinical definitions. The surveillance definitions of catheter-associated BSIs include all BSIs that occur in patients with CVCs, when other sites of infection have been excluded. A more rigorous definition might include only those BSIs for which other sources have been excluded by careful examination of the patient record, and where a culture of the catheter tip has demonstrated substantial colonies of an organism identical to those found in the blood-stream. The Center for Disease Control and Prevention (CDC) [2] and the Joint Commission on Accreditation of Healthcare Organizations (JCAHO) [3] recommend that the rate of catheter-associated BSIs be expressed as the number of catheter associated BSIs per 1,000 CVC days.

The majority of BSIs in children are associated with the use of an intravascular catheter [4]. The types of organisms that most commonly cause hospital-acquired BSIs change over time. The most frequent causes of catheter-related BSIs are coagulase-negative staphylococci (37%) and *Staphylococcus aureus* (12.6%). Gram-negative bacteria account for 25% of BSIs reported in pediatric ICUs, whereas enterococci and *Candida* spp. account for 10% and 9%, respectively [1].

Exposure to lipids has been identified as an independent risk factor for the development of coagulase-negative staphylococcal bacteremia in very low birth weight infants, as well as candidemia in neonatal ICUs [5].

Important pathogenic determinants of catheter-related infection are the material from which the device is made and the intrinsic virulence of the infecting organism. The adherence properties of a given microorganism are also important in the pathogenesis of catheter-related infection. For example, *S. aureus* can adhere to host proteins (fibronectin) commonly present on catheters. Also, coagulase-negative staphylococci adhere to polymer surfaces more readily than do other pathogens (*Escherichia coli* or *S. aureus*). Additionally, certain strains of coagulase-negative staphylococci produce an extracellular polysaccharide often referred to as "slime". *Candida* spp. in the presence of glucose-containing fluids can also produce slime, potentially explaining the increased proportion of BSIs caused by fungal pathogens among patients receiving parenteral nutrition fluids.

Strategies for Prevention of Catheter-Related Infections in Children

Quality Assurance and Continuing Education Well-organized programs or specialized "IV teams" that enable health-care providers to provide, monitor, and evaluate care and to become educated are critical in minimizing the infection risk. Otherwise, infection risk increases with staff reductions below a critical level.

Site of Catheter Insertion The density of the skin flora at the catheter insertion site is a major risk factor for catheter-related BSI. Studies in children have demonstrated that femoral catheters have a low incidence of mechanical complications and might have an equivalent infection rate to that of nonfemoral catheters.

Type of Catheter Material Teflon or polyurethane catheters have been associated with fewer infectious complications than catheters made from polyvinyl chloride or polyethylene.

Hand Hygiene and Aseptic Technique Maximal sterile barrier precautions (cap, mask, sterile gown, sterile gloves, and large sterile drape) during the insertion of CVCs substantially reduces the incidence of catheter-related BSI [6].

Skin Antisepsis A 2% aqueous solution of chlorhexidine gluconate for preparation of the central venous site provides better control of BSI than 10% povidone-iodine or 70% alcohol.

Catheter Site Dressing Regimens Transparent, semipermeable polyurethane dressings are recommended. Transparent dressings reliably secure the device, permit continuous visual inspection of the catheter site, permit the patient to bathe and shower without saturating the dressing, and require less-frequent changes than standard gauze and tape dressings.

In-line Filters No strong recommendation can be made in favor of using in-line filters. They might become blocked, especially with certain solutions (dextran, lipids, and mannitol), thereby increasing the number of line manipulations and decreasing the availability of administered drugs.

Antimicrobial/Antiseptic Impregnated Catheters These catheters have been approved by the FDA for use in patients weighing more than 3 kg. No antiseptic or antimicrobial impregnated catheters are currently available for use in patients weighing less than 3 kg. Catheters coated with chlorhexidine/silver sulfadiazine only on the external luminal surface have been studied and their benefit in reducing catheter-related BSI will be realized within the first 14 days. A second-generation catheter with chlorhexidine coating both the internal and external luminal surfaces is now available and preliminary studies indicate a prolonged anti-infective activity.

Systemic Antibiotic Prophylaxis This is not recommended because the prophylactic use of vancomycin is an independent risk factor for the acquisition of vancomycin-resistant enterococcus (VRE), and the risk of acquiring VRE outweighs the benefit of using prophylactic vancomycin [7].

Antibiotic Ointments Antibiotic ointments applied to the catheter insertion site may increase the rate of catheter colonization with *Candida* spp., especially if the antibiotic ointments used have no fungicidal activity.

Antibiotic Lock Prophylaxis One study involving a limited number of children revealed no difference in rates of catheter-related BSI between children receiving a heparin flush compared with those receiving heparin and vancomycin [8].

Anticoagulants Anticoagulant flush solutions are used widely to prevent catheter thrombosis. Because thrombi and fibrin deposits on catheters might serve as nests for microbial colonization of intravascular catheters, the use of anticoagulants might be useful in the prevention of catheter-related BSI.

Ultrasonography for Catheter Placement in Infants and Children

Performing a successful blind puncture procedure to place a central venous line in neonates and children depends greatly on a correct knowledge of vascular anatomy and clinical experience, that is "experienced hands". The small caliber of central veins and a greater anatomical variation in their position make the success rate of central venous catheterization lower and the complication rate higher in infants and children than in adults, and it is associated with significant morbidity and mortality [9]. The landmark method can fail if there is an anatomic anomaly, if the patient moves, or if there is variability in vessel position.

Although anatomic landmarks are widely used by most physicians, there are a number of different puncture techniques for vascular access. Acoustic Doppler ultrasonography (US) provides accurate guidance for the puncture procedure. The signals on acoustic Doppler US reflect arterial and venous signals on a single A-scan line [10]. Within this line, there is usually either a high-frequency signal from an artery or a low-frequency signal from a vein when the vessel is directly under the A-scan probe.

The US procedure of choice is the two-dimensional scan, or so-called B-scan [11]. A B-scan is the depiction of several A-lines transformed into a signal that is almost identical to an anatomic depiction of the subcutaneous structures. The needle can be guided through the tissue under direct US guidance in real time. A single operator performs the imaging and the vascular access at the same time, holding the US probe with one hand and the needle with the other. Positioning should enable the anesthesiologist to see the entire US picture and the patient's landmarks without moving his or her head. This in-line view of the anatomy and US image is mandatory for hand–eye coordination during the procedure. The US probe has to be disengaged to introduce the guidewire and its intravascular position can be confirmed after its insertion. US gel is required for acoustic coupling between the US probe, the protective sheath, and the skin surface, and it must be sterile. Scanning of the vessels can be longitudinal or cross-sectional. Similarly, the needle can be inserted in either a longitudinal or transverse direction in relation to the US probe. For the IJV, a cross-sectional scan provides a better view of the surrounding structures.

Ultrasonography of the Internal Jugular Vein

The location and successful cannulation of the IJV depend on a number of factors, including the size of the IJV, intravascular volume status, and the pressure exerted by the US probe on the patient [12]. Head rotation and patient positioning are further factors influencing the procedure of cannulation and US detection [13]. Moreover, a large number of anatomic variations in the position of the IJV based on US examinations have been reported.

Ultrasonography of the Subclavian Vein

Children are placed in a light head-down position with their head in a neutral position. For infants, a rolled towel is placed transversally under the shoulders and the head is slightly turned away from the side of venipuncture in order to make room for the US probe. The probe is placed at the supraclavicular level with its foot on the clavicle and the stick directed medially and slightly cranially. Two bony structures are first recognized as bright hyperechoic structures with an acoustic shadow beneath them. The most superficial and lateral structure is the clavicle, whereas the first rib is deeper and more medial. The vascular structures are found passing between these two structures. When the best picture of the subclavian vein is obtained two surface marks are made. The first mark is made at the middle of the foot-end of the US probe, at the infraclavicular level, and this will be the entry point of the needle. The second mark is made at the other end of the probe, and shows the direction to be followed by the needle to reach the vein [14].

In September 2002 the UK National Institute for Clinical Excellence (NICE) published guidelines for central venous catheterization in children and recommend the use of US guidance as the preferred method for elective insertion of CVCs into the IJV in children [15]. The recommendations were based on randomized controlled studies of jugular venous cannulation in infants [16–18]. In these trials, comparing US guidance with a landmark technique, US was associated with a reduction in the risk of failure to place a catheter, a reduction in complications associated with catheter placement, and a reduction in the number of attempts to achieve successful catheterization. However, these recommendations have not been universally accepted. Critics have noted that the trials supporting the use of US in children all had small sample sizes, and in two of the studies CVCs were placed by trainees rather than experienced practitioners. Some anesthesiologists remain unconvinced of the usefulness of US guidance for regular practitioners.

In summary, some clinical trials have shown that US-guided vascular access leads to shorter procedure times, reduces the number of failed puncture attempts, and reduces to a minimum the complications of CVC. It combines the puncture process with diagnosis and detection of anatomic variations, lesions, and complications, which makes it a powerful tool for vascular access. Patients thus benefit from a reduced rate of complications.

Although some trials and recent meta-analyses have shown advantages of US in pediatric practice, more clinical trials are required to prove its effectiveness, especially for access sites other than the IJV. To compare the results of clinical investigations of US in vascular access procedures, not only should the success and complication rates be reported, but also the number of puncture attempts through skin, the number of needle advancements, patient anatomy, positioning of the patient and the US probe, and the number of previous catheterizations. Moreover, the medical materials used for venous cannulation is still not optimized for US visualization in small children [19].

US guidance is therefore likely to provide benefits to patients with a reduction in the risks of the procedure, and they are less likely to have to undergo a prolonged, sometimes uncomfortable and possibly fruitless attempt at CVC. If confirmed by future studies, US could lead to deskilling in the landmark method that may still be required in some emergency situations. Guidance from the NICE in this area states that it is important that "operators maintain their ability to use the landmark method and that the method continues to be taught alongside the 2-D ultrasound guided technique".

Conclusion

- Hundreds of thousands of central venous lines are placed in patients every year in hospitals; complication and failure rates vary, and deaths have been reported.
- Clinical trials have shown that catheterization under two-dimensional US guidance is quicker and safer than the landmark method in both adults and

children, and is more effective than Doppler US guidance for more difficult procedures.

- It is important that "operators maintain their ability to use the landmark method and that the method continues to be taught alongside the 2-D ultrasound guided technique".
- Guidelines for infection control must be provided by each institution to increase the safety in pediatric patients.

References

1. O'Grady NP, Alexander M, Dellinger EP et al (2002) Guidelines for the prevention of intravascular catheter-related infections. Pediatrics 110:e51
2. National Nosocomial Infections Surveillance System (1999) NNIS System report, data summary from January 1990–May 1999, issued June 1999. Am J Infect Control 27:520–532
3. Joint Commission on the Accreditation of Healthcare Organizations (1994) Accreditation manual for hospitals. Joint Commission on the Accreditation of Healthcare Organizations, Chicago, pp 121–140
4. Richards MJ, Edwards JR, Culver DH, Gaynes RP (1999) Nosocomial infections in pediatric intensive care units in the United States: National Nosocomial Infections Surveillance System. Pediatrics 103:103–109
5. Avila-Figueroa C, Goldmann DA, Richardson DK et al (1998) Intravenous lipid emulsions are the major determinant of coagulase-negative staphylococcal bacteremia in very low birth weight newborns. Pediatr Infect Dis J 17:10–17
6. Pittet D, Hugonnet S, Harbath S et al (2000) Effectiveness of a hospital-wide programme to improve compliance with hand hygiene. Lancet 356:1307–1309
7. Centers for Disease Control and Prevention (1995) Recommendations for preventing the spread of vancomycin resistance. Recommendations of the Hospital Infection Control Practices Advisory Committee (HICPAC). MMWR 44(RR12):1–13
8. Rackoff WR, Weiman M, Jakobowski D et al (1995) A randomized, controlled trial of the efficacy of a heparin and vancomycin solution in preventing central venous catheter infections in children. J Pediatr 127:147–151
9. Stenzel JP, Green TP, Fuhrman BP et al (1989) Percutaneous central venous catheterization in a pediatric intensive care unit: a survival analysis of complications. Crit Care Med 17:984–988
10. Macintyre PA, Samra G, Hatch DJ (2000) Preliminary results with the Doppler ultrasound guided vascular access needle in paediatric patients. Paediatr Anaesth 10:361–365
11. Muhm M (2002) Ultrasound guided central venous access: is useful for beginners, in children and when blind cannulation fails. BMJ 325:1373–1374
12. Mallinson C, Bennett J, Hodgson P et al (1999) Position of the internal jugular vein in children. A study of the anatomy using ultrasonography. Paediatr Anaesth 9:111–114
13. Alderson PJ, Burrow FA, Stemp LI et al (1993) Use of ultrasound to evaluate internal jugular vein anatomy and to facilitate central venous cannulation in paediatric patients. Br J Anaesth 70:145–148
14. Merrer J, De Jonghe B, Golliot F et al (2001) Complications of femoral and subclavian venous catheterization in critically ill patients: a randomized controlled trial. JAMA 286:700–707
15. Grebenik CR, Boyce A, Sinclair ME et al (2004) NICE guidelines for central venous catheterization in children. Is the evidence base sufficient? Br J Anaesth 92:827–831
16. Verghese ST, McGill WA, Patel RI et al (1999) Ultrasound-guided internal jugular venous cannulation in infants. Anaesthesiology 91:71–77

17. Verghese ST, McGill WA, Patel RI et al (2000) Comparison of three techniques for internal jugular venous cannulation in infants. Paediatr Anaesth 10:505–511

18. Chiang VW, Baskin MN (2000) Uses and complications of central venous catheters inserted in a pediatric emergency department. Pediatr Emerg Care 16:230–232

19. Nikolaus A, Haas, Silke AH (2003) Central venous catheter techniques in infants and children. Curr Opin Anaesthesiol 16:291–303

Chapter 6

Prevention of Bloodstream Infections

Hendrick K.F. van Saene, Kentigern Thorburn, Andy J. Petros

Sources

Bloodstream infections occur from various sources. Certain microorganisms thrive in different parts of the body or colonize exogenous prosthetic pieces of equipment. Hence the source of a bloodstream infection can almost be predicted according to the microorganism detected. Coagulase-negative staphylococci (CNS) are in general associated with catheter-related bloodstream infections, whereas aerobic Gram-negative bacilli (AGNB) cause bloodstream infections following lymph drainage from the respiratory tract, intraabdominal space and urinary tract. Most bloodstream infections of unknown origin are gut-derived, e.g., fungemia following translocation of *Candida albicans* present as overgrowth in the gut. Table 6.1 shows that the contaminated catheter and the lower airways are leading causes of bloodstream infections [1–4].

Table 6.1 Major sources of bloodstream infections in the intensive care unit (values are percentages)

Source	Pittet et al. [1]	Rello et al. [2]	Edgeworth et al. [3]	Valles et al. [6]
Catheter	18	35	62	37.1
Lower airways	28	10	3	17.5
Intra-abdominal	N/A	9	6.9	6.1
Genitourinary tract	5.4	3.6	2.4	5.9
Surgical wound or soft tissue	8	8	3	2.4
Other	14.5	7	–	2.9
Unknown origin	20	27	22.4	28.1

M. Astuto (ed), *Basics*, Anesthesia, Intensive Care and Pain in Neonates and Children.
ISBN 978-88-470-0654-6 © Springer-Verlag Italia 2009

Systemic Response to Bloodstream Infection

Bloodstream infection and fungemia have been defined as the presence of bacteria or fungi in blood cultures. Four stages of systemic response to infection have been described:

1. *Systemic inflammatory response syndrome (SIRS)*: patients have a combination of simple and readily available clinical signs and symptoms, i.e. fever or hypothermia, tachycardia, tachypnea, and changes in blood leukocyte count.
2. *Sepsis*: patients in whom the SIRS is caused by a documented infection.
3. *Severe sepsis*: patients have dysfunction of the major organs.
4. *Septic shock*: patients have hypotension and organ dysfunction in addition to sepsis.

As sepsis progresses to septic shock, the risk of death increases substantially. Early sepsis is usually reversible, whereas many patients with septic shock succumb despite aggressive therapy.

The presence of microorganisms in the blood is one of the most reliable criteria for characterizing a patient with sepsis or one of its more severe presentations, such as severe sepsis or septic shock.

In a recent multicenter study, Brun-Buisson et al. analyzed the relationship between bloodstream infection and severe sepsis in patients on adult ICUs and in the general wards in 24 hospitals in France [5]. In this study, there were 842 episodes of clinically significant bloodstream infection recorded, of which 162 (20%) occurred in patients receiving intensive care, and 377 (45%) were nosocomial. Their incidence was 12 times greater in ICUs than in wards. The frequency of severe sepsis during bloodstream infection differed markedly between wards and ICUs (17% versus 65%, $p<0.001$). The nosocomial episodes developing on the ICUs represented an incidence of 41 episodes per 1,000 admissions and the incidence of severe sepsis amongst patients with nosocomial bloodstream infection on the ICUs was 24 episodes per 1,000 admissions.

In another recent multicenter study, Valles et al. analyzed exclusively nosocomial bloodstream infections acquired in patients on adult ICUs of 30 hospitals in Spain, and classified their systemic response according to new definitions as sepsis, severe sepsis, and septic shock [6]. Among the 590 episodes of nosocomial bloodstream infection, sepsis developed in 371 episodes (63%), severe sepsis in 109 episodes (18.5%), and septic shock in the remaining 110 (19%). Interestingly, the systemic response differed markedly according to the source of the bloodstream infection. Bloodstream infections associated with intravascular catheters showed the lowest rate of septic shock (13%), whereas those originating from the lower airways or the abdominal cavity showed the highest incidence of severe sepsis and septic shock. In the study by Brun-Buisson et al., in patients requiring intensive care, catheter-related blood infection was also associated with a lower risk of severe sepsis (OR 0.2, 95% CI 0.1–0.5, $p<0.01$) [5].

Similarly, the systemic response may differ according to the microorganism causing the episode of bloodstream infection. AGNB and yeasts were associated with a higher incidence of severe sepsis and septic shock in the multicenter study by Valles et al. [6]. In the multicenter study by Brun-Buisson et al., ICU bloodstream infections were analyzed separately and the episodes caused by CNS were found to be also associated with a reduced risk of severe sepsis (OR 0.2, p=0.02) compared with other microorganisms [5]. These results suggest that the source of infection and probably the type of microorganism causing the infection, especially if a species other than CNS is involved, may be important in the development of severe sepsis and septic shock [7].

Among community-acquired episodes, the incidence of severe sepsis and septic shock is higher than that of nosocomial episodes, in part because the severity of the systemic response is the reason for ICU admission. In the study by Brun-Buisson et al., 75% of the patients with community-acquired bloodstream infections presented with severe sepsis or septic shock on admission to the ICU [5]. In the study by Valles et al., the incidence of severe sepsis and septic shock was identical, at 75% [6]. AGNB and infections of the urinary tract and the abdominal cavity were associated with septic shock.

Classification of Bloodstream Infections According to the Concept of the Carrier State

Practically all bloodstream infections in the critically ill are endogenous, i.e. preceded by the carrier state (Table 6.2) [8]. More than 50% of all bloodstream infections occurring in the ICU are primary endogenous infections. They are

Table 6.2 Control of bloodstream infections. The efficacy and safety of prophylaxis are monitored by surveillance cultures from the throat and rectum

Infection	Potentially pathogenic microorganisms[a]	Timing	Frequency (%)	Maneuver
Primary endogenous	Six 'normal, nine 'abnormal'	<1 week	55	Parenteral antimicrobials
Secondary endogenous	Nine 'abnormal'	>1 week	30	Enteral antimicrobials
Exogenous	Nine 'abnormal'	Any time during ICU treatment	15	Hygiene

[a]Six 'normal' microorganisms are *Streptococcus pneumoniae*, *Haemophilus influenzae*, *Moraxella catarrhalis*, *Candida albicans*, *Staphylococcus aureus*, and *Escherichia coli*; nine 'abnormal' microorganisms are *Klebsiella*, *Proteus*, *Morganella*, *Enterobacter*, *Citrobacter*, *Serratia*, *Acinetobacter*, *Pseudomonas* species, and methicillin-resistant *S. aureus* (MRSA)

caused by both 'normal' and 'abnormal' potential pathogens present in the patient's admission flora, and in general, develop 'early', i.e. during the first week of treatment on the ICU. Approximately one-third of bloodstream infections in ventilated patients are secondary endogenous infections due to 'abnormal' potential pathogens acquired during treatment on the ICU.

Microorganisms are usually transmitted via the hands of carers, and are firstly acquired in the oropharynx, followed by carriage in the digestive tract and overgrowth in the throught and gut [8]. Subsequently, infection of the bloodstream may occur. Secondary endogenous bloodstream infections generally develop 'late', i.e. after one week. Of all bloodstream infections developing on the ICU, some 20% may be of exogenous pathogenesis, that is those not preceded by the carrier state. The causative microorganisms belong to the 'abnormal' flora and are directly introduced into the bloodstream as a consequence of poor hygiene. These infections may occur at any time during treatment on the ICU.

Control of Bloodstream Infections

Only the immediate administration of parenteral antimicrobials can control primary endogenous or 'early' bloodstream infections due to microorganisms present in the patient's admission flora [9–12]. However, parenteral antimicrobials fail to protect against acquisition, carriage and subsequent overgrowth in the throat and gut, as the salivary and bile concentrations of the injected antimicrobial are in general not bactericidal. Only enteral antimicrobials applied in a gel or paste to the buccal cavity and administered via a nasogastric tube into the stomach and gut have been shown to protect against acquisition and subsequent overgrowth of AGNB and methicillin-resistant *Staphylococcus aureus*. Obviously, neither parenteral nor enteral antimicrobials control microorganisms introduced directly into the bloodstream as a result of poor hygiene. High standards of hygiene are required to prevent this type of exogenous infection of the bloodstream.

These three distinct bloodstream infections due to a limited range of potential pathogens each requires a different prophylactic maneuver. Only parenteral antimicrobials are able to control primary endogenous or 'early' bloodstream infections, enteral antimicrobials effectively control secondary endogenous or 'late' bloodstream infections, and high standards of hygiene control exogenous bloodstream infections. Regular surveillance cultures are indispensable to monitor compliance, efficacy and safety of the prophylactic maneuvers. The combination of surveillance cultures, hygiene, and enteral and parenteral antimicrobials is termed the full four-component protocol of selective digestive decontamination (SDD) [12].

Prevention of Bloodstream Infections by Selective Decontamination of the Digestive Tract

SDD usually includes the enteral administration of the antimicrobials polymyxin, tobramycin and amphotericin B applied to the throat and gut throughout the whole treatment period on the ICU, in combination with parenteral cefotaxime for the first 4 days.

During 20 years of clinical SDD research, 56 randomized controlled trials (RCTs) and two meta-analyses assessing the efficacy of SDD in the prevention of bloodstream infections have been published [9, 10]. Of these 56 RCTs, 51 conducted between 1987 and 2005 have been reviewed [10]. These included 8,065 critically ill patients, 4,079 who received SDD and 3,986 controls. SDD significantly reduced overall bloodstream infections (OR 0.73, 0.59–0.90; $p=0.0036$), Gram-negative bloodstream infections (OR 0.39, 0.24–0.63; $p<0.001$) and overall mortality (OR 0.80, 0.69–0.94; $p=0.0064$) but did not affect Gram-positive bloodstream infections (OR 1.06, 0.77–1.47; Fig. 6.1). All fungal infections, but not fungemia, were shown to be significantly reduced in a recent meta-analysis on the impact of the antifungal component of SDD (OR 0.89, 95% CI 0.16–4.95) mainly due to the low event rates in the test and control groups [9]. A subsequent Australian meta-analysis has confirmed these results (RR 0.51; 95% CI 0.17–1.58) [11].

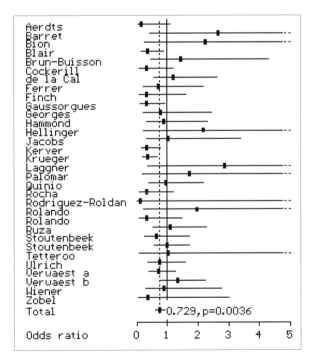

Fig. 6.1 Impact of SDD on overall bloodstream infections [10], with permission

Reduction of Bloodstream Infections Associated with Catheters in Pediatric Intensive Care Units: a Stepwise Approach

Stepwise implementation of the following five interventions leads to a greater than threefold reduction in catheter-related bloodstream infections in the PICU [13, 14]:

1. Maximize barrier precautions for all central venous catheters.
2. Change to antibiotic-impregnated central venous catheters.
3. Introduce annual hand-washing campaigns.
4. Introduce physical barriers between patients' beds.
5. Change the skin disinfectant from povidone-iodine to chlorhexidine.

Figure 6.2 shows the trend over time (1994–2005) in bloodstream infections associated with catheters [14].

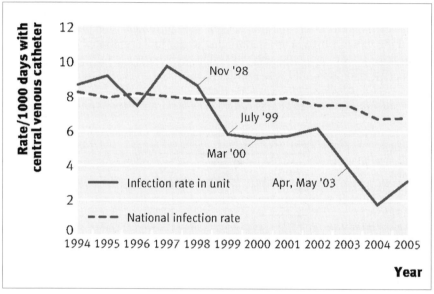

Fig. 6.2 Trend over time (1994–2005) in bloodstream infections associated with catheters in pediatric intensive care units compared with national mean. *Nov '98* introduction of maximal barrier precautions, *July '99* introduction of catheters impregnated with antibiotic, *Mar '00* annual hand-washing campaigns, *April '03* move to new unit with private rooms, *May '03* introduction of skin disinfection with chlorhexidine. (Reproduced from [14] with permission from BMJ Publishing Group)

References

1. Pittet D, Tarara D, Wenzel RP (1994) Nosocomial bloodstream infection in critically ill patients. Excess length of stay, extra costs, and attributable mortality. JAMA 271:1598–1601
2. Rello J, Ricart M, Mirelis B et al (1994) Nosocomial bacteremia in a medical-surgical intensive care unit: epidemiologic characteristics and factors influencing mortality in 111 episodes. Intensive Care Med 20:94–98
3. Edgeworth JD, Treacher DF, Eykyn SJ (1999) A 25 year study of nosocomial bacteremia in an adult intensive care unit. Crit Care Med 27:1421–1428
4. Valles J, Ochagania A, Rue M et al (2000) Critically ill patients with community-acquired bacteremia: characteristics and prognosis. Intensive Care Med 26 [Suppl 3]:222
5. Brun-Buisson C, Doyon F, Carlet J (1996) Bacteremia and severe sepsis in adults: a multicenter prospective study in ICUs and wards of 24 hospitals. French Bacteremia-Sepsis Study Group. Am J Respir Crit Care Med 154:617–624
6. Valles J, Leon C, Alvarez-Lerma F (1997) Nosocomial bacteremia in critically ill patients: a multicenter study evaluating epidemiology and prognosis. Spanish Collaborative Group for Infections in Intensive Care Units of Sociedad Espagnola de Medicina Intensiva y Unidades coronanas (SEMIUC). Clin Infect Dis 24:387–395
7. Thorburn K, Taylor N, Lopez-Rodriguez L et al (2005) High mortality of invasive pneumococcal disease compared with meningococcal disease in critically ill children. Intensive Care Med 31:1550–1557
8. Silvestri L, Petros AJ, Sarginson RE et al (2005) Handwashing in the intensive care unit: a big measure with modest effects. J Hosp Infect 59:172–179
9. Silvestri L, van Saene HKF, Milanese M et al (2005) Impact of selective decontamination of the digestive tract in fungal carriage and infection: systematic review of randomised controlled trials. Intensive Care Med 31:898–910
10. Silvestri L, van Saene HKF, Milanese M et al (2007) Selective decontamination of the digestive tract reduces bacterial bloodstream infection and mortality in critically ill patients. Systematic review of randomised, controlled trials. J Hosp Infect 65:187–203
11. Ho KM, Rochford JA, Dobb GJ (2005) The use of topical non-absorbable gastro-intestinal antifungal prophylaxis to prevent fungal infections in critically ill immunocompetent patients: a meta-analysis. Crit Care Med 33:2383–2392
12. Sarginson RE, Taylor N, Reilly N et al (2004) Infection in prolonged pediatric critical illness: a prospective four-year study based on knowledge of the carrier state. Crit Care Med 32:839–847
13. Hanna H, Raad I (2002) Nosocomial infections related to use of intravascular devices inserted for long-term vascular access. In: Mayhall CG (ed) Hospital epidemiology and infection control, 3rd edn. Lippincott Williams and Wilkins, Philadelphia, pp 241–251
14. Bhutta A, Gilliam G, Honeycutt M et al (2007) Reduction of bloodstream infections associated with catheters in a paediatric intensive care unit: stepwise approach. BMJ 334:362–365

Part III
Perioperative Medicine,
Intensive Care, Pain

Chapter 7

Preoperative Evaluation

Ida Salvo, Anna Camporesi

Introduction

Perioperative morbidity and mortality in pediatric anesthesia have both declined in the last decades due to improvements in perioperative techniques, identification of risk factors and analysis of potentially correctable causes of critical incidents [1–6]. Although the majority of children undergoing anesthesia are healthy, it is essential to identify any risk factor that may lead to an unexpected adverse event in the perioperative period. For this reason, a thorough preoperative assessment is crucial to optimize the child's condition for anesthesia and surgery.

A recent report of the Pediatric Perioperative Cardiac Arrest Registry demonstrates that the most commonly found causes of anesthesia-related cardiac arrests are associated with the cardiovascular system, followed by the respiratory system, medication and equipment (Table 7.1) [7].

However, the position is completely different when analyzing the underlying factors in critical incidents. In contrast with patients who undergo a cardiac arrest, who often present with severe underlying disease [8], the majority of patients who are exposed to a critical incident were previously healthy (80% ASA I and II) and are undergoing elective surgery (73%) [9]. The majority of incidents (80%) occur during the maintenance of anesthesia. Of the total num-

Table 7.1 Causes of anesthesia-related cardiac arrest. Modified from [7]

Causes of cardiac arrest (1998–2004)	No. (% of total), $n=193$
Cardiovascular	79 (41)
Respiratory	53 (27)
Medication	35 (18)
Equipment	9 (5)
Multiple events	3 (2)
Miscellaneous	2 (1)
Unknown	12 (6)

M. Astuto (ed), *Basics*, Anesthesia, Intensive Care and Pain in Neonates and Children.
ISBN 978-88-470-0654-6 © Springer-Verlag Italia 2009

ber of critical incidents, respiratory events account for 77%, while cardiovascular events account for 11%, and equipment and pharmacological problems for only 4% [9]. Comparing pediatric and adult closed-claim law cases with respect to the mechanisms of injury and outcome, respiratory events are more common and have a greater mortality in previously healthy children than in adults [8]. This suggests that a thorough evaluation and potentially the postponement of surgery could have prevented the critical incident, underlying the importance of the preoperative evaluation.

The primary objective of the preanesthetic visit is to assess whether the child is fit for the proposed procedure, identify any disease that may require preoperative treatment and determine which anesthesia regimen is optimal for the child. This period also provides an excellent opportunity for the anesthesiologist to establish a good relationship with the child and family and to allay their anxieties.

The preanesthetic visit should begin with the history of the child. Since most children are not capable of personally giving a medical history, parents should be questioned about it. It is essential to obtain a concise overview of the child's progress since birth, including emotional development. The antenatal and birth history may also be significant in some circumstances. A history of premature birth is particularly important, as these children may have an increased incidence of important diseases during the first years of life. A careful review of the medical record is required, with particular paid attention to previously encountered problems with anesthetics. The airway management techniques used in the past as well as any history of cardiorespiratory diseases and airway anomalies should be reviewed. A history of medical or environmental allergies should be elicited, including questions directed toward evaluating the presence of allergy to latex in children at risk. Results of laboratory tests, when available, should be reviewed. The anesthesiologist must be aware of the child's current therapy and how it may interact with anesthetics. Current drug therapy must also include questions about the use of herbal medications. Many unusual syndromes occur in childhood, which often have multisystem involvement. When a congenital anomaly exists, there is a significant likelihood of anomalies involving other organs.

The symptoms encountered in the preoperative evaluation of a child, their possible underlying diseases and suggested actions prior to surgery are summarized in Table 7.2, and the most commonly found problems encountered are reviewed in the following sections.

Respiratory System

Respiratory adverse events are one of the major causes of morbidity and mortality in pediatric anesthesia. Children have lower oxygen reserves because of the higher tendency for airway collapse leading to decreased functional residual capacity and increased susceptibility to hypoxemia [10]. Difficult intubation accounts for only 13% of all respiratory critical incidents, whereas hypoxia and laryngospasm each account for approximately one-third of the total [9].

Table 7.2 Symptoms encountered during the preoperative assessment, their possible underlying diseases and suggested actions prior to surgery [37]

Symptoms	Possible underlying diseases	Actions
Wheeze; chronic cough; passive smoking	Asthma; bronchial hyperreactivity	Check therapy status (theophylline blood levels, history of corticosteroids, β-agonists); optimize therapy
Snoring; nocturnal apnea	Obstructive sleep apnea syndrome	Consider need for cardiac evaluation or sleep study; consider postoperative monitoring
Prematurity	Bronchopulmonary dysplasia	Consider risk of postoperative apnea; consider cardiac evaluation; optimize respiratory therapy
Non-innocent murmur; cyanosis; sweating; previous heart surgery; enlarged liver	Cardiac malformation	Consider cardiology consultation; ECG; echocardiography; consider need for prophylactic antibiotics
Seizures	Epilepsy	Adequacy of seizure medication; consider possible hepatic dysfunction
Spasticity	Cerebral palsy	Check nutritional status; consider possible chronic infections; check history of chronic aspiration
Enlarged liver/spleen; neurological deficits	Metabolic disease	Consider specialist consultation
Repeated previous surgeries; spina bifida; urinary malformations	Latex allergy	Latex-free environment
Bruising or bleeding	Coagulopathy	Consider further tests; consider preoperative therapy
Death in family during anesthesia	Malignant hyperthermia	Trigger-free anesthesia
Prolonged ventilation in family	Pseudocholinesterase deficiency	Avoid muscle relaxants; consider postoperative monitoring

ECG, electrocardiography

Children should be assessed for asthma, bronchial hyperreactivity, upper respiratory tract infection (URTI) and passive smoking [11, 12]. All these conditions are very common in children and are associated with respiratory adverse events in anesthesia. Age is also an independent risk factor for respiratory adverse events in children. There are two main reason for this. First, the highly compliant chest wall of the infant results in relatively low transpulmonary pressures at end expiration leading to collapse of the small peripheral airways even during normal tidal breathing [13, 14]. Second, infants have a high vagal tone that can rapidly lead to apnea or laryngospasm following vagal stimulation because of irritation of airway receptors by secretions, tracheal intubation or airway suctioning [15].

Airway

Unexpectedly difficult intubation can be encountered in children, although the incidence of the problem is lower than in the adult population [16]. A difficult airway can often be easily predicted in the presence of craniofacial malformations or tumors and syndromes such as Pierre-Robin, Goldenhar, Franceschetti, Cornelia de Lange, mucopolysaccharidoses, Klippel-Feil, and Down. Besides syndromes involving head and neck malformations, a difficult intubation can be expected in the presence of infections (retropharyngeal abscess, adenotonsillitis), musculoskeletal problems (ankylosis of the jaw or cervical spine, unstable vertebrae) or trauma (facial fractures, burns, foreign body aspiration). In general, however, intubation is easier in children than in adults providing the specific anatomy of the infant is well understood and pediatric equipment is readily available.

Every child should be assessed for a potentially difficult airway; the assessment is quick and easy but requires cooperation from the child. The child should be asked to open the mouth wide. In this way it is possible to evaluate the motility of the temporomandibular articulation and the relationship between tongue and mouth. A high arched palate with a narrow mouth opening is likely to be associated with difficult laryngoscopy. The thyromental distance must also be estimated. Its normal range is less defined than in adults (1.5 cm in the newborn and infant, 3 cm in the child), but it can be estimated to be at least the combined width of the child's three middle fingers closed together. The child is then asked to extend the neck. A reduced motility of the atlantooccipital articulation (with an extension less than 35°) or of the cervical spine is seldom present, except in specific syndromes such as Goldenhar or Hurler.

Upper Respiratory Tract Infection

The incidence of URTI in children presenting for anesthesia is very high [17] and anesthesia is often performed in these circumstances, because they occur frequently, especially in children undergoing ear, nose and throat procedures. There is uncertainty as to how long the procedure should be postponed, and also because of the adverse economic and emotional impact associated with cancelling surgery. Deciding whether or not to proceed with elective surgery in a child with a recent URTI is still a controversial issue. Children with an active URTI have more episodes of breath holding, major desaturation and overall adverse respiratory events, but they do not show a higher incidence of laryngospasm or bronchospasm. Independent risk factors for adverse respiratory events in children include the use of an endotracheal tube, history of prematurity, history of reactive airway disease, paternal smoking, and surgery involving the airway.

The patient should be evaluated for fever, dyspnea, productive cough, sputum production, nasal congestion, lethargy and wheezing. Parents should also be interviewed as to the nature of the child's condition, because they may be able to distinguish between infectious and noninfectious conditions, and their opinion has been found to be a better predictor of laryngospasm than reliance on symptom criteria alone [18]. In general, children presenting with symptoms of an uncomplicated URTI and who are afebrile with clear secretions and who appear otherwise healthy should be able to undergo surgery. Children with mucopurulent secretions, productive cough, fever >38°C, lethargy or signs of pulmonary involvement should have their surgery postponed for a minimum of 4 weeks. In any case, the suitability of surgery should be decided considering the risk/benefit ratio, that is, the child's symptoms, comorbid conditions, type of surgery and the frequency of URTI experienced by the child in one year [17]. In a child who experiences more than six URTIs per year, it can be difficult to target the right period for surgery. Another question is the decision as to how long to postpone surgery. Some studies suggest that patients recovering from an URTI have a similar or increased risk of complications compared with those with acute symptoms, and suggest postponement for 4 weeks [19].

Asthma and Bronchial Hyperreactivity

The incidence of asthma is constantly increasing in children [20]. Because bronchial hyperreactivity (BHR) persists for several weeks following an acute asthmatic episode [21], the risk factors for development of perioperative respiratory adverse events are heightened. These risk factors include a recent aggravation of the symptoms, an increase in antiasthma medication, or hospitalization for asthma. Many procedures performed during anesthesia (laryngoscopy, intubation) are potent stimuli that can lead to bronchospasm. In stable asthmatic patients, the perioperative risk is low and is not associated with a significant increase in morbidity [22]. Treatment with corticosteroids prior to surgery reduces adverse events. Treatment should be started at least 48 hours before surgery [23]. Methylprednisolone 1 mg/kg can be beneficial and is not associated with increased wound infection or poor wound healing [24].

Allergies

A history of known medical and environmental allergies should be sought for every patient. Special care must be taken to identify patients with latex allergy [25, 26]. Several predisposing factors are recognized:

- Patients who have a history of atopy; in particular, those with hay fever, asthma, allergies to fruits (pineapple, avocado, banana, chestnut, fig, potato, kiwi, mango, melon, peach, tomato).
- Patients with a history of anaphylaxis of uncertain etiology, especially if associated with previous surgery, hospitalizations or dental visits.
- Patients who have undergone multiple surgical procedures.
- Patients exposed to repeated bladder catheterizations, for instance children with neural tube defects or urogenital malformations.
- Health-care workers.

Only the strict avoidance of latex-containing products can help minimize a child's risk of latex anaphylaxis, as the often-recommended chemoprophylaxis consisting of H1/H2 receptor antagonists is now questioned [27].

Cardiovascular System

Most children (approximately 70%) present with innocent murmurs [28]. If the child has normal growth, normal exercise tolerance and no cyanosis, anesthesia can be expected to be well tolerated. Parents should be asked if the child runs like other children or is calmer or slower, if he turns blue (while feeding or while crying), if he has ever lost consciousness, and in the case of an infant, if he takes long to finish his bottle or sweats during normal care or has swollen eyes in the morning.

Auscultation of the child both standing up and lying down are important. Outflow functional murmurs will be louder in the supine position because of the larger end-diastolic volume and greater stroke volume. Murmurs with an origin in the right heart will be increased in inspiration and those from the left heart during expiration. Further cardiological evaluation is required if murmurs sound pathological (louder than 2/6, diastolic, pansystolic, continuous), if the patient has other symptoms indicating heart disease or associated malformations or recurrent chest infections.

The hemodynamics of intracardiac shunts can significantly change during anesthesia, since most anesthetics decrease both systemic and pulmonary vascular resistances. Left-to-right shunts can invert in direction in the presence of hypoxia, acidosis, hypotension or hypothermia; shunts also allow paradoxical emboli produced by air or thrombi coming from the venous circulation into the systemic circulation.

Pulmonary hypertension is common in the newborn; it is rare in older children and in these cases is generally secondary to airway obstruction, congenital heart disease or chronic pulmonary disease. Hypoxemia and hypercarbia are potent pulmonary vasoconstrictors and should be avoided as they alter the child's hemodynamics. Preoperative assessment of these children should include a thorough evaluation of right heart function.

Neurological Diseases

Neuromuscular or degenerative diseases pose an increased risk because of increased muscle weakness [29]. Children with progressive diseases often present with electrolyte imbalance (especially hyperkalemia), gastroesophageal reflux and cardiorespiratory dysfunction. In the presence of ventriculoperitoneal shunts, their function must be evaluated preoperatively as many anesthetics can raise intracranial pressure because of their vasodilating properties. Anticonvulsive therapy must be optimized because it can be altered by fasting or vomiting in the perioperative period.

Central core disease is associated with malignant hyperthermia (MH). Other neuromuscular diseases react to triggering agents (succinylcholine and volatile agents) leading to a hypermetabolic state. In case of a personal or family history of MH susceptibility or in the presence of a central core disease, the patient should be tested for MH. Genetic testing is even possible from umbilical cord blood [30]. However, in case of a negative genetic result, open muscle biopsy is necessary for the in vitro contracture test.

Obesity

The prevalence of obesity among children has tripled in the last 20 years, paralleling the epidemic increase among adults worldwide [31, 32]. Obese children therefore now represent an increasing proportion of our surgical population. Obesity in adults is defined as a BMI (body mass index) of >30 kg/m^2; defining obesity in children is less straightforward. A definition of childhood obesity has been proposed by Cole et al. [33] using data derived from several international population databases: the cut-off obesity curve is defined as the BMI growth curve which intersects with a projected BMI curve of 30 kg/m^2 at age 18 years.

Anesthetic management of the obese otherwise healthy child has been reported to be associated with a higher incidence of critical incidents [34]. BHR, asthma and respiratory tract infections are more common in obese children, and common pulmonary physiological derangements include decreases in functional residual capacity (FRC), forced vital capacity (FVC) and forced expiratory volume in one second (FEV1) [35]. Obese patients are therefore at risk of rapid oxygen desaturation during periods of apnea and overall increased incidence of respiratory complications during anesthesia. Hypertension, noninsulin-dependent diabetes mellitus, gastroesophageal reflux and potentially delayed gastric emptying times are also more frequent [34].

Moreover, appropriate dosing regimens for obese children rarely exist and most drugs should be given according to lean body weight, which can be difficult to determine. In the perioperative period, an increased risk of respiratory depression and a higher prevalence of obstructive sleep apnea syndrome (OSAS) should be taken into account [35].

Diabetes

The prevalence of diabetes mellitus in the pediatric population is increasing along with obesity. In the great majority of patients, this is a type 1 (insulin-dependent) diabetes. Since anesthesia and surgery result in a typical metabolic stress response characterized by secretion of catabolic hormones and inhibition of insulin secretion, children can be at risk of great fluctuation in blood glucose levels and electrolyte imbalances.

It is good practice to schedule surgery early in the morning in order to avoid long fasting times and provide intravenous infusions of dextrose and insulin in the perioperative period [36].

Long-term Steroid Treatment

The normal daily endogenous production of glucocorticoids is 5–10 mg/m^2, but under stress conditions, it can rise to 100 mg/m^2. It is widely recommended, in spite of lack of evidence, that steroid therapy should be administered to children who are under long-term therapy, at a "stress" dose before surgery and in the perioperative period, according to the degree of substitution and the type of surgery [37].

ASA Status

The American Society of Anesthesiologists physical status (ASA-PS) classification is used worldwide by anesthesia providers as a measure of the preoperative physical status of the patient [38, 39]. This score has been used in policy making, performance evaluation, resource allocation and reimbursement of anesthesia service, and is frequently cited in clinical research. Despite its simplicity, there has been a documented inconsistency in ASA assignment for adult patients by different anesthesia providers [40]. In two recent studies, interobserver consistency in ASA-PS in pediatric patients has been evaluated by pediatric anesthesiologists, with the conclusion that agreement between operators is only moderate [41, 42], but becomes higher if the ASA categories are collapsed from five to three (ASA 1 and 2 for low risk patients; ASA 3 and 4 for high risk patients).

Vaccinations and Anesthesia

Vaccinations can be followed by local swelling, pain, fever, headache, rash, malaise and myalgias, all of which can last for between 1 day and 3 weeks [43]. It is probably reasonable to postpone elective surgery for at least 3 days following a vaccination with killed organisms (pertussis vaccine) and 2 weeks following a vaccination with attenuated live organisms (measles, mumps, rubella and poliovirus vaccine) to reduce the likelihood of the peak systemic reaction to the vaccine occurring at the time of surgery [43].

Herbal Medicines

An increasing proportion of the pediatric population receives or has received herbal preparations [44]. The potential for interaction with anesthesia drugs exists [45]. Many herbal preparations decrease platelet aggregation (e.g. bilberry, brome lain, dong quoi, feverfew, fish oil, garlic, ginger, gingko biloba, grape seed extract) or inhibit clotting (e.g. chamomile, dandelion root, horse chestnut) [46]. The long-term use of Echinacea, which is thought to reduce the duration and severity of URTIs, can result in immunosuppression [47] and can potentially cause anaphylaxis and hepatotoxicity [46]. Another problem is that the majority of parents do not report the use of herbal medications in their children, unless specifically asked. It is therefore important to remember to include this question in the list of questions that compose the preoperative evaluation.

Fasting Times

The purpose of preoperative fasting is to avoid stomach contents being vomited and possibly aspirated, especially during induction of anesthesia. The intake of clear liquids up to 2 hours before anesthesia does not increase the amount and does not alter the pH of the stomach contents. Consumption of clear liquids helps the child to tolerate fasting and avoids perioperative hypoglycemia [48]. For solids and milk, longer fasting periods should be set: 4 hours for breast milk or formula in infants under 6 months of age, and 6 hours for solids and milk in older infants and children.

Inpatient or Outpatient Procedure?

Children gain particular benefit from well-planned and well-conducted day care because separation from parents is reduced. Day surgery regimens can be used for most surgical or diagnostic procedures that require analgesia or anesthesia.

The decision as to whether a surgical procedure should be performed on an inpatient or outpatient basis includes several factors: minimally or well-controlled physiological alterations, a procedure associated with a low rate of surgical or anesthetic complications, a short duration of anesthesia and easily controlled postoperative pain [49]. The majority of procedures in children can be performed on an outpatient basis, and some are listed in Table 7.3 [50, 51].

Ex-premature babies should have reached 60 weeks postconceptional age to be eligible for outpatient surgery because this population has a higher rate of postoperative apnea, periodic breathing and bradycardia.

Table 7.3 Selection criteria for day care. Modified from [37]

Peripheral procedures
Not entering a body cavity
Limited duration
Moderate postoperative pain that can be managed orally/rectally
No major physiological disturbances
No major blood loss
No postoperative fasting necessary
No ex-premature babies (<36 weeks and up to 60 weeks postconceptional age)

Additional Investigations

Hemoglobin Testing

The results of routine preoperative blood testing are abnormal in approximately 2.5–10% of healthy children, but such findings rarely have an impact on scheduled surgery [52, 53]. The most commonly found abnormality is mild anemia, which can be misdiagnosed even with a careful history of the child and a careful physical examination, but which is not associated with increased perioperative risk and does not change the anesthesia management [54, 55]. Laboratory tests should be performed when clinical doubt is present. This approach reduces the costs and patient discomfort that can result from possible false-positive results [56].

Preoperative Coagulation Testing

Routine coagulation tests are often thought to be useful, especially in children who are undergoing a neuraxial blockade, or adenoidectomy or tonsillectomy, or are under 1 year of age and may not have experienced sufficient physical trauma to develop any history of abnormal bleeding episodes. In this situation, a history of prematurity and the neonatal period itself are always considered risk factors for bleeding disorders, since they are often associated with low levels of factor IX from liver immaturity and vitamin K deficiency.

Normal coagulation values do not completely rule out a coagulation disorder [57] and not all children presenting with preoperative abnormalities in coagulation tests will show bleeding problems in the perioperative period and vice versa [58]. It is essential therefore that the tests ordered be supported by a positive history [59].

Preoperative Electrocardiography

Recent reports have attracted attention to the high incidence of congenital long QT syndrome (1:5000) [60] and the possibility that commonly used anesthetics (sevoflurane above all) can cause prolongation of the QT [61, 62]. Since electrocardiography is a noninvasive examination that causes no discomfort to the child and whose cost is acceptable, electrocardiographic evaluation of every child can be recommended, because it will allow the anesthetic management to be changed to reduce the possibility of intraoperative arrhythmias.

Preoperative Chest Radiography

Since this examination involves exposure to radiation, it is widely recommended that chest radiography is ordered only in cases with a clear clinical indication [63].

References

1. Beecher HK, Todd DP (1954) A study of the deaths associated with anesthesia and surgery. Ann Surg 140:2–34
2. Clifton BS, Hotten WI (1963) Deaths associated with anaesthesia. Br J Anaesth 35:250–259
3. Graff TD, Phillips OC, Benson DW, Kelley E (1964) Baltimore Anesthesia Study Committee: factors in pediatric anesthesia mortality. Anesth Analg 43:407–414
4. Tiret L, Nivoche Y, Hatton F et al (1988) Complications related to anaesthesia in infants and children. A prospective survey of 40240 anaesthetics. Br J Anaesth 61:263–269
5. Cohen MM, Cameron CB, Duncan PG (1990) Pediatric anesthesia morbidity and mortality in the perioperative period. Anesth Analg 70:160–167
6. Morray JP, Geidushek JM, Ramamoorthy C et al (2000) Anesthesia-related cardiac arrest in children: initial findings of the Pediatric Perioperative Cardiac Arrest (POCA) Registry. Anesthesiology 93:6–14
7. Bhananker SM, Ramamoorty C, Geidushek JM et al (2007) Anesthesia-related cardiac arrest in children: update from the Pediatric Perioperative Cardiac Arrest Registry. Anesth Analg 102:344–350

8. Morray JP, Geidushek JM, Caplan RA et al (1993) A comparison of pediatric and adult anesthesia closed malpractice claims. Anesthesiology 78:461–467
9. Tay CL, Tan GM, Ng SB (2001) Critical incidents in pediatric anaesthesia: an audit of 10,000 anaesthetics in Singapore. Paediatr Anaesth 11:711–718
10. Bancalari E, Clausen J (1988) Pathophysiology of changes in absolute lung volumes. Eur Resp J 12:248–258
11. Tait AR, Malviya S, Voepel-Lewis T et al (2001) Risk factors for perioperative respiratory adverse events in children with upper respiratory tract infections. Anesthesiology 95:299–306
12. Skolnick ET, Vomvolakis MA, Buck KA et al (1998) Exposure to environmental tobacco smoke and the risk of adverse respiratory events in children receiving general anesthesia. Anesthesiology 88:1144–1153
13. Stocks J (1999) Respiratory physiology during early life. Monaldi Arch Chest Dis 54:358–364
14. Papastamelos C, Panitch HB, England SE et al (1995) Developmental changes in chest wall compliance in infancy and early childhood. J Appl Physiol 78:179–184
15. Nishino T, Tagaito Y, Isono S (1996) Cough and other reflexes on irritation of airway mucosa in man. Pulm Pharmacol 9:285–292
16. Gruppo di Studio SIAARTI "Vie Aeree Difficili", Frova G, Guarino A, Petrini F et al (2006) Recommendations for airway control and difficult airway management in paediatric patients. Minerva Anestesiol 72:723–748
17. Tait AR, Malviya S (2005) Anesthesia for the child with an upper respiratory tract infection: still a dilemma? Anesth Analg 100:59–65
18. Schreiner MS, O'Hara I, Markakis DA, Politis GD (1996) Do children who experience laryngospasm have an increased risk of upper respiratory tract infection? Anesthesiology 85:475–480
19. Skolnick ET, Vomvolakis M, Buck KA (1998) A prospective evaluation of children with upper respiratory infections undergoing a standardized anesthetic and the incidence of adverse respiratory events. Anesthesiology 89:A1309
20. Joseph-Bowen J, de Klerk NH, Firth MJ et al (2004) Lung function, bronchial responsiveness, and asthma in a community cohort of 6-year-old children. Am J Respir Crit Care Med 169:850–854
21. Warner DO, Warner MA, Barnes RD et al (1996) Perioperative respiratory complications in patients with asthma. Anesthesiology 85:460–467
22. Rock P, Passannante A (2004) Preoperative assessment: pulmonary. Anesthesiol Clin North America 22:77–91
23. Maxwell LG (2004) Age-associated issues in preoperative evaluation, testing and planning: pediatrics. Anesthesiol Clin North America 22:27–43
24. Kabalin CS, Yarnold PR, Grammer LC (1995) Low complication rate of corticosteroid-treated asthmatics undergoing surgical procedures. Arch Intern Med 155:1379–1384
25. Hollnberger H, Gruber E, Frank B (2002) Severe anaphylactic shock without exanthema in a case of unknown latex allergy and review of the literature. Paediatr Anaesth 12:544–551
26. Società di Anestesia e Rianimazione Neonatale e Pediatrica Italiana (2008) Linee Guida: Suggerimenti per un percorso intraospedaliero latex-safe. www.sarnepi.it
27. Sussman G, Gold M (1996) guidelines for the management of latex allergies and latex safe use in health care facilities. American College of Allergy, Asthma and Immunology Arlington Heights
28. Roy DL (1989) Heart sounds and murmurs – innocent or organic? Med Clin North Am 73:153–162
29. Allison KR (2007) Muscular dystrophy versus mitochondrial myopathy: the dilemma of the undiagnosed hypotonic child. Paediatr Anaesth 17:1–6
30. Girard T, Treves S, Voronkov E et al (2004) Molecular genetic testing for malignant hyperthermia susceptibility. Anesthesiology 100:1076–1080
31. Hedley AA, Ogden CL, Johnson CL et al (2004) Prevalence of overweight and obesity among US children, adolescents and adults, 1999–2002. JAMA 291:2847–2858

32. Yoshinaga M, Shimago A, Koriyama C et al (2004) Rapid increase in the prevalence of obesity in elementary school children. Int J Obes Relat Metab Disord 28:494–499

33. Cole TJ, Bellizzi MC, Flegal KM et al (2000) Establishing a standard definition for child overweight and obesity worldwide: international survey. BMJ 320:1240–1243

34. Smith HL, Meldrum DJ, Brennan LJ (2002) Childhood obesity: a challenge for the anaesthetist? Paediatr Anaesth 12:750–761

35. Lazarus R, Colditz G, Berkey CS et al (1997) Effects of body fat on ventilatory function in children and adolescents: cross-sectional findings from a random population sample of school children. Pediatr Pulmonol 24:187–194

36. Chadwick V, Wilkinson KA (2004) Diabetes mellitus and the pediatric anesthetist. Paediatr Anaesth 14:716–723

37. von Ungern-Sternberg BS, Habre W (2007) Pediatric anesthesia – potential risks and their assessment: part II. Paediatr Anaesth 17:311–320

38. Saklad M (1941) Grading of patients for surgical procedures. Anesthesiology 2:281–284

39. American Society of Anesthesiologists (1936) New classification of physical status (editorial). Anesthesiology 24:111

40. Haynes SR, Lawler PGP (1995) An assessment of consistency of ASA physical status classification allocation. Anesthesia 50:195–199

41. Jacqueline R, Malviya S, Burke C et al (2006) An assessment of interrater variability of the ASA physical status classification in pediatric surgical patients. Paediatr Anaesth 16:928–931

42. Burgoyne LL, Smeltzer MP, Pereiras LA et al (2007) How well do pediatric anesthesiologists agree when assigning ASA physical status classifications to their patients? Paediatr Anaesth 17:956–962

43. Van der Walt JH, Roberton DM (1996) Anesthesia and recently vaccinated children. Paediatr Anaesth 6:135–141

44. Crowe S, Lyons B (2004) Herbal medicine use by children presenting for ambulatory anesthesia and surgery. Paediatr Anaesth 14:916–919

45. Davis MP, Darden PM (2003) Use of complementary and alternative medicine by children in the United States. Arch Pediatr Adolesc Med 157:393–396

46. Kaye AD, Clarke RC, Sabar R (2004) Perioperative anesthesia clinical considerations of alternative medicines. Anesthesiol Clin North America 22:125–139

47. Boullata JI, Nace AM (2000) Safety issues with herbal medicine. Pharmacotherapy 20:257–269

48. Splinter WM, Schreiner MS (1999) Preoperative fasting in children. Anesth Analg 90:80–89

49. Lonnqvist PA, Morton NS (2006) Paediatric day-case anaesthesia and pain control. Curr Opin Anaesthesiol 19:617–621

50. Fishkin S, Litman RS (2003) Current issues in pediatric ambulatory anesthesia. Anesthesiol Clin North America 21:305–311

51. Solca M, Bettelli G, Leucci M et al (2000) Clinical-organizational recommendations for anesthesia in day surgery of the SIAARTI/AAROI Commission on Day Surgery (in Italian). Minerva Anestesiol 66:915–926

52. Macpherson DS (1993) Preoperative laboratory testing: should any test be "routine" before surgery? Med Clin North Am 77:289–308

53. Meneghini L, Zadra N, Zanette G et al (1998) The usefulness of routine preoperative laboratory tests for one-day surgery in healthy children. Paediatr Anaesth 8:11–15

54. Steward DJ (1991) Screening tests before surgery in children. Can J Anaesth 38:693–695

55. Consensus conference (1988) Perioperative red blood cell transfusion. JAMA 260:2700–2703

56. Hannallah RS (1995) Preoperative investigations. Paediatr Anaesth 5:325–329

57. Windfuhr JP, Chen YS, Remmert S (2004) Unidentified coagulation disorders in post-tonsillectomy hemorrhage. Ear Nose Throat J 83:28–32

58. Suchman AL, Mushlin AI (1986) How well does the activated partial thromboplastin time predict postoperative hemorrhage? JAMA 256:750–753

59. Le Roux C, Lejus C, Surbleb M et al (2002) Is hemostasis biological screening always use-
     ful before performing a neuraxial blockade in children? Paediatr Anaesth 12:118–123
60. Collins KK, Van Hare GF (2006) Advances in congenital long QT syndrome. Curr Opin
     Pediatr 18:497–502
61. Gurcan Y, Canatay H, Agaodiken A et al (2003) Effects of halothane and sevoflurane on QT
     dispersion in pediatric patients. Paediatr Anaesth 13:223–227
62. Kleinsasser A, Kuenszberg E, Loeckinger A et al (2000) Sevoflurane, but not propofol, sig-
     nificantly prolongs the QT interval. Anesth Analg 90:25–27
63. American Academy of Pediatrics, Committee on Hospital Care (1983) Preoperative chest
     radiographs. Pediatrics 71:858

Chapter 8

Anesthesia Induction

Marinella Astuto, Daniela Lauretta

Definition

Induction is the transition from an awake state to an anesthetized state. In this process not only the anesthesiologist but also obviously the child and the parents are involved. Anesthesia induction in children may be associated with significant stress for all those involved. When we speak about anesthesia induction, we should not think only of the classic definition of induction. In the past, the role of anesthesiologists was limited to the operating room, and they had little or no contact with the patient nor the family. Today anesthesiologists are involved in "total patient care" during the perioperative period which includes the pre-, intra-, and postoperative periods.

Pediatric anesthesiologists learn to divide their attention appropriately between the technical aspects of induction, the central nervous system and the cardiorespiratory responses of the patient, and the provision of psychological support to the child and/or parent. With regular practice, however, pediatric inductions are generally safe and smooth, if not fun and easy. This is what we define as a "good induction".

The Basis for a Good Induction

Several elements play an important role in achieving a "good induction":
- The calm baby
- The environment
- The presence of parents
- Pharmacological and nonpharmacological premedication
- The anesthesiologist
- Monitoring.

M. Astuto (ed), *Basics*, Anesthesia, Intensive Care and Pain in Neonates and Children.
ISBN 978-88-470-0654-6 © Springer-Verlag Italia 2009

The Calm Baby

A calm patient facilitates the work of the anesthesiologist in allowing a smooth and rapid induction in a patient who is fearful. The anesthesiologist can obtain this result acting on the environment, and using premedication with and without drugs.

The Environment

Children are often quite anxious when confronted with a strange hospital environment and the necessity for a surgical procedure. This is the reason why many hospitals have established preoperative clinics and programs that allow children and their parents to visit the hospital and receive information about what to expect on the day of the surgery and to receive information, as well as to familiarize themselves with the location and personnel [1].

The first contact with the child and the parents must be in a reassuring place, adapted for children if possible. Moreover, it has been demonstrated that the presence of people other than health-care personnel (for example clowns) who make the child laugh can reduce anxiety [2, 3]. In many hospitals the presence of people external to the operating team is not allowed; there are many reasons for this, but it is worth mentioning in this context that in the past the presence of parents was not well accepted, while it is now considered routine. For the anesthesiologist the parents' presence is not always useful. Adverse parental reactions may result in a prolonged induction and may put additional stress on the anesthesiologist, and sometimes the anxiety state of the parent, transmitted to the child, means that the operation has to be called off and rescheduled [4]. This is a cost/time disadvantage. Thus desirability of the presence of a parent must be carefully evaluated.

The Presence of Parents

Anesthesia in a child affects not only the patient but also the parents.

Parents experience increased stress during separation from their child at the start of surgery, whether or not they are present at anesthesia induction [5]. Although this may be a universal response, preparing and allowing parents to be present for anesthesia induction can decrease this stress. A study has shown that the majority of parents (92.8%) believe their presence at induction was helpful to the child, and many parents believe their presence was also helpful to the anesthesiologist [6]. Psychological support is most easily provided by the anesthesiologist who has met and established a relationship with the family well in advance of the procedure. In modern practice, this ideal is not always possible. Emotional support is now more often provided by informed parents and by an anesthesiologist who has gained the patient's confidence in the preoperative holding or waiting area. One useful technique involves beginning a conversation about a favorite toy or experience in the holding area and then continuing the discussion during anesthetic induction. It is also often helpful to encourage the child to bring a favorite toy or "comfort blanket" to the induction area.

The very common fear of the unknown is largely alleviated by simple, honest communication colored by appropriate positive suggestion. The time spent with the patient and the family is, in many cases, proportional to the compliance with the environment. It is very important to choose the best method for communicating with the family, the correct time and, if necessary, to repeat any explanations. The explanation can include a tour of the operating room and other areas that the family will see during the operation; this means that both the child and, especially the parents, will be familiar with these areas. It has been shown that showing parents a video of the operating room can reduce their anxiety, thus producing a calm child [7].

However, the presence of a parent during induction is a controversial topic. A study investigated children's responses to induction with a parent present [1, 8]. There were significantly fewer "very upset" or "turbulent" children during the preinduction and induction periods among those whose parents were present than among a control group of children whose parents were not present. A limitation of this study was that intravenous induction was employed rather than the standard inhalation technique that most anesthesiologists use in children. Despite this limitation, the authors of the study suggest that the amount of premedication required may be less in some preschool children if a parent is present during anesthesia induction [9, 10].

If parents are appropriately informed and calm, they can be of great benefit to their children. In one study, however, anxious parents who were not adequately prepared increased their children's anxiety levels [11]. The authors of this study found that parents with high anxiety levels who were present for their child's induction became even more anxious after induction. Conversely, parents with low anxiety levels who were present for induction became even less anxious after induction. The children experienced higher anxiety levels if anxious parents accompanied them. The authors of the study suggest that nurses allow parents to be present if they want to, but they should not force this practice on unwilling and anxious parents.

To solve the controversy about the presence of parents it is necessary to evaluate the characteristics of the little patients.

Which Children Will Benefit from Parental Presence?

A child's stress level is affected by multiple factors, including his or her age and the anxiety level of the parents. In a randomized controlled study, factors that could predict which children would benefit from parental presence during anesthesia induction were examined [10]. Serum cortisol concentrations were decreased in even-tempered children older than 4 years when accompanying parents had low baseline anxiety. Although some health-care providers have expressed concern that parental presence prolongs induction time and increases the incidence of nausea and vomiting, postoperative analgesic use, and time to discharge, differences did not exist in this study between children whose parents were present and those whose parents were not present. These findings suggest that some, but not all, children will benefit from the presence of a parent at induction; the decision must be made on an individual basis depending on careful preoperative assessment by the nurse. There are some data from Italian studies that have shown that the presence of a parent is important, especially that of the mother who may be a relaxing influence [12]. An older calm child who understands what is to happen and knows the environment often needs no parental support.

There are several factors that may predict a child's level of non-cooperation: age, sex, fear, behavioral problems, previous hospital experiences and reactions to vaccinations [13].

Premedication

In selected cases, especially if a parent will not be present for induction, or if the patient is particularly turbulent, pharmacological and/or nonpharmacological (hypnosis) premedication may be helpful.

Pharmacological Premedication

Premedication is sometimes the only method to have a calm child. Separation anxiety starts at approximately 9 months of age. In a child under 6 months of age premedication is obviously not useful.

Midazolam (0.5 mg/kg) is the most common drug used for premedication (it is also a good amnestic), followed by fentanyl and ketamine. Children have been shown to have fewer nightmares and negative behavior after surgery if midazolam is given. It is contraindicated in children with previous adverse reactions or obstructive sleep apnea. Table 8.1 shows dosages and routes of administration of midazolam.

Table 8.1 Dosages and routes of administration of midazolam

Route	Dose (mg/ml)	Onset (min)	Duration of effect (min)
Oral/rectal	0.5–0.75 (max 20)	20–30	90
Nasal drops/spray	0.2–0.5	10–20	90
Intravenous	0.5–5 years: 0.05–0.1	2–3	45–60
	>5 years: 0.025–05		

The use of premedication was greater in the past when the states of mind of the child and parents were not taken into consideration. Parents were happier to see their child go into the operating room already asleep [14, 15].

Pharmacological Side Effects

Adverse psychotropic effects of midazolam, including disinhibition, can occur at any dose, and higher doses may be associated with dysphoria. Ketamine at high doses is effective, but may provoke emesis. A combination of these oral premedication drugs at lower doses may be advantageous, such as midazolam 0.25 mg/kg and ketamine 3 mg/kg. Oral premedication with antihistamine, phenothiazine, barbiturates or even alcohol can also be effective, but may produce unacceptable side effects [16, 17].

Nonpharmacological Premedication: Hypnosis

Hypnosis is a state of concentrated attention to the suggestion of the hypnotizer. It represents a useful, additional tool that anesthesiologists may find valuable in everyday practice. Amnesia, absence of postoperative nausea and vomiting or pain are the typical suggestions used. Children are good hypnotic subjects because they have a natural power of playing, and an imaginary world is close and accessible. Many anesthesiologists use this technique when trying to calm the child for induction [18, 19]. Many experienced pediatric anesthesiologists use hypnotic language in their daily working lives, frequently without realizing they are doing so. They often do this when attempting to encourage the cooperation of children to facilitate smooth inhalational induction, or to place an intravenous cannula. The age of the child and the cooperation of everyone in the anesthetic and surgical teams is fundamental to achieve a good hypnotic state. Patients less than 4 years old are not able to concentrate. A noisy and chaotic operating room is not a suitable environment in which to perform this technique.

A study by Fukumoto et al. in which an intentional troposmia was induced so that the child perceived the smell of sevoflurane as a desirable smell demonstrated that troposmia might promote children's participation in anesthesia induction and facilitate inhalational induction [19]. Cyna et al. used a self-hypnosis technique to facilitate intravenous cannula placement in a 5-year-old patient in which oral premedication with midazolam and ketamine was unsatisfactory [20].

Anesthesiologist

Anesthesiologists practice their art as psychologists, physiologists and pharmacologists, and thus they must have the possibility to choose the technique in which they are most skilled, even if it is not the most popular! Multiple factors linked to the patient influence the choice of technique: age, American Society of Anesthesiologists physical status, preexisting illness, kind of surgery, cooperation, presence of parents, previous intravenous line, skills of the anesthesiologist.

There are several methods to induce anesthesia in children:

- Inhalational
- Intravenous
- Others (intramuscular, rectal).

Inhalation Induction

Inhalation mask induction is a cornerstone of pediatric anesthesia. It has gained even more popularity since the introduction of sevoflurane into clinical practice [21]. Induction of anesthesia by mask is a widely used and generally accepted technique. Because of a natural aversion to needles, healthy children are usually anesthetized by mask prior to intravenous cannula insertion to avoid causing pain. Anesthesia is commonly induced in infants and children by means of a "gas induction". This is less commonly the case with adults, leading some anesthesiologists to be unfamiliar or lacking in confidence with this method. Infants may be very hard to cannulate prior to an intravenous induction, so that a gas induction becomes preferable. Neonates may lie on the operating table and breathe from an anesthetic mask attached to a T piece, or similar, low-resistance anesthetic circuit. Various games may be employed to distract children enough for them to receive a gas induction. "Blowing up the balloon" will be familiar to most anesthesiologists and is a very effective way of persuading a child to "breathe the gas". Another useful technique is to use a strong-smelling food substance and rub it in the face mask.

Once the child is asleep, any parent present should be asked to leave. The child should be disturbed as little as possible. Once asleep, the patient goes through an excitatory phase. Moving the child, for example to remove clothing, is often the stimulus that provokes airway reflexes. The anesthesiologist should continue holding the face mask and the child's airway, maintaining a clear airway and good ventilation using oxygen and a high concentration of the volatile anesthetic agent, until a deeply anesthetized state is reached. At this point, the child may be moved to insert an intravenous cannula, be undressed, or have other monitoring applied to facilitate surgery. If an intravenous cannula is needed, this is the time to insert it. Another anesthesiologist or a nurse can help to insert the cannula while the anesthesiologist is maintaining the airway [22]. Inhalational induction involves a basic dilemma for the pediatric anesthesiologist: while the early establishment of an intravenous line provides a means for administering drugs, it can induce coughing, movement, laryngospasm and desaturation. It is important to wait for two minutes following the loss of lid reflex before attempting intravenous cannula placement in children receiving an inhalation induction with sevoflurane.

The obvious question is what to do about any adverse events that occur before an intravenous cannula is inserted. However, with the exception of airway obstruction, problems are exceptionally rare. With the anesthesiologist holding the patient's airway, he/she is ideally placed to diagnose and treat airway obstruction if it occurs. Hypoventilation is noted by decreased excursion of the breathing reservoir bag. Airway obstruction may be revealed by noisy breathing or increased work of breathing (increased chest excursion with decreased bag excursion). Correcting the position of the patient's head normally corrects hypoventilation. Noisy breathing is often due to upper airway collapse during expiration and a small amount of continuous positive airway pressure (CPAP) will resolve it. This is generally applied by keeping tension on the reservoir bag with one hand. If hypoxia occurs, as evidenced by the pulse oximeter trace or by cyanosis, check that a maximum concentration of oxygen is being given increase the CPAP. Occasionally, an oropharyngeal airway is helpful but care should be taken that this is not inserted under too light anesthesia. It is rare that serious laryngospasm cannot be overcome with patience, CPAP, 100% oxygen and correct positioning. If the situation does not resolve, consider other causes of airway obstruction and consider applying suction to the pharynx to clear any secretions which may be in the larynx.

If it becomes necessary to paralyze the patient, after anesthesia has been reached, but before an intravenous cannula is inserted, remember that suxamethonium may be given intramuscularly (5 mg/kg) and will work within two or three minutes. Many anesthesiologists prefer to intubate patients once they are deeply anesthetized with a volatile anesthetic agent alone. It has been advocated that suxamethonium may be given intramuscularly into the tongue. There are some circumstances when inhalational anesthetic induction is not the method of choice. If a child already has a cannula in situ, perhaps for maintenance fluid therapy, then it is more appropriate to use this cannula. Many children express a preference for intravenous anesthetic induction. There are also numerous occasions where a rapid sequence induction is indicated and here inhalational induction is inappropriate.

Inhalational induction has advantages and disadvantages. To know them allows the anesthesiologist to reduce complications.

- *Advantages*:
  - Children, understandably, are reluctant to have a "needle" to put them to sleep. Many are aware of an alternative and will prefer this method
  - Blood/gas and tissue/gas partition coefficients are lower in children, so induction and awakening are more rapid
  - Inhaled anesthetics allow breath-by-breath monitoring of the individual pharmacokinetics
- *Disadvantages*:
  - The most problematic disadvantage of inhalational induction is laryngospasm. During induction with sevoflurane the incidence of laryngospasm is higher with early placement of an intravenous line [22]
  - Coughing

-   Postoperative vomiting
-   Emergence delirium
-   Interaction with Duchenne's muscular dystrophy (DMD).

There are several clinical and experimental reports suggesting a correlation between exposure to sevoflurane and generalized clonic or tonic seizure activity. A child with emergence agitation needs considerable nursing time in the recovery room because of possible injury, damage to surgical dressings or dislodgement of venous access [23]. The incidence of emergence delirium varies between inhalation agents: sevoflurane as well as desflurane induce delirium more often than isoflurane, and isoflurane more than halothane. There is, however, a possible solution to this problem. It has been shown that maintenance with desflurane [24] or isoflurane [25] decreases delirium, while midazolam [26] has no effect.

Reports are still discordant about the use of gaseous induction in children with DMD. It would seem reasonable to consider other anesthetic agents in young males and a risk of cardiomyopathy and myocardial depression in adolescents with DMD [27, 28].

Sevoflurane

Sevoflurane has been used in Japan since the 1970s. It is a volatile agent with a minimum alveolar concentration (MAC) of 2.3 in infants and 1.8 in adults. Its major advantage is that it has a smell which is nonpungent and it is possible to induce anesthesia with high concentrations from the outset. It preserves a good cardiocirculatory and respiratory performance and it has no arrhythmogenic effect. When compared to halothane, higher concentrations may be used earlier in induction, without complaint. Therefore, it appears to cause a swifter onset of anesthesia. Moreover, it has a low hepatic toxicity. Together with desflurane for maintenance, it is replacing isoflurane and halothane in modern anesthesiology. After desflurane, it is the volatile anesthetic with the fastest onset and recovery. A disadvantage is that it is a more potent respiratory depressant than halothane and therefore breath holding may occur before a truly deep stage of anesthesia is reached. The other major disadvantage of this agent is its high cost.

Techniques of gaseous induction with sevoflurane include the tidal volume technique, the single-breath vital capacity technique, incremental sevoflurane, and immediate 8–12%. Tidal volume is commonly used in pediatric anesthesia, while the single-breath technique [29–31], generally reserved for adults, has been shown to be tolerated and is efficient for inducing anesthesia in children older than 5 or 6 years. For problematic, unstable, or very young patients the incremental technique with immediate 8% is the most used (it reduces excitation during early anesthesia), while 12% offers a smoother anesthesia induction in children aged 5–10 years with no additional consequences for the cardiovascular system. Probably 12% will be used more in the future.

Desflurane

Desflurane seems to be inappropriate for mask induction, as it may provoke complications during inhalational induction in children resulting in breath-holding, laryngospasm, and coughing [32].

Intravenous Induction

The availability of venous access is a prerequisite for intravenous induction. The choice could be based on the preference of the child, but many anesthesiologists believe it better, and safer, to have venous access available before induction and thus prefer, when possible, intravenous induction. The main problems with intravenous induction are pain on insertion of the cannula, a natural aversion of children to "needles", and difficulty in insertion. These are all relevant to adults, but we can reason with an adult and explain why it is necessary and why the cannula may be hard to place.

Children as young as 5 years may well understand the reasons for needing a cannula and may even understand that sometimes a cannula is not easy to insert and a second go might be required. Whatever the reasoning ability of the child, the process may be made much less unpleasant by the application of a topical anesthetic to prevent the child feeling the cannula needle. EMLA (eutectic mixture of local anesthetics) takes about 40 minutes to become effective. If placed over a cannulation site for an adequate amount of time, it is very effective. Amethocaine gel works quickly [33]. Unfortunately, these drugs are not uniformly available and sometimes the only sensible plan is to explain why a cannula is needed and to use the smallest gauge possible. If nitrous oxide is available, the child may breathe a mixture of nitrous oxide and oxygen whilst the cannula is inserted, but this technique often seems to combine the worst aspects of both intravenous and inhalational techniques, the child getting a "nasty mask" and a "horrible needle"!

Insertion of a venous cannula may be easy if the veins are obvious. Sometimes this is a difficult procedure. The task is harder when the child has a large amount of subcutaneous fat, a common situation in toddlers. Veins become smaller in cold, dehydrated and frightened children. A warm, well-hydrated, comfortable child should be our aim and parental presence or premedication may well help.

After insertion of an intravenous cannula, suitable monitoring can be attached and an intravenous induction agent injected. The choice of agent is described above, and a list of drugs together with suggested dosages is presented in Table 8.2, but in a healthy child, the normal choice is between sodium thiopentone and propofol. Propofol undeniably results in less "hang-over" in the postoperative period. However, after one hour, the difference between sodium thiopentone and propofol becomes very subtle in children. Pain on injection is a considerable problem, especially when we have gone to such lengths to secure

Table 8.2 Anesthetic drugs and doses

Drug	Neonate Dose	Ref.	Infant Dose	Ref.
Propofol	2 mg/kg	[45]	4 mg/kg	[34–38]
	35 mg/kg/h	[48]	5 µg/ml	[39]
			2.5–3.0 mg/kg	[35, 41]
			2–3 mg/kg	[43]
			2.5–4.0 mg/kg	[44]
			Induction 2.5 mg/kg, maintenance 200 µg/kg/min	[46]
			Induction 2 mg/kg, maintenance 10 mg/kg/h	[47]
Thiopentone			5.23 mg/kg (±0.37 mg/kg)	[41]
			5 mg/kg age 1–10 years	[42]
			3–5 mg/kg i.v.	[43]
Midazolam	0.1 mg/kg i.v. bolus, 0.1–0.3 mg/kg/h	[36]	0.3–0.5 mg/kg 0.1–0.3 mg/kg/h	[34]
			0.5 mg/kg	[35]
			0.1 mg/kg i.v. bolus, 0.1–0.3 mg/kg/h	[36]
Ketamine	1–2 mg/kg, infusion 25–75 µg/kg/min	[35]	0.5 mg/ml	[34]
			1–2 mg/kg infusion, 25–150 µg/kg/min	[36]
			1.5 mg/kg with additional 0.5–1 mg/kg	[37, 43]
			0.5–2 mg/kg, infusion 10–50 µg/kg/min	[38]
			5 mg/kg/h	[39]
			2 mg/kg or 1 mg/kg	[40]
			0.5–1 mg/kg	[41]
			4 mg/kg i.m.	[42]
			Induction 1–1.2 mg/kg, infusion 16.7 µg/kg/h, addiction 0.25–0.5 mg/kg (ASA II–III)	[44]
			1 mg/kg, addiction 0.5–1 mg/kg	[45]
			1 mg/kg caudal	[46]

painless venous access. Therefore, unless immediate postoperative discharge is needed, sodium thiopentone may still be preferred. This drug is injected as a single bolus of 5–6 mg/kg, the child painlessly goes to sleep and after the briefest pause, begins to breathe. Maintenance with a volatile agent may then be substituted without recourse to a period of positive pressure ventilation, with a bag and mask, as generally is the case when propofol is used.

The advantages and disadvantages of, and problems with, intravenous induction can be summarized as follows:

- *Advantages*:
  - The process is rapid
  - The use of a face mask can be eliminated
  - There is no excitatory phase
  - There is no risk of laryngospasm
- *Disadvantages*:
  - Fear and aversion to needles
  - Pain on needle insertion
  - Bradycardia
  - Difficulties in dosing the individual patient
  - Pain on injection of propofol [49–52]. Currently new mixtures are being tested to reduce pain on propofol injection. This may lead to a change in clinical practice to avoid unnecessary pain [53–55]
- *Problems*:
  - Paravenous infusion [56]
  - Pump dysfunction.

Monitoring

A careful monitoring of the patient's condition is mandatory. In a healthy infant or child observation alone can give invaluable information (skin color, chest wall movements, breath sounds); so the most important—the best—monitor is the anesthesiologist.

During induction the patient is at one of the most vulnerable points in his or her perioperative care. Experience gives the anesthesiologist the tools to evaluate the situation: listening, observing, comparing, and anticipating. The experienced pediatric anesthesiologist will often recognize and correct problems before a pulse-oximeter has demonstrated any change. However, observation of the patient is not infallible, so electronic monitoring is fundamental and should be in place as soon as possible. It gives us another pair of ears and eyes.

The basic monitoring of a sick infant or child, especially if unstable, includes:

- Respiratory function: airway pressure, flow/volume curve, SpO_2, end-tidal CO_2
- Cardiocirculatory function: heart rate, ECG, noninvasive blood pressure
- Body temperature.

It is important that all anesthetic equipment is working correctly. This is the point at which equipment errors may put the patient at high risk of harm, for example, through compromising the airway, causing circulatory problems, preventing satisfactory oxygenation or even causing death.

Rapid Sequence Induction

The indication for a rapid sequence induction is the same in adults and children. If a risk of aspiration of gastric contents is foreseen, a rapid sequence induction should be performed. The procedure is the same in children as in adults. A working intravenous cannula is mandatory. The patient should be monitored and positioned on a tilting trolley with suction readily available. Oxygen is administered via a close-fitting mask for 3 minutes and anesthesia is induced. As the induction agent works, an assistant applies pressure to the cricoid ring, with one hand supporting the patient's neck. This maneuver completely closes the esophagus and prevents material from the stomach and esophagus reaching the pharynx. The traditional agents are sodium thiopentone 5 mg/kg and suxamethonium 2–3 mg/kg.

In practice, there are several problems with this procedure and it is rare to achieve as good preoxygenation in a child as in an adult. A good relationship and explanation works in many children, but in the younger or less cooperative, three or four good screams into the oxygen mask is often all that can be managed. In this situation, it seems sensible to delay administration of the short-acting depolarizing muscle relaxant until a few breaths of oxygen have been taken. In this technique, an attempt is made to preoxygenate the child before induction. Thiopentone or propofol is administered and sleep induced. Cricoid pressure is applied and the mask put on. The child should take a breath quite soon after administration of the hypnotic, and once this is seen, suxamethonium administered. Suxamethonium (0.2 mg/kg) is effective more quickly than in adults at this dose. It is possible to also use mivacurium (0.2 mg/kg), or rocuronium (0.9–1.2 mg/kg).

A difficult situation is when a child who cannot be cannulated needs emergency surgery and has a full stomach. Although not ideal, the most practical way forwards here is, probably, to induce anesthesia by volatile induction with the patient in the lateral position [57]. Once anesthesia is induced, it should be easier to secure intravenous access, apply cricoid pressure, turn the patient supine and perform intubation.

Rapid sequence induction is associated with a high risk of complications. This is related to the period of apnea between induction and tracheal intubation and to the fact that a neuromuscular blocking agent is given before the possibility of mask ventilation has been ensured. In infants and obese patients, apnea, even for less than one minute, may lead to hypoxemia and, and in a worst case scenario, neither mask ventilation nor tracheal intubation is possible.

Other problems with rapid sequence induction are circulatory depression and complications caused by the use of succinylcholine, such as hyperkalemia and malignant hyperthermia.

It is important to be aware of the increased risk associated with the procedure. The anesthetist should limit the use of rapid sequence induction to patients in whom a true benefit may be obtained [58, 59].

Conclusion

Both inhalational and intravenous induction have advantages and drawbacks. Because experience in small children is very limited, it is important to continually reevaluate our practice with a critical eye. The debates over which drugs and which methods are "best" to use to anesthetize infants and children are popular at meetings of pediatric anesthesiologists. The fact that these debates occur indicates that there are no simple answers. The skilled, confident anesthesiologist, who is prepared to react flexibly and to adopt methods to suit the opportunities presented by a child and his/her parents, will have most success.

References

1. Chan CS, Malassiotis A (2002) The effect of an educational programme on the anxiety and satisfaction level of parents having parent present induction and visitation in a postanesthesia care unit. Paediatr Anaesth 12:131–139
2. Vagnoli L, Caprilli S, Robiglio A, Messeri A (2005) Clown doctors as a treatment for preoperative anxiety in children: a randomized, prospective study. Pediatrics 116:563–567
3. Astuto M, Rosano G, Rizzo G et al (2006) Preoperative parental information and parents' presence at induction of anaesthesia. Minerva Anestesiol 72:461–465
4. McCann ME, Kain ZN (2001) The management of preoperative anxiety in children: an update. Anesth Analg 93:98–105
5. Shirley PJ, Thompson N, Kenward M, Johnston G (1998) Parental anxiety before elective surgery in children. A British perspective. Anaesthesia 53:956–959
6. Ryder IG, Spargo PM (1991) Parents in the anaesthetic room. A questionnaire survey of parents' reactions. Anaesthesia 46:977–979
7. McEwen A, Moorthy C, Quantock C et al (2007) The effect of videotaped preoperative information on parental anxiety during anesthesia induction for elective pediatric procedures. Paediatr Anaesth 17:534–539
8. Rieker M (2007) Con: Should parents be present during their child's anesthesia induction? MCN Am J Matern Child Nurs 32:73
9. Kam PC, Voss TJ, Gold PD et al (1998) Behaviour of children associated with parental participation during induction of general anaesthesia. J Paediatr Child Health 34:29–31
10. Kain ZN, Mayes LC, Caramico LA et al (1996) Parental presence during induction of anesthesia. A randomized controlled trial. Anesthesiology 84:1060–1067
11. Bellew M, Atkinson KR, Dixon G, Yates A (2002) The introduction of a paediatric anaesthesia information leaflet: an audit on its impact on parental anxiety and satisfaction. Paediatr Anaesth 12:124–130
12. Messeri A, Caprilli S, Busoni P (2004) Anaesthesia induction in children: a psychological evaluation of the efficiency of parents' presence. Paediatr Anaesth 14:551–556
13. Proczkowska-Björklund M, Svedin CG (2004) Child related background factors affecting compliance with induction of anaesthesia. Paediatr Anaesth 14:225–223
14. Arai YC, Ito H, Kandatsu N et al (2007) Parental presence during induction enhances the effect of oral midazolam on emergence behavior of children undergoing general anesthesia. Acta Anaesthesiol Scand 51:858–861
15. Kain ZN, Mayes LC, Wang SM et al (2000) Parental presence and sedative premedication for children undergoing surgery: a hierarchical study. Anesthesiology 92:939–946
16. Singh N, Pandey RK, Saksena AK, Jaiswal JN (2002) A comparative evaluation of oral midazolam with other sedatives as premedication in pediatric dentistry. J Clin Pediatr Dent 26:161–164

17. Dallman JA, Ignelzi MA Jr, Briskie DM (2001) Comparing the safety, efficacy and recovery of intranasal midazolam vs. oral chloral hydrate and promethazine. J Clin Pediatr Dent 23:424–430
18. Lucas-Polomeni MM (2004) Hypnosis: a new anesthetic technique! Paediatr Anaesth 14:975–976
19. Fukumoto M, Arima H, Ito S et al (2005) Distorted perception of smell by volatile agents facilitated inhalational induction of anesthesia. Paediatr Anaesth 15:98–101
20. Cyna AM, Tomkins D, Maddock T, Barker D (2007) Brief hypnosis for severe needle phobia using switch-wire imagery in a 5-year old. Paediatr Anaesth 17:800–804
21. Lerman J (2007) Inhalation agents in pediatric anaesthesia – an update. Curr Opin Anaesthesiol 20:221–226
22. Schwartz D, Connelly NR, Gutta S et al (2004) Early intravenous cannulation in children during sevoflurane induction. Paediatr Anaesth 14:820–824
23. Akeson J, Didriksson I (2004) Convulsions on anaesthetic induction with sevoflurane in young children. Acta Anaesthesiol Scand 48:405–407
24. Mayer J, Boldt J, Rohm KD et al (2006) Desflurane anesthesia after sevoflurane inhaled induction reduces severity of emergence agitation in children undergoing minor ear-nose-throat surgery compared with sevoflurane induction and maintenance. Anesth Analg 102:400–404
25. Bortone L, Ingelmo P, Grossi S et al (2006) Emergence agitation in preschool children: double-blind, randomized, controlled trial comparing sevoflurane and isoflurane anesthesia. Paediatr Anaesth 16:1138–1143
26. Breschan C, Platzer M, Jost R et al (2007) Midazolam does not reduce emergence of delirium after sevoflurane anesthesia in children. Paediatr Anaesth 17:347–352
27. Girshin M, Mukherjee J, Clowney R et al (2006) The postoperative cardiovascular arrest of a 5-year-old male: an initial presentation of Duchenne's muscular dystrophy. Paediatr Anaesth 16:170–173
28. Yemen TA, McClain C (2006) Muscular dystrophy, anesthesia and the safety of inhalational agents revisited; again. Paediatr Anaesth 16:105–108
29. Fernandez M, Lejus C, Rivault O, Bazin V (2005) Single-breath vital capacity rapid inhalation induction with sevoflurane: feasibility in children. Paediatr Anaesth 15:307–313
30. Chawathe M, Zatman T, Hall JE et al (2005) Sevoflurane (12% and 8%) inhalational induction in children. Paediatr Anaesth 15:470–475
31. Baum VC, Yemen TA (1997) Immediate 8% sevoflurane induction in children: a comparison with incremental sevoflurane and incremental halothane. Anesth Analg 85:313–316
32. Lee J, Oh Y, Kim C et al (2006) Fentanyl reduces desflurane-induced airway irritability following thiopental administration in children. Acta Anaesthesiol Scand 50:1161–1164
33. Speirs AF, Taylor KH, Joanes DN, Girdler NM (2001) A randomised, double-blind, placebo-controlled, comparative study of topical skin analgesics and the anxiety and discomfort associated with venous cannulation. Br Dent J 190:444–449
34. Murat I, Billard V, Vernois J et al (1996) Pharmacokinetics of propofol after a single dose in children aged 1–3 years with minor burns: comparison of three data analysis approaches. Anesthesiology 84:526–532
35. Raoof AA, Van Obbergh IJ, Verbeeck RK (1995) Propofol pharmacokinetics in children with biliary atresia. Br J Anaesth 74:46–49
36. Marsh B, White M, Morton N, Kenny GN (1991) Pharmacokinetic model driven infusion of propofol in children. Br J Anaesth 67:41–48
37. Gepts E, Camu F, Cockshott ID, Douglas EJ (1987) Disposition of propofol administered as constant rate intravenous infusions in humans. Anesth Analg 66:1256–1263
38. Rigby-Jones AE, Nolan JA, Priston MJ et al (2002) Pharmacokinetics of propofol infusions in critically ill neonates, infants, and children in an intensive care unit. Anesthesiology 97:1393–1400
39. Absalom A, Amutike D, Lal A et al (2003) Accuracy of the 'Paedfusor' in children undergoing cardiac surgery or catheterization. Br J Anaesth 91:507–513

40. Schuttler J, Ihmsen H (2000) Population pharmacokinetics of propofol: a multicenter study. Anesthesiology 92:727–738
41. Harling DW, Harrison DA, Dorman T, Barker I (1997) A comparison of thiopentone-isoflurane anaesthesia vs propofol infusion in children having repeat minor haematological procedures. Paediatr Anaesth 7:19–23
42. Morley-Forster P, McAllister JD, Vandenberghe H et al (1997) Does thiopentone delay recovery in children premedicated with midazolam? Paediatr Anaesth 7:279–285
43. Amantéa SL, Piva JP, Zanella MI et al (2003) Rapid airway access. J Pediatr (Rio J) 79 [Suppl 2]:S127–S138
44. Morton NS (1998) Total intravenous anaesthesia (TIVA) in paediatrics: advantages and disadvantages. Paediatr Anaesth 8:189–194
45. Davis PJ, Galinkin J, McGowan FX et al (2001) A randomized multicenter study of remifentanil compared with halothane in neonates and infants undergoing pyloromyotomy. I. Emergence and recovery profiles. Anesth Analg 93:1380–1386
46. Davis PJ, Lerman J, Suresh S et al (1997) A randomized multicenter study of remifentanil compared with alfentanil, isoflurane, or propofol in anesthetized pediatric patients undergoing elective strabismus surgery. Anesth Analg 84:982–989
47. Ganidagli S, Cengiz M, Baysal Z (2003) Remifentanil vs alfentanil in the total intravenous anaesthesia for paediatric abdominal surgery. Paediatr Anaesth 13:695–700
48. Eyres R (2004) Update on TIVA. Paediatr Anaesth 14:374–379
49. Wax D (2007) Ketamine for reducing propofol-induced pain. Anesth Analg 105:540
50. Pollard RC, Makky S, McFadzean J et al (2002) An admixture of 3 mg x kg(-1) of propofol and 3 mg x kg(-1) of thiopentone reduces pain on injection in pediatric anesthesia. Can J Anaesth 49:1064–1069
51. Kaabachi O, Chettaoui O, Abdelaziz AB et al (2007) A ketamine-propofol admixture does not reduce the pain on injection compared with a lidocaine-propofol admixture. Paediatr Anaesth 17:734–737
52. Liljeroth E, Karlsson A, Lagerkranser M, Akeson J (2007) Low dose propofol reduces the incidence of moderate to severe local pain induced by the main dose. Acta Anaesthesiol Scand 51:460–463
53. Mallick A, Elliot SC, Krishnan K, Vucevic M (2007) Lidocaine is more efficient than the choice of propofol formulations to reduce incidence of pain on induction. Eur J Anaesthesiol 24:403–407
54. Nyman Y, Von Hofsten K, Palm C et al (2006) Etomidate-Lipuro is associated with considerably less injection pain in children compared with propofol with added lidocaine. Br J Anaesth 97:536–539
55. Soltész S, Silomon M, Gräf G et al (2007) Effect of a 0.5% dilution of propofol on pain on injection during induction of anesthesia in children. Anesthesiology 106:80–84
56. Roth W, Eschertzhuber S, Gardetto A, Keller C (2006) Extravasation of propofol is associated with tissue necrosis in small children. Paediatr Anaesth 16:887–889
57. Sharma KR (2007) A new technique of holding the anesthesia face mask. Acta Anaesthesiol Scand 51:384–385
58. Zelicof-Paul A, Smith-Lockridge A, Schnadower D et al (2005) Controversies in rapid sequence intubation in children. Curr Opin Pediatr 17:355–362
59. Rasmussen LS, Viby-Mogensen J (2007) Rapid sequence intubation – how? Acta Anaesthesiol Scand 51:787–788

Chapter 9

Monitoring the Level of Anesthesia and Sedation in Children – An Overview

Nicola Disma, Andrew J. Davidson, Marinella Astuto

Introduction

Anesthesia is a balance between the amount of anesthetic drugs administered and the state of arousal of the patient. A large number of variables can interfere with the conduction of anesthesia, such as age, concomitant disease or therapies, physiological parameters and human variability. Moreover, clinical signs, such as blood pressure and heart rate, are routinely used by anesthesiologists to monitor anesthetic depth, but such methods are unreliable. Furthermore, patient movement in response to noxious stimulation remains an important sign of inadequate anesthetic dosage, but is unreliable and is suppressed by paralysis. As a consequence, an imbalance between anesthetic requirement and anesthetic drug administration is not uncommon. Under-dosing of anesthetic drugs may be caused by equipment failure or error. Conversely, over-dosing of the hypnotic components, leading to an excessive depth of anesthesia, might compromise patient outcome. How can the "depth of anesthesia" be measured and monitored? Several devices tested in adults with promising results have been recently introduced in clinical practice. Much more difficult is monitoring in the pediatric age group and the interpretation of data derived from such monitoring.

Application of Electroencephalography-based Monitors

Throughout the history of anesthesia anesthesiologists have used clinical signs to identify the correct level of hypnotic state. The recently introduced anesthesia depth monitors based on electroencephalography (EEG) have substantially modified this approach. Many clinical trials have been performed to verify the feasibility of these monitors during anesthesia in adults, and pediatric data are usually an extrapolation from adult data. However, ethical and physiological considerations are important in interpreting the results. The transfer of a technology from one population to another requires a clear understanding of the physiology and the principles behind the technology applied. The particular

M. Astuto (ed), *Basics*, Anesthesia, Intensive Care and Pain in Neonates and Children.
ISBN 978-88-470-0654-6 © Springer-Verlag Italia 2009

characteristics of the physiology and neuroanatomy of infants and of the technology mean that monitoring the depth of anesthesia is not straightforward.

Neuroanatomy of Consciousness

Consciousness is defined as "the ability to respond to the environment in a coordinated intentional manner," and it is dependent on the activity of both cerebral hemispheres as well as the ascending arousal system. The state of sedation is characterized by blunting of higher cortical function. Otherwise, unconsciousness can be produced by either diffuse injury to the cerebral cortex, or a lesion in the ascending arousal system.

The *ascending arousal system* compsises an ascending monoaminergic pathway that passes from the brainstem and hypothalamus to the cortex and thalamus to increase wakefulness and vigilance. Cholinergic pathways from pedunculopontine and laterodorsal tegmental nuclei and input from the parabranchial nucleus through the paramedian midbrain reticular formation also join this pathway. The arousal system divides. One branch enters the thalamus activating and modulating thalamic relay nuclei, and other thalamic nuclei with extensive and diffuse cortical projections. The other branch travels through the lateral thalamic area where it is joined by basal forebrain and hypothalamic ascending pathways. Together, these diffusely innervate the cortex. Lesions in either branch will impair consciousness.

Model of Anesthesia

To measure anesthesia we can use a model. There are four principal clinical aims of anesthesia; these are:
1. Loss of consciousness
2. Amnesia
3. Lack of movement
4. Reduction of autonomic reflexes.

These clinical signs are linked to varying degrees, and the drugs are the specific link. Some drugs have very specific clinical actions, but other drugs have more complex effects on the different components of anesthesia. For example, neuromuscular blockers act at specific sites of action. Opioids are effective in reducing nociceptive stimuli but they can, in large doses, produce unconsciousness. In synthesis, some drugs may act on a component of anesthesia, but may interfere with the other components. Similarly measuring one component may or may not be a reliable reflection of another component.

A balance between arousal and the concentration of various anesthetic drugs determines the state of anesthesia. In turn, a balance of between drug concentration and nociceptive stimulus also determines the degree of arousal. Finally, the degree of nociceptive stimulus may also be directly influenced by drug concentration. Anesthetic drugs can have direct and indirect effects at many points.

The concept of arousal is to some extent an abstract construct. We do not know anatomically where arousal is located; however, it may act in parallel in the reticular system or other activating systems in the brainstem and thalamus.

Can We "Measure" Anesthesia?

A profound understanding of "what anesthesia is" is a necessary background to determine what we want to measure using anesthesia depth monitors. After having established a model of anesthesia, the two spontaneous questions are: What do we want to measure? and How should a measure of anesthesia be represented?

If anesthesia is a binary phenomenon, it should be defined as 'adequate' or 'not adequate'. The word "depth" implies a surface and a linear extension below the surface. Thus a graded scale can be applied. If the component has ordinal or continuous characteristics then the measure may be represented as a scale or number that correlates with the effect. This is a key concept when assessing anesthesia depth monitor output.

Memory and *consciousness* are two components of arousal, but they are very difficult to measure and to reproduce on an ordinal scale. Explicit memory is described as the most sensitive to increasing doses of anesthesia, followed by implicit memory, and lastly consciousness. A measure of consciousness depends on the definition. In anesthesia measures of consciousness are usually measures of response to applied stimuli. Unconsciousness may be defined as no coordinated intentional response to a stimulus. In this respect, consciousness is a binary phenomenon; a person is either conscious or unconscious! The issue becomes confused when scales use graded stimuli. The Observer's Assessment of Alertness/Sedation Scale (OAA/S), the University of Michigan Sedation Scale (UMSS), the Glasgow Coma Scale and other measures of consciousness use increasingly intense stimuli to elicit a response. The deeply unconscious patient does not respond to an intense painful stimulus. A less deeply unconscious patient responds to an intense painful stimulus but not the human voice. Both patients are unconscious. In conclusion, what the scale is actually measuring is arousal, not consciousness. A low level of arousal results in no response. A higher level of arousal results in response with a lesser stimulus.

In summary, anesthesia and sedation are dependent on:
- Balances of arousal
- Concentration of drug
- Strength of stimuli.

Arousal can be measured indirectly by gauging the response to a stimulus. As response varies with the strength of the stimulus, arousal may be regarded as an abstract but basically linear construct. In conclusion, *it is arousal that sits most comfortably as a linear scale.*

EEG and Anesthesia

Von Marxow was the first to study the effects of anesthesia on brain waves in 1890 and Berger demonstrated the effect of anesthesia on the EEG in 1933. The EEG rhythm is derived from thalamocortical pathways and direct activity of the cortex; anesthesia may slow the EEG by actions in the thalamocortical component of the ascending arousal system and produce decreases in arousal or unconsciousness, or by actions directly on the cortex. The differential effect depends on the drug, dose and the kind of anesthesia performed.

Thus, from a physiological point of view it is reasonable to assume some link between the EEG and a measure of anesthesia. As mentioned above, the component of anesthesia that would be most amenable to measurement is arousal. However, such a link would have a degree of uncertainty and not be applicable to all situations.

The normal awake EEG changes with brain maturation. With increasing age the frequency of the awake dominant background activity increases:
- 6 months: 5 Hz
- 9–18 months: 6–7 Hz
- 2 years: 7–8 Hz
- 7 years: 9 Hz
- 15 years: 10 Hz (adult level).

Children less than 5 years old also have specific EEG patterns associated with the transition to and from sleep and drowsiness. Increasing the dose of a volatile anesthetic first increases the amplitude of the signal, then with increasing dose the amplitude decreases and the predominant frequencies become slower. After further increases in anesthetic an isoelectric EEG is achieved. During anesthesia, there is a characteristic activation of the EEG then a slowing of the EEG.
- Anesthesia may slow the EEG by actions in the thalamocortical component of the ascending arousal system, or by actions directly on the cortex. The differential effect may depend on drug and dose.
- Anesthesia may produce decreases in arousal or unconsciousness by actions in the thalamocortical component of the ascending arousal system or by actions directly on the cortex.

Uses of EEG-derived Anesthesia Depth Monitors

In essence, there are two ways to use an EEG-derived anesthesia depth monitor. First, as a machine that quantifies a component of anesthesia, and second as a guide, or arbitrary scale, to guide the anesthesiologist through anesthesia using particular drugs. *The component of anesthesia most likely to be represented by the EEG-derived monitor is arousal.*

In measuring arousal, a monitor can give a fair indication of the possibility that a patient may be conscious or may switch to the conscious state with the appropriate stimulus. The mean values associated with consciousness are higher than those associated with unconsciousness, but there is a significant degree of imprecision and overlap. There is other indirect evidence that monitors give a measure of arousal. At constant levels of stimulation, the values will change with anesthesia concentration and, with constant drug concentration, the values will change with stimulus. However, arousal is not a well-defined phenomenon so it is not surprising that it is unclear exactly what the numbers represent in a clinical setting. When a monitor is used for physiological studies this uncertainty must always be highlighted. Similarly, as the scales do not represent any defined physiological phenomenon, it is more appropriate to regard the data as on an ordinal rather than a linear or interval scale.

If a patient is unrousable, even with maximal stimulation, then the degree of arousal might be regarded as zero. However, the brain concentration of anesthetic drug may still rise resulting in further change in the EEG. This change in EEG is still useful information as, the higher the brain concentration, the further it must fall before any measurable degree of arousal. At high concentrations of anesthetic and low levels of arousal, it is difficult to determine if the changes seen in the EEG are related to changes in arousal or to the direct effects of the anesthetic agent on the thalamic or cortical neurons producing the EEG. This is particularly the case when *burst suppression* is occurring.

Aim of Anesthesia in Neonates and Children

The aim of sedation, anxiolysis, and various forms of hypnosis is the reduction of the humoral stress response, pain, anxiety, and emotional distress. In contrast, general anesthesia also aims to produce unconsciousness and amnesia. Unconsciousness is the complete lack of perception of any experience thus guaranteeing lack of any pain, anxiety, or distress. Immobility or the provision of surgical relaxation is another separate aim of general and regional anesthesia.

What is the evidence that the neonate is actually aware of the cold, incision or other painful stimulus? The issue becomes even more uncertain when one asks if the neonate can ever remember a distressing event. The discussion surrounding evidence of consciousness is profoundly philosophical. When we try to accurately measure unconsciousness and amnesia, the question of the development of consciousness and memory becomes far more practical. For infants to benefit from the precise delivery of anesthetic drugs, we need to understand exactly what we are hoping to achieve with these drugs in terms of unconsciousness and amnesia. In other words, what are the actual aims of general anesthesia in a neonate and what end-point do we use as adequate? No movement, no crying, no humoral stress response, no memory, or no consciousness? The question has an even greater relevance if these drugs are indeed found to be more toxic to the developing neonatal brain!

However, one thing is clear: measuring or guiding the effect of anesthesia in infants using adult-derived definitions of consciousness and amnesia is a difficult and perhaps futile exercise. When choosing a drug or a drug dose, adult models of the effect of anesthesia on memory and consciousness have only limited usefulness. In many circumstances, we have no idea if we are giving too little or too much. There is much room for further thought and investigation. Progress in understanding the physiology of consciousness and memory will become increasingly relevant not only to philosophers and psychologists, but also to pediatric anesthesiologists.

EEG-derived Devices

Do they work in children? Simply put, an anesthetic depth monitor is "working" if it is monitoring anesthetic depth, but what exactly do we mean by "anesthetic depth" in children? If a monitor "works" in adults, can we assume it would work in children? These devices have all been derived from adult EEG data. In adults the difference between the EEG when awake and the EEG when anesthetized is obvious. The EEG in awake children is well described and steadily changes with maturation, but our knowledge of the EEG during anesthesia in children is scant and, at this stage, too limited to make any assumptions about extrapolating adult data to children. Therefore, monitors ought to be assessed specifically in children.

Davidson et al. studied the effects of age on EEG during routine clinical anesthesia [1]. This physiological study provided important findings on the EEG characteristics during general anesthesia in infants and children. The power (area under the curve of EEG of the power frequency spectrum in 4-s epochs) has been noted to increase with age at equilibrium. Moreover, at equilibrium and gas-off a greater spread in power values was found in the younger than in older children. The amplitude encephalogram (aEEG) was also generated in these patients. The height of the aEEG was considered as an indicator of amplitude while the width of the band indicated the variability in the amplitude with time. Interestingly, the results showed that infants had a wide band width and a large fluctuation in amplitude during emergence from anesthesia. This occurred as a result of burst-like patterns that persisted from deep anesthesia to emergence. The burst-like pattern described by Davidson et al. is similar to the discontinuous pattern typical of neonatal physiological neurology. On the contrary, burst suppression after a bolus of propofol has been described in adolescents. It is of great relevance to underline that the burst-like pattern in infants is different from the burst suppression associated with overdose in adolescents. The latter has been described as periods of high activity interrupted by a sudden period of isoelectric activity, while the neonatal burst-like pattern is like a spindle with a smooth transition from near isoelectric to high amplitude activity.

In summary, infants have a typical EEG during general anesthesia characterized by a low power during anesthesia and no changes during emergence. Furthermore, a discontinuous pattern has been described during emergence. EEG of older children has been described with a high power that falls during emergence. As described in adults, burst suppression occurs after a propofol overdose.

Bispectral Index

The Bispectral Index (BIS) monitor was approved in 1996 by the US Food and Drug Administration for use in the setting of general anesthesia to aid in assessing the depth of anesthesia in adults. Traditional power spectral analysis decomposes raw EEG signal into a function of power (amplitude) and frequency. The BIS incorporates the phase-coupling relationship (bispectral analysis) into a conventional frequency/power analysis of the EEG. The BIS Monitoring System is designed to monitor the hypnotic state of the brain of the patient based on acquisition and processing of EEG signals. It processes raw EEG signals to produce a single number, the BIS, which correlates with the patient's level of hypnosis.

Early studies have demonstrated the correlation between BIS and responsiveness in children. BIS significantly decreases with 3% sevoflurane compared with 0.5% sevoflurane [2]. Recent studies have also found a correlation between BIS and predicted propofol concentration [3]. Rodriguez et al. showed that the sensitivity of BIS to detect consciousness was between 81% and 71% at emergence, and the positive predictive value of BIS to predict consciousness was between 53% and 63% [4]. Several other recent studies have demonstrated an influence of neuraxial blockade on the BIS [5]. The BIS falls with caudal block during general anesthesia (in older children, but not in infants) and falls during spinal anesthesia in infants.

Entropy

There are a number of concepts and analytical techniques directed at quantifying the irregularity of the EEG. One such concept is entropy. Entropy, when considered as a physical concept is related to the amount of 'disorder' in a system. Entropy is an intuitive parameter in the sense that one can visually distinguish a regular signal from an irregular one. Entropy also has the property of being independent of absolute scales such as the amplitude or the frequency of the signal: a simple sine wave is perfectly regular, whether it is fast or slow. The starting point of the algorithm applied in the Datex-Ohmeda Entropy Module (Datex-Ohmeda Division, Instrumentarium, Helsinki, Finland) is the spectral entropy, which has the particular advantage that contributions to entropy from any particular frequency range can be explicitly separated.

Davidson et al. performed a pilot study comparing BIS and response entropy/state entropy [6]. They were low during anesthesia and rose on awakening and a significant difference between values awake and during anesthesia was found for all age groups and monitors. Klockars et al. found a reasonable correlation between sevoflurane and spectral entropy and BIS in older children, but a less clear correlation between sevoflurane and the indices in infants [7].

Narcotrend

The Narcotrend (Monitor Technik, Bad Bramstedt, Germany) is an EEG monitor designed to measure the depth of anesthesia. It was developed at the University Medical School of Hannover, Germany, and it has received US Food and Drug Administration approval. The Narcotrend algorithm is based on pattern recognition of the raw EEG and classifies the EEG traces into different stages from A (awake) to F (increasing burst suppression down to electrical silence). The newest Narcotrend software version includes a Narcotrend index from 100 (awake) to 0 (electrical silence). There are several recent studies evaluating the Narcotrend as a measure of anesthetic depth in children. Weber et al. showed a strong correlation between the Narcotrend index and sevoflurane concentration, both during induction of anesthesia and from anesthesia to return of consciousness [8].

A-line ARX Index

The A-line ARX index (AAI) generated from the A-line monitor extracts the mid-latency auditory evoked potentials with an autoregressive model. This version of the AAI has now been superseded by the AAI-1.6, which incorporated passive EEG measures at deeper levels of anesthesia.

Cerebral State Index

The Cerebral State Index (CSI) is a recently introduced EEG-derived monitor. The CSI calculates an index from the raw EEG signals using an algorithm based on power analysis of the beta, alpha and beta-alpha ratio. The monitor also evaluates the amount of instantaneous burst suppression in each 30-s period of EEG, that is expressed as a percentage. There has been a limited evaluation of the CSI in children. Disma et al. compared the CSI and the AAI with the UMSS in children aged from 8 months to 7 years. Both CSI and AAI decreased with induction and rose with emergence. There was also a strong correlation between CSI and sedation scores and AAI and sedation scores [9].

Depth of Anesthesia Monitors and the Impact on Outcome in Children

This is the crucial point in the future application of these devices. Although the monitors are imprecise measures, it is incorrect to conclude that they are without use. Indeed, outcome studies have provided increasing evidence of their value in preventing awareness [10] and improving recovery times [11]. In a recent clinical trial, Myles et al. [10] demonstrated that BIS-guided anesthesia is able to reduce the incidence of awareness in high-risk patients. Much more difficult would be to transfer this result to a pediatric population, considering that awareness is not a clearly defined phenomenon in children. Davidson et al. [12] underlined that, like adults, children are at risk of awareness. Andrade et al. [13], in a trial in a large pediatric population, found that the incidence of awareness in children is eight times that measured in adults. Although the cause of awareness in children remains unclear, anesthesiologists should be alert to the possibility of this adverse event, bearing in mind that the utility of EEG-derived monitors to prevent awareness in children is still unknown.

In spite of uncertainty surrounding maturational changes in the EEG, and the paucity of data about EEG changes during anesthesia in children, there are several physiological studies indicating that EEG-derived anesthesia monitors give some measure of arousal in children [14]. The differences in infants may be due to the immaturity of the EEG or it may be that the nature of arousal in an infant differs from that in adults. For example, infants may have a more marked 'switch' in the transition from anesthesia to emergence. If the relationship between arousal and consciousness is different in infants, then the relationship between the monitor and consciousness will also be different in infants. There are therefore several possible clinical benefits derived from measuring the EEG, such as improved recovery and reduced awareness [12]. An improved recovery has been demonstrated with a shorter time to discharge with BIS-guided anesthesia in older children, but not in younger children [15]. To the best of our knowledge, there are no studies evaluating EEG-derived monitors and the incidence of postoperative nausea and vomiting. Some trials have investigated a possible relationship between depth of anesthesia and laryngospasm with both sevoflurane and halothane, and have shown a strong relationship with the latter agent. Finally, no clear correlation has been found between BIS and complications during laryngeal mask insertion and removal [16].

In conclusion, further clinical trials are needed to prove the real benefits in terms of outcome derived from the use of these devices, particularly in children.

Areas of Application

A large number of articles have been published on the clinical use of anesthesia depth monitors during anesthesia, procedural sedation and sedation in intensive care.

During *procedural sedation,* the anesthesia depth monitors have a well-established role in improving safety, quality of sedation and recovery period. Sadhasivam et al. performed a validation study on BIS during sedation for invasive and noninvasive procedures [17]. They concluded that BIS strongly correlates with sedation scales and it can be considered a quantitative, nondisruptive and easy to use depth of sedation monitor in children. Powers et al. demonstrated that the BIS can be a useful monitoring guide for the titration of propofol to achieve deep sedation in children undergoing painful procedures [18].

Concerning the use of anesthesia depth monitors in pediatric intensive care, there are some trials that have shown correlations between BIS and commonly used clinical sedation scoring systems, such as the COMFORT score with a moderate correlation [19]. Crain et al. studied the impact of BIS in sedated and mechanically ventilated children. They concluded that BIS can be considered useful to identify and prevent oversedation [20]. Moreover, a specific area of use could be in those patients sedated and receiving neuromuscular blocking, with the aim of preventing inadequate sedation in paralysed patients. Aneja et al. performed a trial and highlighted the inadequacy of clinical scoring systems and the ability of BIS to detect children who were at risk of awareness and recall [21].

The real impact on outcome will be the special topic of future trials. At the moment, the UK Paediatric Intensive Care Society Sedation and Analgesia and Neuromuscular Blockade Working Group do not recommend the routine use of anesthesia depth monitors in the pediatric intensive care unit, because of the heterogeneity of the samples and results, and the lack of gold standard sedation protocols [22].

Conclusion

In recent years a large variety of studies has been published on the clinical use of anesthesia depth monitors in children, and the BIS is the most studied. Some interesting conclusions have been reported on the uses of these monitors, but the real benefits on outcome will be obtained after future well-designed trials. In any case, the increasing evidence is that this monitors work in older children, with possible and desirable effects on outcome. Which monitor is the most suitable in the different areas of use is a further topic of future trials.

References

1. Davidson AJ, Sale SM, Wong C et al (2007) The electroencephalograph during anesthesia and emergence in infants and children. Pediatr Anesth 18:60–70
2. Brosius KK, Bannister CF (2001) Effect of oral midazolam premedication on the awakening concentration of sevoflurane, recovery times and bispectral index in children. Paediatr Anaesth 11:585–590
3. Park H, Kim YL, Kim CS et al (2007) Changes in bispectral index during recovery from general anesthesia with 2% propofol and remifentanil in children. Pediatr Anesth 17:353–357
4. Rodriguez RA, Hall LE, Duggan S, Splinter WM (2004) The bispectral index does not correlate with clinical signs of inhalational anesthesia during sevoflurane induction and arousal in children. Can J Anaesth 51:472–480
5. Davidson AJ, Ironfield CM, Skinner AV, Frawley GP (2006) The effects of caudal local anesthesia blockade on the bispectral Index during general anesthesia in children. Paediatr Anaesth 16:828–833
6. Davidson AJ, Kim MJ, Sangolt GK (2004) Entropy and bispectral index during anaesthesia in children. Anaesth Intensive Care 32:485–493
7. Klockars JG, Hiller A, Ranta S et al (2006) Spectral entropy as a measure of hypnosis in

children. Anesthesiology 104:708–717

8. Weber F, Hollnberger H, Gruber M et al (2004) Narcotrend depth of anesthesia monitoring in infants and children. Can J Anaesth 51:855–856

9. Disma N, Lauretta D, Palermo F et al (2007) Level of sedation evaluation with Cerebral State Index and A-Line Arx in children undergoing diagnostic procedures. Pediatr Anesth 17:445–451

10. Myles PS, Leslie K, McNeil J et al (2004) Bispectral index monitoring to prevent awareness during anaesthesia: the B-Aware randomised controlled trial. Lancet 363:1757–1763

11. Gan TJ, Glass PS, Windsor A et al (1997) Bispectral index monitoring allows faster emergence and improved recovery from propofol, alfentanil, and nitrous oxide anesthesia. BIS Utility Study Group. Anesthesiology 87:808–815

12. Davidson AJ, Huang GH, Czarnecki C et al (2005) Awareness during anesthesia in children: a prospective cohort study. Anesth Analg 100:653–661

13. Andrade J, Deeprose C, Barker I (2008) Awareness and memory function during paediatric anaesthesia. Br J Anaesth 100:389–396

14. Murat I, Constant I (2005) Bispectral index in pediatrics: fashion or a new tool? Pediatr Anesth 15:177–180

15. Bannister CF, Brosius KK, Sigl JC et al (2001) The effect of bispectral index monitoring on anesthetic use and recovery in children anesthetized with sevoflurane in nitrous oxide. Anesth Analg 92:877–881

16. Davidson A (2004) The correlation between bispectral index and airway reflexes with sevoflurane and halothane anaesthesia. Pediatr Anesth 14:241–246

17. Sadhasivam S, Ganesh A, Robison A et al (2006) Validation of the bispectral index monitor for measuring the depth of sedation in children. Anesth Analg 102:383–388

18. Powers KS, Nazarian EB, Tapyrik SA et al (2005) Bispectral index as a guide for titration of propofol during procedural sedation among children. Pediatrics 115:1666–1674

19. Triltsch AE, Nestmann G, Orawa H et al (2005) Bispectral index versus COMFORT score to determine the level of sedation in pediatric intensive care unit patients: a prospective study. Crit Care 9:R9–R17

20. Crain N, Slonim A, Pollack MM (2002) Assessing sedation in the pediatric intensive care unit by using BIS and the COMFORT scale. Pediatr Crit Care Med 3:11–14

21. Aneja R, Heard AM, Fletcher JE, Heard CM (2003) Sedation monitoring of children by the bispectral index in the pediatric intensive care unit. Pediatr Crit Care Med 4:60–64

22. Playfor S, Jenkins I, Boyles C et al (2006) Consensus guidelines on sedation and analgesia in critically ill children. Intensive Care Med 32:1125–1136

Chapter 10
Locoregional Anesthesia in Children

Marinella Astuto

Introduction

The last decade has seen many advances in the management of neonates, which are based upon an increased understanding of the neurophysiology of pain, combined with the development of clinical pain services, analgesic delivery devices, and monitoring protocols.

The nervous system of neonates is characterized by the absence of full myelination and by poorly myelinated thalamocortical radiations. These elements must be considered as a reflection of immaturity but not as an indication of lack of function. The immaturity of the nociceptive system implies that young patients cannot localize pain as accurately as adults, and the corresponding perception of nociceptive sensation may be more widespread. The differences in subclasses of opioid receptors in neonates may contribute to a reduced ability to modulate nociceptive transmission.

Painful experiences in very low-weight infants may result in significantly higher somatization scores. This increased understanding of pain transmission and the long-term consequences of pain [1] underlines the need for a wide spectrum of strategies to achieve optimal patient pain relief. Regional anesthesia is commonly used as an adjunct to general anesthesia or, most commonly, as a means of providing postoperative analgesia. Peripheral (both continuous and single-shot) and central blocks (epidural or spinal) and the choice of new low-toxicity local anesthetics, eventually combined with nonopioid additives, are current strategies for multimodal analgesia in neonates. These procedures for performing blocks have to take into consideration the anatomical and physiological differences between neonates and children.

Anatomical and Physiological Considerations

A good knowledge of pediatric anatomy is mandatory for regional anesthesia. Physiology in newborns and infants differs from that in older children and

M. Astuto (ed), *Basics*, Anesthesia, Intensive Care and Pain in Neonates and Children. ISBN 978-88-470-0654-6 © Springer-Verlag Italia 2009

adults. The metabolism and clearance of drugs, including local anesthetics, are reduced so that we have a narrow therapeutic window and an increased toxicity [2].

The spinal cord at birth and in term babies ends at the level of the third lumbar vertebra and the dural sac ends at the fourth sacral foramen. Only after the first years of life do they reach their definitive anatomical position (the dural sac at the level of the second or third foramen and the spinal cord at the level of the first lumbar vertebra). The intercristal line crosses the midline at the S1 interspace in neonates, and at the L5 interspace in older children. The distance between the skin and the dural sac depends on age and weight [3, 4]. In the neonate it is about 1.4 cm (14 mm), and in the child aged 2 years and above it can be estimated from the expression: distance in millimeters = (age in years x2) + 10. The distance between the dural sac and the hiatus varies, but it must be born in mind that it is only a few millimeters, less than 10 mm in the newborn. Moreover, the sacral hiatus in the child is in a more cephalad position. These anatomical differences between neonates and children are summarized in Table 10.1.

The volume of cerebrospinal fluid (CSF) is 4 ml/kg in children (<15 kg) while in adults it is 2 ml/kg. The effect of this is higher drug dilution and, in addition to the higher blood flow in children, a higher uptake.

In conclusion, in preterm, term and older infants the dosage of local anesthetics is higher than that in adults and the duration of intrathecal analgesia is shorter. In neonates, plasma levels of albumin and alpha-1 glycoprotein are lower

Table 10.1 Anatomical differences between neonates and children of relevance to locoregional anesthesia

	Neonates	Children (>1 year of age)
Dural sac	S4	S2–S3
Spinal cord	L3	L1
Intercristal space	L5–S1	L5
Lumbar lordosis	Absent	Present (acquired upright position)
CSF volume	4 ml/kg (50% in spinal canal)	4 ml/kg
Plasma levels of albumin and alpha-1 glycoprotein	Very low	Low
Nerve fibers	Small	Small
	Amyelinated	Amyelinated
	Smaller distance between	Smaller distance between
	Ranvier nodes	Ranvier nodes
Distance between skin and dural sac (mm)	14	(age in years x2) + 10

CSF, cerebrospinal fluid

than in adults and in older children, thus the binding capacity of local anesthetics is reduced and the amount of unbound local anesthetics is higher.

The nerve fibers are relatively smaller and the distance between the nodes of Ranvier is shorter so that large volumes and low concentrations is the key to obtain an adequate sensorial block in children.

Another important factor that can explain the different dosage of local anesthetics in children is the different area of the spinal cord where the drugs take effect: in term babies the length of the spinal cord is about 20 cm (in adults 65–70 cm). This means that the length to weight ratio is four or five times higher in newborns than in adults.

The epidural space contains gelatinous fat, connective tissue, blood and lymph vessels. In children aged less than 8 years the low concentrations of gelatinous fat allow a more rapid reabsorption of local anesthetics from the epidural space. This means that drugs can reach higher plasma levels.

The epidural veins are without valves and have a thin wall that allows the absorption of drugs or gas without puncturing the vein.

The hemodynamic responses to sympathetic block due to local anesthetics depend on age. Children aged less than 7 years have no hemodynamic responses after spinal or epidural block except for thoracic block up to fourth thoracic vertebra. This difference could be due to the lower sympathetic tone in children. In children, during central blocks, the systemic blood pressure and cardiac output remain steady if the child is normovolemic, in which case it is not necessary to fill with solution before the block.

Peripheral Nerve Blocks

Standard peripheral blocks, such as paraumbilical, axillary, intercostal, inguinal, penile and femoral blocks and those of the fascia iliaca compartment, are the mainstay of analgesic management in neonatal surgery. Peripheral nerve blocks may avoid the risks inherent in central blockade and also its side effects. Other advantages are higher safety, less nausea/vomiting, less urinary retention, good postoperative analgesia that is long-lasting, and the option of performing it even in anticoagulated or febrile patients. However, peripheral nerve blocks require multiple injections and larger volumes of anesthetic solution and have a longer onset time. Moreover, their limited effects in cavity surgery (thoracotomy/laparotomy) and their relatively short duration of action means that they are less well suited to more major surgery.

A *single-shot peripheral block* means a single injection of local anesthetic. This technique is now widely used in infants, but can provide analgesia for only a few hours. Another drawback of these blocks is the relatively high failure rate. For example, although inguinal hernia repair is one of the most common surgical procedures performed in neonates and premature infants, the precise anatomical positions of both the ilioinguinal and the iliohypogastric nerves are still not identified in this age group, and the relatively high failure rate of 10–25%, even when the technique is performed by an experienced practitioner, could be due to a lack of specific spatial knowledge of the anatomy of these nerves in infants and neonates [5].

Direct ultrasonographic (US) visualization of the inguinal and iliohypogastric nerves might improve the quality of the block and reduce the risk of complications. The use of real-time imaging makes it possible to detect the precise location of the needle tip between the ilioinguinal and iliohypogastric nerves and to observe the spread of the local anesthetic around both nerves. This allows the use of a significantly smaller amount of local anesthetic while still achieving a clinically effective block. This is particularly relevant for neonates, who are at risk of local anesthetic toxicity and higher free plasma concentrations of local anesthetic agents in view of their lower plasma concentration of the binding protein alpha-1 acid glycoprotein.

The results of a recent study are encouraging and demonstrate a further application of the use of US in pediatric regional anesthesia [6]; it is important, however, to underline that US in neonates should be considered an important and ongoing part of training in regional pediatric anesthesia, as it is a way of demonstrating the relevant anatomical differences in this age group and many of the structures that regional anesthesiologists seek to avoid are clearly shown: the pleura, arteries and veins. It is for this reason that the availability of US may lead to changes in regional neonatal anesthetic practice.

A *continuous peripheral nerve block* (CPNB) means a continuous infusion of local anesthetics. CPNBs are even safer than central ones and are very effective for long-term pain control.

Prolonged analgesia with CPNBs in the treatment of pediatric postoperative limb pain, sometimes with patient-controlled regional analgesia, should be preferred instead of continuous epidural analgesia. Many published studies demonstrate the efficacy and safety of analgesia via a peripheral catheter; no complications or side effects linked to long-term infusions, and few accidental removals and little drug leakage have been described. CPNBs are at least as efficient as epidural analgesia, but produce fewer side effects [7].

The use of ropivacaine and levobupivacaine for CPNBs is particularly interesting in neonates because of the lower cardiac and central nervous system (CNS) toxicity and differential sensory/motor blockade duration with these agents [8]. Ropivacaine is the drug of choice; it has the potential to produce differential neural blockade with less pronounced motor block and induces less myotoxicity than bupivacaine [9]. Conversely, continuous infusion of these new local anesthetics offers the safest therapeutic index, especially in infants. Many adjuncts have been used, but clonidine offers clear advantages [10].

There has so far been a lack of specific equipment for performing such techniques in neonates, and practitioners have used radial artery catheterization sets, epidural kits, and central venous catheter sets. A specially designed set for pediatric CPNB has recently been developed. It is composed of a 20-G beveled (15°) conducting needle 33 or 55 mm long sheathed in a plastic cannula and a 22-G, catheter 400 mm long with a wire.

Data in the literature suggest that the starting bolus dose administered before a continuous infusion depends on the objective. Generally, 0.4–0.6 ml/kg of a low concentration (e.g. 0.2% ropivacaine) is used for intraoperative pain control and for postoperative analgesia. Lidocaine 1.5% can be added to the bolus of 0.2% ropivacaine. A continuous infusion is then administered using 0.125–0.25% bupivacaine or 0.2% ropivacaine at 0.1–0.3 ml/kg per hour, which is equivalent to 0.2–0.4 mg/kg per hour. A 25–30% reduction in local anesthetic is recommended for infants <6 months of age [11]. Ivani et al. [12] demonstrated better postoperative analgesia when 2 µg/kg clonidine was added to ropivacaine for an ilioinguinal–iliohypogastric nerve block, but this observation was not supported by the results of a study by Kaabachi et al. [13], which, in fact, failed to demonstrate better postoperative analgesia following the addition of 1 µg/kg clonidine to 0.25% bupivacaine for ilioinguinal–iliohypogastric nerve blocks. These different effects of a small dose of clonidine on the efficacy of a nerve block may be explained by differences in the type of nerve block, the mixture injected, and the technique used, which probably influence the rate of absorption of the anesthetic solutions injected [14].

US-guided blocks will probably become the reference technique for local anesthetic injection and regional anesthesia catheter placement; new training in this field should be available in the near future.

Central Blocks

Epidural

The performance of regional blocks in anesthetized patients is generally contraindicated in adults but acceptable in children. Performance of a block during anesthesia is safer than when performed in an awake child. Epidural analgesia in combination with light general anesthesia is a useful alternative for neonates undergoing major surgery; it avoids the adverse effects related to systemic administration of opioids and other agents. Apart from providing good intraoperative and postoperative analgesia, epidural blockade has beneficial effects on the humoral, metabolic, and hemodynamic responses to surgery and may improve postoperative respiratory performance.

In experienced hands, the complication rate of epidural analgesia is low. Serious complications have been described in small infants, including paraplegia and death. In most cases direct trauma is reported, and it seems probable that it is a result of difficulty in performing the procedure. Many authors share the opinion that only anesthesiologists who are experienced in the technique should perform epidural anesthesia in small infants and neonates.

In neonates and infants, the straighter column and less-dense packing of the extradural space by fat and fibrous tissue allows catheters to be placed via the sacral hiatus, then threaded to the thoracic region. This provides segmental thoracic analgesia, yet avoids the hazards associated with direct needling of the thoracic extradural space. Catheters may also be passed to low lumbar levels for lumbar blocks, so that the large doses of local anesthetic needed when the injection is performed at the sacral hiatus are avoided. Correct cannula placement and catheter level should be checked to avoid high blocks and respiratory compromise or low blocks and inadequate analgesia. A number of techniques have been described for the confirmation of correct or intravascular placement, but the novel use of US to visualize the epidural catheter has a particularly high potential for improving safety and providing better quality analgesia [15, 16].

The toxicity of local anesthetics affects the heart and the brain and is commonly produced as a result of inadvertent intravascular administration or administration of an excessive bolus dose. Moreover, there is a risk of inadvertent intravascular injection and this can be minimized only with adequate monitoring during the block. Owing to the lower levels of plasma protein α1-acid glycoprotein and albumin, and lower bicarbonate reserves, neonates have a high risk of bupivacaine toxicity, such as cardiac dysrhythmia or respiratory arrest, which are a more likely to occur in neonates and infants than convulsions [17]. This can be avoided using bolus doses and infusion rates that are within recommended guidelines and by taking account of the pharmacokinetics of local anesthetics in neonates. Pharmacokinetic studies of several local anesthetics have been performed in neonates and have led to important information on the safe use of local anesthetics in neonates (Table 10.2) [18].

Pharmacokinetic studies on bupivacaine have shown a reduction in clearance in neonates which reaches mature values by 4–6 months of age. An infusion rate of 0.2 mg/kg per hour induces a continuous increase in plasma concentrations, which rise to the threshold for toxicity in about 72 hours. Therefore, bupivacaine infusion rates of 0.3–0.4 mg/kg per hour are safe in infants aged more than 6 months, but infusion rates in neonates should be no faster than 0.2 mg/kg per hour. Suggested concentrations of local anesthetics for continuous infusion are shown in Table 10.3 [19].

Table 10.2 Suggested doses (mg/kg) for local anesthetics for single-shot administration

Local anesthetic	Thoracic block	Lumbar block	Transacral block
Bupivacaine 0.25%	1–1.2	2	2
Ropivacaine 0.2%	0.8–1	1.4	1.4
Levobupivacaine 0.2–0.25%	0.8–1.2	1.4–2	1.4–2

Table 10.3 Suggested concentrations of local anesthetics for continuous infusion

Local anesthetic	Concentration (%)
Bupivacaine	0.125
Ropivacaine	0.1
Levobupivacaine	0.125

Ropivacaine has a number of advantages that could be considered important in neonates. These include lower cardiotoxicity than is associated with equal concentrations of racemic bupivacaine and a higher threshold for CNS toxicity of the unbound concentration. The greater degree of block in nerve fibers of pain transmission than of motor function for a given concentration [20] would be of further benefit. Plasma concentrations of unbound ropivacaine are expected to level off during an epidural infusion as ropivacaine is eliminated by liver metabolism with an intermediate to low hepatic extraction ratio (in adults as well as in children and neonates). Consequently, the plasma concentrations of unbound ropivacaine at steady-state will depend on clearance of unbound ropivacaine. As a consequence of the age-related variations in clearance, the plasma concentrations of unbound ropivacaine are higher in neonates than in older age groups [21].

A study by Bösenberg et al. [22] showed that plasma concentrations of unbound ropivacaine level off after 24 hour of infusion in all age groups, including neonates. This is important and suggests that long-term epidural infusions of ropivacaine may be administered to both infants and neonates. Furthermore, continuous epidural infusion of ropivacaine 0.2% (0.2–0.4 mg/kg per hour) for 48–72 hours provided satisfactory postoperative pain relief in infants aged 0–362 days. Notwithstanding the use of different doses in different age groups, no age-related differences were found in the need for supplementary analgesia. A dose of 0.4 mg/kg per hour of ropivacaine is generally recommended for continuous epidural infusion in children, but no studies have been performed to define the minimum effective infusion rate. However, because of the wider variability of plasma concentrations of ropivacaine in neonates, extreme caution should be exercised whenever neonates undergo surgery during the first week of life [22].

Finally, levobupivacaine is the newest local anesthetic to be introduced into clinical practice. An open-label study by Chalkiadis et al. [23] using 2 mg/kg of 0.25% levobupivacaine in infants showed that there is a direct link between the immaturity of P450 CYP3A4 and CYP1A2 enzyme isoforms that metabolize this local anesthetic in infants and a lower clearance than in adults. This lower clearance delays peak plasma concentration, which was noted to occur approximately 50 min after administration of caudal epidural levobupivacaine. The low intrinsic toxicity of levobupivacaine makes it ideal as a local anesthetic for pediatric use, but there are no data describing its pharmacokinetics in infants after caudal administration.

Various agents are currently being used as adjuncts to regional anesthesia. Combination of these additives with local anesthetics prolongs the duration of the block with improves postoperative analgesia, as shown in several clinical trials. Various studies have demonstrated a prolonged duration of analgesia in children when clonidine is combined with local anesthetics. The addition of 1–2 µg/kg of clonidine given via the epidural route increases the duration of analgesia by 1–2 h compared with local anesthetics alone. In a recent clinical trial the effects of adding three different doses of clonidine (1, 1.5 and 2 µg/kg) to 0.125% bupivacaine were compared. After the dose of 2 µg/kg dose a significantly longer period of analgesia was demonstrated, with no significant respiratory or hemo-dynamic side effects. Clonidine at 1–2ia by approximately 5–10 h when com-bined with bupivacaine 0.1–0.25% or ropivacaine 0.08–0.2%.

Although clonidine-induced respiratory depression is uncommon in the dose range normally used (1–2 µg/kg), clonidine reduces the ventilatory response to carbon dioxide [24]. The consequent respiratory depression has been associated with differential recruitment of upper airway muscles and continuous activation of laryngeal and pharyngeal muscles in animal studies. Clonidine has been shown to stimulate central alpha-2 adrenoceptors with a differential effect on the baroreflex heart rate and vasomotor regulation. Alpha-2 adrenoceptor stimula-tion greatly augments baroreflex-mediated bradycardia and exerts a tonic inhibitory influence on respiratory rhythm in the awake goat. These effects can be reversed by selective alpha-2 adrenoceptor blockade [25].

Clonidine has other potential benefits, including reduced postoperative agita-tion, shivering and vomiting. On the other hand, administration of higher dosages of clonidine is associated with a potential risk of apnea, particularly in neonates [26]. Finally, a pharmacokinetic study was performed that demonstrated that epidural and intramuscular administration of the same dose is followed by a sim-ilar peak plasma concentration, but no correlation was found between the anal-gesic effects produced by epidural administration and systemic absorption.

Another study has demonstrated that (S)-ketamine 0.5 mg/kg when added to 0.2% caudal ropivacaine provides better postoperative analgesia than clonidine without any clinically significant side effects [27]. Ketamine has been used as the sole agent to produce caudal block in children. Moreover, as demonstrated by Hager et al. [28], the addition of 1–2 µg/kg of clonidine to 1 mg/kg of (S)-ketamine via the caudal route significantly prolongs analgesia for 24 hours. De Negri et al. [27] have shown that the addition of 0.5 mg/kg of (S)-ketamine to caudal ropivacaine 0.2% prolongs the duration of postoperative analgesia in children significantly beyond that attained with ropivacaine plus clonidine 2 µg/kg or ropivacaine alone. At the higher dosage levels both agents are associ-ated with a greater risk of sedation, apnea (particularly in neonates and infants) and nausea.

Fentanyl, in contrast, does not prolong the duration of analgesia when added to 'single-shot' caudal block, but does significantly increase the incidence of nausea and vomiting. Other agents, such as buprenorphine, tramadol neostig-mine, and midazolam, are associated with an unacceptably high incidence of nausea and vomiting with minimal added benefit [29]. Drugs used as adjuncts in regional anesthesia and their doses and sites of action are shown in Table 10.4.

The Lumbar Block

This is usually performed at the L5–S1 or L4–L5 level, with a midline approach. The Tuohy needle (i.e. Portex 19 G or Bbraun 20 G) is an appropriate age-suit-able needle. The technique used to perform a lumbar block requires the position-

Table 10.4 Drugs used as adjuncts in regional anesthesia

Drug	Dose	Site of action	Side effects
Clonidine	1–2 µg/kg	Agonist of µ2-adrenergic receptor	Sedation, respiratory depression
(S)-Ketamine	0.5 mg/kg	NMDA receptor blocker	Rare
Midazolam	50 µg/kg	GABA receptor agonist	Sedation
Neostigmine	2 µg/kg	Muscarinic receptor	Nausea, vomiting

ing of the needle almost perpendicularly in the midline with the bevel pointing cephalad, then after crossing the superficial planes, the stylet is removed and a syringe is connected as soon as a loss of resistance (LOR) is perceived when, after the yellow ligament, the epidural space is reached (Fig. 10.1). The LOR technique can be performed with air or with saline solution or CO_2. There are different opinions that support one or the other technique [30]. If an epidural catheter is required, the Tuohy needle should be inserted correctly, close to the target area for block, to avoid excessive postoperative infusion of the drug (Figs. 10.2 and 10.3).

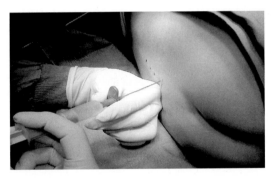

Fig. 10.1 Lumbar block with Tuohy needle and loss of resistance (LOR) technique

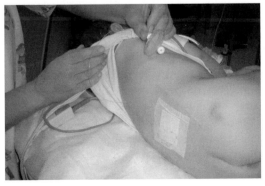

Fig. 10.2 Correct positioning of epidural catheter

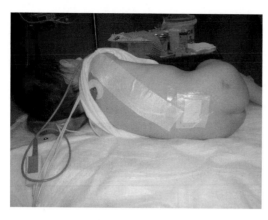

Fig. 10.3 Correct positioning of epidural catheter

The Thoracic Block

The technique is similar to that used for the lumbar block, but the needle should be inserted more obliquely because the spinous processes are more oblique than at the lumbar level.

The level of the block depends on the surgical site (Table 10.5). If an epidural catheter is required it should be inserted, like a lumbar catheter, close to the target area, only 3–4 cm within the epidural space.

Table 10.5 Levels of thoracic block for different surgical sites

Surgical site	Level of block
Pectus excavatum	T3–T5
Upper abdominal surgery	T6–T7
Nephrectomy	T7–T8
Lower abdominal surgery	T8–T10
Pelvis	T10–T12

The Transacral Block

The transacral block was described in 1987 by Busoni and Sarti as "epidural persacral block". The landmarks are the posterior iliac spines, the line connecting the spines across S2. In this block both the S1–S2 level and the S2–S3 level can be used. The needle is inserted perpendicularly in the midline or at 45° or more. This technique can be used thanks to the lower resistance of tissues in children and to the incomplete fusion and ossification of the spines of the sacral vertebrae.

Generally the transacral block is used when it is impossible to perform a caudal or epidural block, particularly for surgery if the lower abdominal, pelvis or lower limbs. This technique is also important because it can be used for training for epidural lumbar or thoracic anesthesia. The indications and contraindications are similar to those for the caudal block with a lower incidence of infections.

The Caudal Block

Caudal epidural anesthesia remains the most frequently performed regional anesthesia technique in infants and children. This is a popular single-shot technique characterized by a high level of efficacy and safety. This block has the lowest incidence of complications of all central blocks (0.7/1,000 cases) [31]. A disadvantage of the caudal blockade is the relatively short duration of postoperative analgesia. The caudal block provides a good state of anesthesia with low concentrations of inhalation agents, allows rapid and comfortable recovery, allows maintenance of spontaneous breathing, and is associated with a shorter time in the postanesthetic care unit.

The caudal block is the technique of choice for surgery up to level T8 lasting no longer than 60–90 minutes in children aged less than 7 years. The majority of routine operations on the lower abdomen and lower limbs in children can be performed with this method (i.e. inguinal hernia, hydrocele, testicular torsion, hypospadias, and diseases affecting the hips, pelvis or anorectum).

The usual contraindications to caudal block are:
- Infection or skin lesion at site of puncture
- Coagulation disorders
- Platelet count <50,000/mm^3
- Inflammatory or infectious lesion of the CNS
- Sacral malformations (myelomeningocele)
- Uncontrolled seizures
- Uncontrolled hypovolemia.

The positioning of the child is very important for correctly performance of a caudal block. As for other epidural approaches, the anesthetized child should be positioned on his/her side with legs and knees flexed 90°. At birth, the sacral hiatus, determined by lack of fusion of the posterior arches of the fifth and fourth sacral vertebrae, is present and tends to close around 7–8 years of age. The landmark is the tip of an upside down equilateral triangle where the upper angles are the posterior iliac spines (Fig. 10.4).

Several tools can be used for pediatric caudal block aesthesia, but in practice it can be safely performed only with a small number of instruments. The needle should always have a stylet because the risk of transporting epithelial cells into the subarachnoid space is well documented, although rare, with the possibility of seeding the space itself and favoring the growth of an epidermoid tumor [32]. The needle should not be too thin (lack of blood or CSF reflux), nor too long (the dural sac is very close). A good choice is a 22 or 25 G metallic needle with a stylet and short bevel (B. Braun), specifically designed for caudal use.

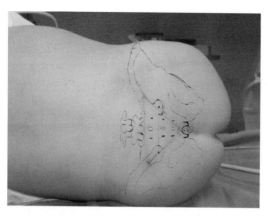

Fig. 10.4 Landmarks for caudal block

The technique described and commonly used by the author is as follows. After having applied the usual sterile conditions (clots, gloves and disinfectants) due to the vicinity of the anus and after having identified the sacral hiatus, the needle, on the midline, is inserted at 60° to the sacral plane (Fig. 10.5). After crossing the ligament (a characteristic LOR is felt when passing the sacrococcygeal membrane), the needle with the bevel facing anteriorly is lowered 20° cephalad and advanced 2–3 mm forward to introduce the bevel completely into the sacral canal. Whatever the technique used, safety rules must be observed after reaching the space. An aspiration test should be repeated often during anesthetic administrations to check for possible presence of CSF or blood. Furthermore, the presence of eventual subcutaneous pomphi due to incorrect needle placement should also be checked.

For the calculation for the solution volume, Armitage's plan can be used in its modified form as it is simple, safe and easy to remember. The maximum recommended volume is 1 ml/kg with a maximum volume of 20 ml. Examples of procedures for which caudal block is appropriate and the doses of anesthetic used are shown in Table 10.6.

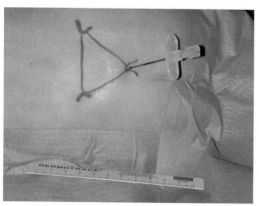

Fig. 10.5 Landmarks and needle position for caudal block

Table 10.6 Examples of procedures for which caudal block is appropriate and the doses of anesthetic used

Anesthetic level	Dosage (ml/kg)	Example
Sacral or lower lumbar (L4–L5)	0.5	Phimosis, hypospadias, perianal fistula
Lower thorax (T9–10) and lumbar	1	Inguinal hernia, cryptorchidism, lower limb surgery

The following anesthetic solutions are used:

- Children less than 10 kg: ropivacaine 0.2%, bupivacaine/levobupivacaine 0.125– 0.25%
- Children more than 10 kg: ropivacaine 0.2%, bupivacaine/levobupivacaine 0.2–0.25%

It is possible to distinguish three types of complication:

1. Complications due to devices
2. Complications due to toxicity of the drug
3. Complications due to intravascular or intraosseous injection.

Other complications, fortunately rare, such as perforation of the rectum or other viscera, are mainly due to lack of experience.

Spinal Anesthesia

Owing to improvements in neonatal care, increasing numbers of premature infants are surviving and could require surgical procedures [33]. Apnea of prematurity (AOP) is a concurrent issue for pediatric anesthesiologists and is attributed to immaturity of the respiratory and CNS. Numerous authors have provided case reports and case series detailing their experiences with spinal anesthesia as an alternative to general anesthesia to avoid the risk of AOP [34]. By far the largest number of spinal anesthesia procedures are performed in infants who were born prematurely. The safety of the procedure and the high rate of success have extended the application of this anesthetic technique to a wide variety of surgical procedures, such as pyloromyotomy, gastrostomy placement, myelomeningocele repair, cardiac surgery, and genitourinary procedures. Moreover, spinal anesthesia has been successfully used in high-risk infants and for cardiac catheterization, as documented by several case reports [35–38]. Studies comparing general and spinal anesthesia are available only for inguinal herniorrhaphy. The outcomes of interest have focused on the need for prolonged mechanical ventilation, apneic and/or bradycardic episodes and length of hospital stay.

Relatively larger doses of local anesthetics are required for spinal anesthesia in infants than in adults and older children. The physiological/anatomical explanation for this is that the volume of CSF is larger in neonates than children (4 versus 2 ml/kg) and the spinal cord and nerve roots have a relatively greater diameter in neonates. Moreover, there is a proportionally greater blood flow to the infant's spinal cord, leading to faster drug uptake from the subarachnoid space [39].

Lumbar puncture can be safely performed at the L4–L5 or L5–S1 interspaces. The conus medularis terminates at the L3 level in neonates (Table 10.1). Cutting-point needles (e.g. 22 or 25 G Quincke) are the ones most frequently used by pediatric specialists. For neonates, a spinal needle length of 25 mm is sufficient.

Spinal anesthesia in neonates has been associated with minimal respiratory and hemodynamic changes [40, 41]. Dohi et al. [42] studied hemodynamic stability during spinal anesthesia in young children and premature infants and found little or no change in blood pressure or heart rate in response to sympathectomy. It was postulated that the lack of hemodynamic changes was due to the immaturity of the sympathetic nervous system in young children. The relatively smaller blood volume of the lower extremities compared with those of adults may account for the lesser degree of lower extremity venous pooling during sympathectomy and thus fewer cardiovascular changes [40]. As in adults, certain associated conditions remain contraindications to spinal anesthesia, including patient or parent refusal, uncorrected hypovolemia, infection at the insertion site, untreated systemic sepsis, and increased intracranial pressure [43]. Spinal anesthesia is characterized by a high success rate of more than 80% [44].

Bupivacaine is a widely used local anesthetic for neonates and has been used for spinal anesthesia in neonates in some clinical trials [45]. The use of hyperbaric bupivacaine is suggested by the study of Kokki et al. [46]. They reported a greater success rate of the block when they used bupivacaine in 8% glucose than with isobaric bupivacaine in 0.9% saline. Frawley et al. [47] suggest an administration dose of 0.8 mg/kg of levobupivacaine. Ropivacaine and levobupivacaine have recently been introduced, but their safety in spinal anesthesia has still not been fully confirmed. Doses ranging between 0.75 and 1.25 mg/kg of isobaric solution of levobupivacaine are suggested by the same dose range-finding study [47].

Investigators have used tetracaine 0.5% in dextrose 5% (0.4–1 mg/kg), bupivacaine 0.5% (0.6–1 mg/kg), and bupivacaine 0.75% in dextrose 8.25% (0.6–1 mg/kg) for infants with a body weight of less than 5 kg. These dosing regimens will provide approximately 60–80 min of operating time. Return of hip flexion is observed within 2 h. The addition of adrenaline (epinephrine; 20–50 mg) to tetracaine solutions can prolong spinal anesthesia by approximately 20 min [33].

Even though a review by Craven et al. recently published in The Cochrane Database of Systematic Reviews [48] found no reliable evidence of the effects of spinal anesthesia compared to general anesthesia on the incidence of apnea, bradycardia, or oxygen desaturation in children born as preterm infants, we can consider spinal anesthesia a safe procedure that avoids the risk associated with general anesthesia.

A major drawback of neonatal spinal anesthesia is its short duration. The addition of clonidine has been proved to prolong bupivacaine spinal anesthesia with no immediate deleterious side effects, but clonidine has not been reported in neonatal spinal anesthesia except in the recent study by Rochette et al. [49]. This observational study evaluated the clinical acceptability of clonidine in neonatal spinal anesthesia, which was induced by injection of 0.2 ml/kg of a solution prepared with the addition of 100 µg clonidine to 20 ml 0.5% bupivacaine over 30 s, so that isobaric bupivacaine 1 mg/kg and clonidine 1 µg/kg were given. The results showed that clonidine-related complications may be acceptable with careful monitoring, and encourage a prospective, comparative study to evaluate the risk-benefit ratio of clonidine spinal anesthesia in newborns, underlining that clonidine may not affect postoperative desaturation in neonates [49].

Suggested anesthetic agents and doses for spinal anesthesia in neonates, infants and children are shown in Table 10.7, and the doses used by the author are shown in Table 10.8. It is important to add the volume of dead needle space to the total dosage; for example, 25 G spinal needle, dead space = 0.1 ml

Table 10.7 Suggested dosing regimens for spinal anesthesia in neonates, infants and children

Ref.	Age range	Agent	Dose (mg/kg)
[50]	Less than one year	Tetracaine	0.22–0.32
[35]	Less than 7 months	Tetracaine	0.5
[51]	7 weeks to 13 years	Tetracaine	0–3 months: 0.4–0.5
			3–24 months: 0.3–0.4
			>24 months: 0.2–0.3
		Bupivacaine	0–24 months: 0.3–0.4
			>24 months: 0.3
[52]	Neonate	Tetracaine	0.6
[53]	Neonate	Tetracaine	0.6
[54]	2 to 5 years	Bupivacaine	0.5
[55]	2 months to 17 years	Lidocaine	2–3
		Bupivacaine	0.3–0.4
[56]	0.5 months to 15 years	Lidocaine	1.5–2.5
[57]	Less than 6 months	Bupivacaine	0.6
[58]	1–12 months	Lidocaine	3
		Tetracaine	0.4
[59]	1 day to 12 months	Tetracaine	0.5
[60]	9 days to 12 months	Bupivacaine	0.5–0.6

Table 10.8 Doses used by the author

Weight (kg)	Bupivacaine (mg/kg)	Ropivacaine (mg/kg)	Levobupivacaine (mg/kg)
<5	0.8	1	1
5–15	0.5	0.5	0.5
16–35	0.4	0.5	0.3

Technique

The patient without preanesthesia is monitored (EKG, SpO$_2$, noninvasive blood pressure) and has an intravenous line inserted. Preterm infants or neonates under 5 kg are seated with their head resting forward and neck extended, helped by a nurse from the front (Figs. 10.6, 10.7 and 10.8). In older children, the position is more frequently lateral decubitus with hips flexed about 90° and neck partially extended.

Lumbar puncture can be safely performed at the L4–L5 or L5–S1 interspaces. The conus medularis terminates at the L3 level in neonates (Table 10.1). Cutting-point needles (e.g. 22 or 25 G Quincke) are the ones most frequently used by pediatric specialists. The use of thinner needles (29 G) is less effective in localizing the subarachnoid space, with a higher failure rate [61]. For neonates, a spinal needle length of 25 mm is sufficient. Local anesthetics should be administered slowly (20–30 s). There is a correlation between injection time and duration of anesthesia. In fact, the longer the injection the wider the diffusion of the anesthetic and the shorter the duration of anesthesia. Moreover, a rapid injection may cause a high level block due to reduced distance between segments.

Immediately after the block the patient is positioned according to the type of operation and baricity of the anesthetic. Patient positioning is very important, especially when administering hyperbaric anesthetics since this determines the block level. In fact, high-level spinal anesthesia may occur especially after maneuvers immediately following the block, such as positioning of electrocautery grounding pads. The onset of the block is immediate and the duration of spinal anesthesia is shorter in young children than in older children and adults; for this reason the surgeon must start the operation immediately.

In neonates, during spinal anesthesia, cardiovascular activity is stable and there are no arterial pressure variations. Moreover, the postdural headache is not frequent and does not require specific treatment.

Among the main contraindications already observed for other central block techniques, emphasis has to be given to the lack of experience of the anesthesiologists and collaborators.

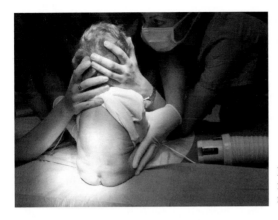

Fig. 10.6 Sitting position for performance of spinal anesthesia in a neonate

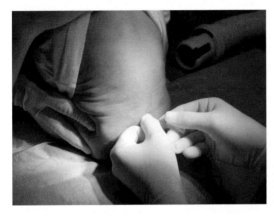

Fig. 10.7 Spinal needle is inserted in the midline between the spinous processes

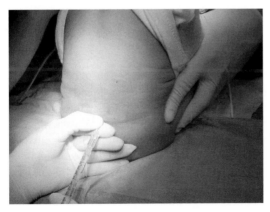

Fig. 10.8 Local anesthetic is injected slowly after free flow of CSF has confirmed the correct position

Ultrasonography and Pediatric Regional Anesthesia

The key requirement for successful regional anesthetic blocks is the distribution of local anesthetic around the nerve structures. Morgan affirmed, in a personal communication, that regional anesthesia always works if the anesthesiologist "put the right dose of the right drug in the right place".

The LOR technique is usually used to check needle-tip penetration into the epidural space, and catheter insertion is traditionally achieved blind. US can be used to identify neuraxial structures during insertion and placement of epidural catheters and to identify peripheral nerves. Moreover, US can be particularly useful for teaching trainees who are inexperienced in anesthesia. During the performance of caudal block the ultrasound probe can be positioned cephalad to the injection site in the transverse plane, approximately at the tip of the needle. Dilatation of the caudal space and localized turbulence are noted on the US monitor when placement is successful. Roberts et al. [16] studied 60 caudal blocks in children monitored by US and concluded that US is a reliable indicator of correct performance of caudal block. They found that US was safe, quick to perform, and useful insofar as it provided additional information on anatomy.

Similarly, US guidance of peripheral nerve blocks of both the upper and the lower extremities reduces the number of complications and improves the quality of the blocks. Willschke et al. [6] demonstrated that US-guided ilioinguinal/iliohypogastric nerve blocks can be achieved with significantly smaller volumes of local anesthetic and that the intra- and postoperative requirements for additional analgesia are significantly lower than with conventional methods.

In summary, direct visualization of the distribution of local anesthetics with the aid of US can improve the quality of the block and avoid the complications of upper/lower extremity nerve blocks and neuraxial techniques in real time. Thus nerve stimulation and LOR procedures are significant, particularly in children [62]. Considering their enormous potential, these techniques should have a role in the future training of anesthesiologists.

Conclusion

Although considerable progress has been made in studying the safety, efficacy, dose–response relationships, and clinical outcomes associated with the use of analgesics and anesthetics in neonates, there are still major gaps in our knowledge that hinder optimal clinical practice. Multicenter clinical trials with adequate sample sizes are needed to assess the occurrence of uncommon adverse effects and examine safety concerns. Ethical constraints demand development of designs that permit immediate rescue while allowing examination of efficacy and dose–response relationships. Future studies should examine whether optimal application of multimodal analgesia, as in adults, can improve clinical outcomes in neonates undergoing major surgery.

References

1. Peters JW, Schouw R, Anand KJ et al (2005) Does neonatal surgery lead to increased pain sensitivity in later childhood? Pain 114:444–454
2. Kodric N (2003) Regional anesthesia in children. Med Arch 57:61–64
3. Busoni P, Sarti A (1987) Sacral intervertebral epidural block. Anesthesiology 67:993–995
4. Bösenberg AT, Gouws E (1995) Skin-epidural distance in children. Anaesthesia 50:895–897
5. Van Schoor AN, Boon JM, Bosenberg AT (2005) Anatomical considerations of the pediatric ilioinguinal/iliohypogastric nerve block. Paediatr Anaesth 15:371–377
6. Willschke H, Marhofer P, Bösenberg A et al (2005) Ultrasonography for ilioinguinal/iliohypogastric nerve blocks in children. Br J Anaesth 95:226–230
7. Ivani G, Mossetti V (2005) Continuous peripheral nerve blocks. Paediatr Anaesth 15:87–90
8. Gunter JB (2002) Benefit and risks of local anesthetics in infants and children. Pediatr Drugs 4:649–672
9. Dadure C, Capdevila X (2005) Continuous peripheral nerve blocks in children. Best Pract Res Clin Anaesthesiol 19:309–321
10. Ecoffey C (2007) Pediatric regional anesthesia – update. Curr Opin Anaesthesiol 20:232–235
11. Sciard D, Matuszczak M, Gebhard R (2001) Continuous posterior lumbar plexus block for acute postoperative pain control in infants. Anesthesiology 95:1521–1523
12. Ivani G, Conio A, De Negri P et al (2002) Spinal versus peripheral effects of adjunct clonidine: comparison of the analgesic effect of a ropivacaine-clonidine mixture when administered as a caudal or ilioinguinal-iliohypogastric nerve blockage for inguinal surgery in children. Paediatr Anaesth 12:680–684
13. Kaabachi O, Zerelli Z, Methamem M (2005) Clonidine administered as adjuvant for bupivacaine in ilioinguinal-iliohypogastric nerve block does not prolong postoperative analgesia. Paediatr Anaesth 15:586–590
14. Ivani G, Mossetti V (2008) Regional anesthesia for postoperative pain control in children: focus on continuous central and perineural infusions. Paediatr Drugs 10:107–114
15. Chawathe MS, Jones RM, Gildersleve CD et al (2003) Detection of epidural catheters with ultrasound in children. Paediatr Anaesth 13:681–684
16. Roberts SA, Guruswamy V, Galvez I (2005) Caudal injectate can be reliably imaged using portable ultrasound – a preliminary study. Paediatr Anaesth 15:948–952
17. Lloyd-Thomas AR (1999) Modern concepts of paediatric analgesia. Pharmacol Ther 83:1–20
18. Larsson BA, Lonnqvist PA, Olsson GL (1997) Plasma concentrations of bupivacaine in neonates after continuous epidural infusion. Anesth Analg 84:501–505
19. Bösenberg A (1998) Epidural analgesia for major neonatal surgery. Paediatr Anaesth 8:479–483
20. McClellan KJ, Faulds D (2000) Ropivacaine: an update of its use in regional anaesthesia. Drugs 60:1065–1093
21. Rapp HJ, Molnar V, Austin S et al (2004) Ropivacaine in neonates and infants – a population pharmacokinetic evaluation following single caudal block. Paediatr Anaesth 14:724–732
22. Bösenberg AT, Thomas J, Cronje L et al (2005) Pharmacokinetics and efficacy of ropivacaine for continuous epidural infusion in neonates and infants. Paediatr Anaesth 15:739–749
23. Chalkiadis GA, Anderson BJ, Tay M et al (2005) Pharmacokinetics of levobupivacaine after caudal epidural administration in infants less than 3 month of age. Br J Anaesth 95:524–529
24. Ooi R, Pattison J, Feldman SA (1991) The effects of intravenous clonidine on ventilation. Anaesthesia 46:632–633
25. O'Halloran KD, Herman JK, Bisgard GE (2000) Ventilatory effects of alpha2-adrenoceptor blockade in awake goats. Respir Physiol 126:29–41
26. Fellmann C, Gerber AC, Weiss M (2002) Apnoea in a former preterm infant after caudal bupivacaine with clonidine for inguinal herniorrhaphy. Paediatr Anaesth 12:637–640

27. De Negri P, Ivani G, Visconti C, De Vivo P (2001) How to prolong postoperative analgesia after caudal anaesthesia with ropivacaine in children: S-ketamine versus clonidine. Paediatr Anaesth 11:679–683

28. Hager H, Marhofer P, Sitzwohl C et al (2002) Caudal clonidine prolongs analgesia from caudal S(+)-ketamine in children. Anesth Analg 94:1169–1172

29. Bösenberg A (2004) Pediatric regional anesthesia update. Paediatr Anaesth 14:398–402

30. Scott DB (1997) Identification of the epidural space: loss of resistance to air or saline? Reg Anesth 22(1):1–2

31. Broadman L, Ivani G (1999) Caudal block. Techn Reg Anaesth Pain Manage 3:150–156

32. Broadman LM (1997) Where should advocacy for pediatric patients end and concerns for patient safety begin? Reg Anesth 22:205–208

33. Lederhaas G (2003) Spinal anaesthesia in paediatrics. Best Pract Res Clin Anaesthesiol 17:365–376

34. Nickel US, Meyer RR, Brambrink AM (2005) Spinal anesthesia in an extremely low birth weight infant. Paediatr Anaesth 15:58–62

35. Sartorelli KH, Abajian JC, Kreutz JM et al (1992) Improved outcome utilizing spinal anesthesia in high-risk infants. J Pediatr Surg 27:1022–1025

36. Astuto M, Sapienza D, Di Benedetto V, Disma N (2007) Spinal anesthesia for inguinal hernia repair in an infant with Williams syndrome: case report. Paediatr Anaesth 17:193–195

37. Puncuh F, Lampugnani E, Kokki H (2004) Use of spinal anaesthesia in paediatric patients: a single centre experience with 1132 cases. Paediatr Anaesth 14:564–567

38. Katznelson R, Mishaly D, Hegesh T et al (2005) Spinal anesthesia for diagnostic cardiac catheterization in high-risk infants. Paediatr Anaesth 15:50–53

39. Saint-Maurice C (1995) Spinal anesthesia. In: Dalens B (ed) Regional anesthesia in infants, children and adolescents, 1st edn. Williams and Wilkins, Baltimore, pp 261–273

40. Finkel JC, Boltz MG, Conran AM (2003) Haemodynamic changes during high spinal anaesthesia in children having open heart surgery. Paediatr Anaesth 13:48–52

41. Oberlander TF, Berde CB, Lam KH et al (1995) Infants tolerate spinal anesthesia with minimal overall autonomic changes: analysis of heart rate variability in former premature infants undergoing hernia repair. Anesth Analg 80:20–27

42. Dohi S, Naito H, Takahashi T (1979) Age-related changes in blood pressure and duration of motor block in spinal anaesthesia. Anesthesiology 50:319–323

43. Tobias JD (2000) Spinal anaesthesia in infants and children. Paediatr Anaesth 10:5–16

44. Shenkman Z, Hoppenstein D, Litmanowitz I et al (2002) Spinal anesthesia in 62 premature, former-premature or young infants – technical aspects and pitfalls. Can J Anaesth 49:262–269

45. Mahe V, Ecoffey C (1988) Spinal anesthesia with isobaric bupivacaine in infants. Anesthesiology 68:601–603

46. Kokki H, Touvinen K, Hendolin H (1998) Spinal anaesthesia for paediatric day-case surgery: a double-blind, randomized, parallel group, prospective comparison of isobaric and hyperbaric bupivacaine. Br J Anaesth 81:502–506

47. Frawley G, Farrell T, Smith S (2004) Levobupivacaine spinal anesthesia in neonates: a dose range finding study. Paediatr Anaesth 14:838–844

48. Craven PD, Badawi N, Henderson-Smart DJ et al (2003) Regional (spinal, epidural, caudal) versus general anaesthesia in preterm infants undergoing inguinal herniorrhaphy in early infancy. The Cochrane Database of Systematic Reviews, Issue 3, Art. No. CD003669

49. Rochette A, Troncin R, Raux O (2005) Clonidine added to bupivacaine in neonatal spinal anesthesia: a prospective comparison in 124 preterm and term infants. Paediatr Anaesth 15:1072–1077

50. Abajian JC, Mellish RW, Browne AF et al (1984) Spinal anesthesia for surgery in the high-risk infant. Anesth Analg 63:359–362

51. Blaise GA, Roy WL (1986) Spinal anaesthesia for minor paediatric surgery. Can Anaesth Soc J 33:227–230

52. Tobias JD, Flannagan J, Brock J et al (1993) Neonatal regional anesthesia: alternative to

general anesthesia for urologic surgery. Urology 41:362–365

53. Tobias JD, Flannagan J (1992) Regional anesthesia in the preterm neonate. Clin Pediatr 31:668–671

54. Kokki H, Hendolin H, Vainio J et al (1992) Operationen im vorschulalter: vergleich von spinalanasthesie und allgemeinanasthesie. Anaesthetist 41:765–768

55. Kokki H, Hendolin H (1995) Comparison of spinal anaesthesia with epidural anaesthesia in paediatric surgery. Acta Anaesthesiol Scand 39:896–900

56. Melman E, Penuelas J, Marrufo J (1975) Regional anesthesia in children. Anesth Analg 54:387–390

57. Parkinson SK, Little WL, Malley RA et al (1990) Use of hyperbaric bupivacaine with epinephrine for spinal anesthesia in infants. Reg Anesth 15:86–88

58. Rice LJ, DeMars PD, Whalen TV et al (1994) Duration of spinal anesthesia in infants less than one year of age. Reg Anesth 19:325–329

59. Aronsson DD, Gemery JM, Abajian JC (1996) Spinal anesthesia for spine and lower extremity surgery in infants. J Pediatr Orthop 16:259–263

60. Tobias JD, Mencio GA (1998) Regional anesthesia for clubfoot repair in children. Am J Ther 5:273–277

61. Kokki H, Hedolin H (1996) comparison of 25G and 29G Quincke spinal needle in paediatric day case surgery. A prospective randomized study of the puncture characteristics, success rate and postoperative complaints. Paediatr Anaesth 6:115–119

62. Marhofer P, Greher M, Kapral S (2005) Ultrasound guidance in regional anaesthesia. Br J Anaesth 94:7–17

Chapter 11
Perioperative Fluid Management

Davinia E. Withington

Introduction

Correct management of perioperative fluids can make the difference between good and bad outcomes in pediatric anesthesia. Effective correction of preoperative fluid deficits, including those due to hemorrhage or vomiting, combined with careful maintenance and replacement of ongoing losses, will ensure that a stable child arrives in the recovery room or pediatric intensive care unit (PICU).

Fluid management must be based on sound physiological principles. These are discussed in detail elsewhere in this volume and are briefly summarized as follows [1]:

- The fetus is 93–80% water, decreasing as term approaches.
- Total body water decreases from 80% body weight at birth approximating adult values (about 60%) at around 12 years of age.
- Antenatally and until 4 months of age extracellular fluid volume > intracellular fluid volume.
- In the neonate body weight is 45% extracellular fluid volume and 35% intracellular fluid volume.
- Sodium is the principal extracellular cation, and potassium the principal intracellular cation.
- Fluid and electrolyte homeostasis are controlled by the renin-angiotensin-aldosterone axis, atrial natriuretic peptide, ADH.
- Glomeruli are formed by 34–35 weeks' gestation; tubules are immature at term.
- The neonatal kidney may only concentrate to 500–600 mosmol/l in the first week.

Perioperative fluids can be divided into:
1. Deficit replacement
   - Preoperative fasting
   - Acute losses
2. Replacement of ongoing losses
3. Maintenance.

The two latter fluid calculations should be continued into the postoperative period.

M. Astuto (ed), *Basics*, Anesthesia, Intensive Care and Pain in Neonates and Children.
ISBN 978-88-470-0654-6 © Springer-Verlag Italia 2009

Deficit Replacement

Preoperative Fasting

Policies have become more liberal in the last two decades. It has been recognized that a child distressed by starvation and thirst is less likely to have a smooth induction of anesthesia and can also become seriously dehydrated when fasting times are unduly prolonged. Infants less than 6 months of age are at particular risk of dehydration if fasting is prolonged. This can lead to difficulties achieving intravenous access at induction and may predispose to hemodynamic instability.

According to the current recommendations of the Canadian Anesthesiologists Society (CAS), before elective procedures, the minimum duration of fasting should be:

- 8 hours after a meal that includes meat, fried or fatty foods
- 6 hours after a light meal (such as toast and a clear fluid), or after ingestion of infant formula or nonhuman milk
- 4 hours after ingestion of breast milk
- 2 hours after ingestion of clear fluids.

The Association of Pediatric Anaesthetists of Great Britain and Ireland has recently published a new guideline [2] addressing perioperative fluid management. This is a consensus document and although their recommendations are the same as those of the CAS it was noted that consensus was not obtained on the safe starvation time for infants given breast milk or formula. The time deemed by the participating experts to be safe between a breast milk feed and anesthesia was from 3 to 4 hours or from 4 to 6 hours for formula. Some participants felt that a 4-hour fast after breast milk should only be applied to infants less than 6 months of age.

These guidelines should be modified by certain conditions. Any situation which will predispose to delayed gastric emptying such as gastrointestinal disease, intracranial pathology or administration of drugs, such as opiates, which decrease gastrointestinal motility, should lead to a more prolonged fast or to the use of rapid sequence induction with intubation for airway protection.

In the elective patient it is as important to emphasize to parents that fasting should not be prolonged beyond the recommended times as it is to ensure that the guidelines are understood and adhered to [3]. Replacement of deficits incurred by preoperative fasting can be calculated by multiplying the hourly maintenance rate (Table 10.1) by the number of hours since the last oral intake:

Table 10.1 Maintenance fluid requirements of children

Weight (kg)	Hourly
<10	4 ml/kg
10–20	40 ml + 2 ml/kg for every kilogram >10 kg
>20	60 ml + 1 ml/kg for every kilogram >20 kg

for example, a 5-kg infant fasted for 3 hours has a calculated deficit of 4 ml/kg x 5 kg x 3 h = 60 ml. This can be replaced over 2–3 hours along with the intra-operative maintenance fluid.

Replacement of Acute Losses

Children may arrive in the operating room in shock or compensated shock from hemorrhage or dehydration. These deficits need to be assessed and corrected appropriately and promptly. Paediatric Advanced Life Support guidelines [4] are useful for assessment of such children and to guide therapy. Physiological differences between infants/children and adults are again extremely important. Infants maintain cardiac output by increasing heart rate and may present with a normal blood pressure until relatively late in their progression to uncompensated shock. Thus a significant tachycardia with other signs of decreased perfusion and a cause of fluid loss should be treated aggressively, even with a normal blood pressure.

Blood Loss

Blood volume, like total body water, varies with age. Preterm babies have a blood volume at delivery of 90–100 ml/kg, term babies of 80–90 ml/kg. At 3 months this will have fallen to 70–80 ml/kg and to 70 ml/kg at 1 year of age. Hemoglobin concentration also changes with age, falling to a nadir of 9–11 g/dl at 8–12 weeks in the term infant but lower and earlier in the premature infant. A knowledge of these changes is essential to make informed decisions about transfusion in the acute situation.

Using this information an acceptable maximum blood loss can be calculated preoperatively along with the correct blood volume to be transfused to correct the hematocrit (Hct) to a desired level. The maximum blood loss can be calculated as:

EBV x (patient Hct x lowest acceptable Hct)/patient Hct

and replacement volume as:

EBV x (desired Hct x current Hct)/Hct of blood product

where EBV is the estimated blood volume.

The decision to transfuse must not rest on absolute values of Hct alone but also on the likelihood of ongoing blood losses and on hemodynamic parameters. Transfusion at a higher Hct than that initially chosen as a threshold would be triggered by physiological perturbations which are not normalized by rapid infusion of crystalloid or colloid. These include a combination of elevated heart rate, lower blood pressure and central venous pressure or changes in ST segments on the electrocardiogram or low mixed venous oxygen concentration. An acceptable Hct would also be higher, triggering earlier transfusion, in patients with cyanotic heart disease and in others with a high baseline Hct or with significant oxygen need.

In general blood loss should be replaced with blood and blood products. However, losses of less than 30% blood volume can usually be safely replaced with plasma expanders, either albumin, substituted starches or dextrans. The discussion of strategies to minimize intraoperative blood loss and allogenic blood transfusion such as preoperative autologous blood donation, acute normovolemic hemodilution, cell salvage, antifibrinolytic agents and recombinant activated factor VII are beyond the scope of this chapter, but are well reviewed elsewhere [5].

Directed blood donation has been advocated as a method of decreasing the patient's exposure to donor blood. However, despite the popularity of this technique with many parents, studies have failed to show a reduction in adverse events, including infection rates. A retrospective study from 2001 at a tertiary care pediatric hospital in Canada found that refusal of units due to detection of infectious disease markers, malaria and high-risk activities was at least tenfold higher for units from directed donors than from volunteer donors [6]. There was no evidence of improved safety and blood wastage was significantly greater than with volunteer donation (63.6% vs. 7%). Indeed although there continues to be public concern about the risk of transmission through blood transfusion of human immunodeficiency virus and hepatitis C, this risk was estimated to be 1 in 752,000 and 1 in 225,000 donations, respectively, in a study of the Canadian blood supply between 1987 and 1996 [7].

The decision of when to transfuse in the non-acute setting has been based on set hemoglobin concentrations. Surveys of pediatric intensive care practice, however, have demonstrated a wide range of values used in clinical practice [8]. In order to rationalize this situation the TRIPICU study with the Canadian Critical Care Trials Group enrolled 637 stable critically ill children and randomized them to two different thresholds for blood transfusion [9]. The primary outcome of multiple organ dysfunction was no difference between groups transfused when their hemoglobin fell below 7 g/dl compared to those transfused at a threshold of 9.5 g/dl. Use of these data will decrease the utilization of blood and minimize the exposure of children to allogenic blood transfusions. However, management in the intensive care situation must always be individualized taking into account situations mentioned above such as the cyanotic infant after cardiac surgery in whom a higher threshold is required to ensure adequate oxygen carriage.

Research on alternatives to blood transfusion continues. These artificial oxygen carriers are either hemoglobin-based oxygen carriers (HBOC) or perfluorocarbon emulsions. Neither group has been approved for use in Europe or North America although hemoglobin glutamer 250 (HBOC-201) and a perfluorocarbon product have been approved in South Africa [10]. Concerns relate to side effects caused by extravasation of HBOCs into peripheral tissues, particularly pulmonary and systemic vasoconstriction, and also the adverse effects of perfluorocarbons on neurological outcomes. The value of these alternatives to blood would be in situations of blood shortage and for management of patients refusing blood transfusions, especially Jehovah's Witnesses.

Albumin 5% is a commonly used fluid for volume expansion in children, although a 1998 Cochrane review [11] found that its use in critically ill adults was associated with an increased mortality rate. This systematic review was heavily criticized for its methodology [12] and for lack of pediatric evidence [13]. Of the four pediatric studies analyzed three were of premature infants or neonates and only one dealt with the use of albumin as a resuscitation fluid for hypovolemia. It provoked a huge media reaction and much heated correspondence. Since its publication the SAFE trial from New Zealand and Australia compared albumin with normal saline in over 6,000 adults and demonstrated that albumin can be safely used for volume resuscitation in the critically ill [14]. A recent update by the Cochrane Collaboration [15] has taken these data into account and revised its recommendations. Trials in children are still lacking. However, a recent publication from the Dutch Pediatric Society, examining the latest Cochrane review from the pediatric perspective, recommends that in neonates and children with hypovolemia the first-choice fluid for resuscitation should be isotonic saline [16].

Albumin is a human-derived product and although it now carries an extremely small risk of infection, another problem is limitation of supply. Alternatives are dextrans and hydroxyethyl starches (HES). Newer HES, such as the latest third-generation low molecular weight (130 kDa) small degree of substitution (0.4) product seem to offer greater flexibility in volume resuscitation with a significantly lower risk of interference with platelet function than older products [17]. This allows greater volumes to be infused, eliminating the limitation to 20 ml/kg prescribed for the older HES products. Pediatric studies are, however, unavailable. There are recent animal studies suggesting an antiinflammatory role for HES although the benefits and uses of this effect remain to be elucidated in humans [18].

Finally, in considering the need for transfusion, the requirements for other blood products must be evaluated. Massive blood transfusion will dilute coagulation factors unless fresh whole blood (<48 hours old) is provided. In the majority of hospitals most blood is transfused in the form of packed red cells and so plasma should be provided if more than one and a half times blood volume has been transfused or if the prothrombin time or partial thromboplastin time is prolonged by more than one and a half times normal. Frozen plasma (15–20 ml/kg) will be indicated earlier in situations where there is a known disturbance of coagulation such as hepatic insufficiency. Cryoprecipitate 0.5 U/kg is indicated where there is known factor VIII or fibrinogen deficiency. Fresh whole blood will also improve platelet preservation. Platelets should be administered if the level falls below $50 \times 10^9/l$ or below $100 \times 10^9/l$ if there is ongoing bleeding.

Infusion of 1 U per 5 kg will raise the platelet count effectively. In the special situation of cardiopulmonary bypass, platelets are often used automatically when the cardiopulmonary bypass time is long (more than 2 hours) or there are multiple suture lines.

Crystalloid Deficits

The replacement fluid should approximate the composition of the fluid lost as closely as is feasible. Vomiting leads to a hypochloremic metabolic alkalosis, the hallmark of pyloric stenosis, one of the commonest acute surgical problems in the first three months of life. Resuscitation with normal saline or Ringer's lactate will correct this situation. Acid–base status should be normalized before surgery. Conversely, persistent diarrhea will lead to loss of bicarbonate and, if prolonged, metabolic acidosis may develop requiring the addition of bicarbonate for correction.

The assessment of fluid deficits cannot be based on measured losses alone as these are very inaccurate. Hemodynamic status must be evaluated including heart rate, capillary refill, urine output and, if available, central venous pressure. Infants and children maintain their cardiac output by increasing heart rate and therefore blood pressure alone is a poor index of hemodynamic status although diastolic pressure can be helpful in states of vasodilated preshock.

Acute infections, including diarrhea, illnesses, are a major cause of illness and death in children worldwide. In Africa, 50% of in-hospital deaths of children occur within 24 hours of admission, and shock complicates many cases. The WHO [19] guidelines for fluid replacement in this setting have come under recent scrutiny. The use of hypotonic solutions (e.g., half-strength Darrow's solution with 5% glucose[1]), has been advocated by WHO owing to concern about sodium overload in the treatment of shock in patients with severe malnutrition. This approach may be appropriate when the primary problem is depletion of intracellular volume due to dehydration. However, hypotonic solutions should never be used for the correction of shock. The circulating volume must be restored with isotonic solutions or colloids. In children with hypernatremic dehydration (clinically identifiable by a doughy feel to the skin and by irritability), the serum sodium concentration may be alarmingly high, and sodium-rich fluids should then be avoided [20].

Replacement of Ongoing Intraoperative Losses

If during surgery significant blood losses are anticipated, fluid conservation strategies such as normovolemic hemodilution and intraoperative cell salvage

---

[1] Darrow's solution: sodium, 61 mmol; potassium, 17 mmol; chloride, 52 mmol; lactate, 27 mmol; glucose, 50 g; calories, 200 per liter

may be employed. If crystalloid is used as volume replacement, the volume infused should be at least three times the blood lost since for every 100 ml of crystalloid infused the plasma volume will be expanded by 30 ml only because of distribution between intracellular and extracellular spaces. The same considerations apply to the use of blood, blood products and plasma expanders as to the replacement of acute losses. However, if large volumes of citrate-phosphate-dextrose stored blood are to be transfused, calcium may be needed to prevent or correct hypocalcemia caused by the chelation of calcium with citrate. Citrate metabolism is primarily hepatic, so hepatic disease or dysfunction can cause this effect to be more pronounced. If more than a blood volume is transfused per hour, it is likely that intravenous calcium supplementation will be required to counteract citrate toxicity.

Other acute complications of large-volume transfusion include hypothermia due to inadequate warming of refrigerated blood, hyperkalemia from blood stored for more than 7 days (especially if irradiated), acid–base disturbances and dilution of coagulation factors and platelets.

Increased fluid losses may be anticipated during abdominal surgery due to "third spacing" into the intestinal lumen and interstitial space and to increased transudate from exposed intestinal surfaces. Greater losses can also be predicted if the patient is febrile: a 12% increase in fluid requirement has been measured per degree Celsius above 38°C [21]. Berry suggests an increased infusion rate for thoracic and abdominal surgery: 4 ml/kg/h for "simple" surgery without significant tissue damage, 4–6 ml/kg/h for thoracic or neurosurgical procedures, and 8–10 ml/kg/h for abdominal surgery [22].

Maintenance

Parenteral fluid therapy was first reported in the cholera epidemic of 1830–1831 and in 1879 Claude Bernard described the concept of the "milieu internale": the maintenance of body fluid homeostasis. However, parenteral fluid therapy did not become commonplace until the twentieth century. Maintenance fluids should be considered in terms of volume and type of fluid. During surgery, maintenance fluids are frequently provided as Ringer's lactate or Hartmann's solution with glucose-containing solutions added in specific circumstances, such as for premature infants or newborns, or during prolonged surgery. Postoperatively these are frequently replaced with hypotonic solutions.

Standard recommendations have been based on work carried out in the 1950s, including that by Holliday and Segar [23], on which their well-known formula was based. Berry modified this to include ongoing intraoperative losses; however, the Holliday and Segar formula is one of the commonest in use worldwide and therefore requires careful consideration (Table 10.1). Despite half a century of use the discussion of maintenance fluids is currently one of the most contentious areas in perioperative management, complicated for the physician, and potentially perilous for the patient.

Water

Basal metabolic rate (BMR) in children was originally derived by Talbot [24] based on water loss. The concept was extended by Crawford et al. [25] who evaluated BMR plus energy for growth and activity, and related this to body surface area. Holliday and Segar indexed energy expenditure to body weight, an immediately available parameter. The derivation of Holliday and Segar's formula is from studies of resting energy expenditure in hospitalized, breast-fed infants and of children of different weights and levels of activity, and measurement of electrolyte content of breast and cows' milk. They concluded that the energy expenditure of children on bed rest was mid-way between total energy expenditure of healthy active children and BMR. This produced the result of 1 ml water per 1 calorie of energy, giving an energy requirement of 120 kcal/kg/day for a 10-kg child [23].

There are several problems with this approach. Firstly, metabolic rate changes with state of health. In acute illness or in the perioperative period energy expenditure measured by calorimetry will be close to the BMR calculated by Talbot as 50–60 kcal/kg/day [24, 26–28]. This is due to the combined effects of catabolism, immobility and medication producing sedation and muscle relaxation. Anesthetic agents depress metabolism [29]. The allowance of almost 50% of the proposed caloric intake for growth further overestimates requirements since this is an unreasonable goal in the acutely ill child.

Lindahl [30] evaluated energy expenditure, fluid and electrolyte requirements in ASA 1 children undergoing halothane anesthesia for minor surgery, and found an energy expenditure of 50% below previously obtained values. However, due to an unexplained finding of a higher water requirement per calorie (1.66 ml/kcal), he derived a formula for fluid requirements (2.4 x weight in kilograms + 10 = milliliters per hour) with correlation coefficient (r) of 0.96, which is very close to that of Holliday and Segar.

A second problem is that it has been demonstrated [31] that resting energy expenditure is closely linked to fat-free mass rather than total body weight. Fat-free mass is largely accounted for by muscle, heart, liver, kidneys and brain, the main sites of metabolic activity. However, these organs account for only 7% of total body weight, which will lead to a serious overestimate of caloric requirements. Comparing Holliday and Segar's weight-based calculations with those of Crawford et al., the latter surface area method gives values, on average, 14% lower in infants.

A further issue is water requirements. These take into account insensible and measurable losses. Heeley and Talbot [32] in 1955 estimated 930 ml/m^2/day (27 ml/kg/day) for losses from skin and respiratory tract. More recent work has provided significantly lower values: 250 ml/m^2/day (7 ml/kg/day) from skin and 170 ml/m^2 per day (5 ml/kg/day) from the respiratory tract [33]. In the perioperative period or in intensive care, other factors including a thermoneutral environment and the use of humidifiers on ventilators will further reduce these losses. Indeed in catabolic patients in acute renal failure, insensible water losses of 10 ml/kg/day have been demonstrated [34], along with an increased production of water of oxidation: 15 ml/100 kcal expended.

The formula of Holliday and Segar incorporated urinary losses: 50–60 ml/kg based on measurements in 28 infants and 25 children given intravenous dextrose solutions [35]. However, in acute illness antidiuretic hormone (ADH) will have a major effect on urine output, resulting in the production of a low volume of concentrated urine. Output may be less than half that measured in healthy children. Stress, pain, nausea and drugs including morphine, barbiturates and nonsteroidal antiinflammatory agents are among the nonhemodynamic stimuli to ADH release. Pulmonary and cerebral pathology are also potent stimuli, and all may result in the syndrome of inappropriate ADH secretion, so called because the hormone is not released in response to hypovolemia or other hemodynamic stimuli. Thus, there are many factors in the perioperative period or during critical illness that may lead to ADH secretion and consequent water retention.

It is therefore clear that due to the wide variability in factors influencing water requirement in the acutely ill child (resting energy expenditure 60 vs. 120 kcal/kg/day, insensible losses 12 vs. 27 ml/kg/day, urinary losses 25 vs. 50 ml/kg/day), the original calculations may seriously overestimate the child's actual water requirements.

Sodium

Another issue is the type of fluid to be infused. The recommendation by Holliday and Segar of hypotonic solutions such as 4% dextrose with 0.2% or 0.18% saline is also determined by calculations in healthy infants. Thus the guideline that 1–3 mmol/kg/day of sodium and potassium are required per 100 kcal expended is somewhat arbitrary, but reflects the electrolyte composition of human breast milk and cows' milk. It is also based on the premise that sodium intake should balance loss. Holliday and Segar [23] derived a sodium requirement of 30 mmol/kg/h for the 10-kg child, whereas Lindahl [30] found a requirement of 15 mmol/kg/h. The same discrepancy was found for potassium requirements.

Most concerns about sodium intake relate to the neonate. The ability of the neonatal kidney to dilute and concentrate urine and to excrete a sodium load is not fully developed. With the inability to excrete a sodium load the neonate is at increased risk of becoming over-hydrated and hypernatremic. However, the kidney's vascular resistance decreases and renal blood flow increases shortly after birth, with a capacity to both concentrate the urine and excrete a water load being well developed by 4–5 days of life. Furthermore, recent work has demonstrated benefits to neurodevelopment of doubling usual sodium intake in the premature newborn, without evidence of hypernatremia. While commenting on the demonstrated risk of cerebral palsy in very low birthweight infants with hyponatremia [36]. The new APAGBI guidelines [2] note that term (>36 weeks gestational age) infants normally lose 10–15% of their body weight in the first few days of life and recommend a reduction in the first 48 hours to 2–3 ml/kg/h or 40–80 ml/kg/day given as 10% dextrose, with no consensus on type or volume of fluid from day 3 of life. Neonatologists continue to favor 0.18% saline in 10% dextrose at 4 ml/kg/h. However, it is a universal truth that infusion of hypotonic fluids to infants or children *in the presence of ADH secretion* will produce hyponatremia.

Glucose

Dextrose is included in maintenance solutions to provide at least the minimal amount of energy to avoid catabolism: 3 g/kg glucose per day. This is provided by 4% dextrose if given in the volumes calculated to provide adequate water intake. A major concern has been the potential development of intraoperative hypoglycemia, which may remain undiagnosed in the anesthetized infant and lead to devastating neurological consequences. In newborns the formula 4–6 mg/kg/min may be used to calculate glucose needs.

In certain settings it may be preferable to use glucose-free solutions because of the potential for ischemia and the dangers of hyperglycemia in this setting, e.g. cardiac and neurosurgery. Even outside these specialized situations hyperglycemia may be detrimental to outcome by production of osmotic diuresis affecting fluid balance and, at least theoretically, can interfere with wound healing and increase risk of infection. Other patient groups are at increased risk of hypoglycemia and should routinely be given glucose-containing solutions, albeit with careful monitoring of plasma glucose. These include infants and children receiving total parenteral nutrition, premature babies, and those undergoing prolonged surgery especially under regional anesthesia which will blunt the stress response. Regular measurement of glucose during surgery will prevent prolonged hypoglycemia and avoid hyperglycemia.

The incidence of unexpected hypoglycemia in fasting children varies enormously between reports: 0.5–28% [37]. However, the lower figure is probably more representative of current practice employing reduced fasting periods. Indeed Welborn et al. have shown that 10 ml/kg of apple juice given 2 hours before induction abolishes the risk of hypoglycemia in children 1–10 years old [38]. Reviewing four studies using lactated Ringer's solution with or without 1% dextrose Dubois et al. [37] found that all children who received solutions without dextrose had increased plasma glucose after induction and the only instances of hypoglycemia at induction were in patients who had undergone prolonged periods of fasting. These latter children all showed an increase in their plasma glucose whether or not they received dextrose. None was hyperglycemic.

The Current Debate

In the acutely ill child in the presence of ADH secretion, strict adherence to the traditional Holliday and Segar formula [23] using 4% dextrose and 0.2% saline is likely to provide inadequate sodium to maintain plasma tonicity, but excessive water, and will result in hyponatremia. Free water will distribute proportionately between intracellular and extracellular spaces (two-thirds:one-third in older children and adults) whereas isotonic solutions will expand the extracellular compartment. There is a strong inverse relationship between plasma sodium and intracellular volume because sodium controls fluid shifts across membranes. Thus the infusion of hypotonic solutions will increase intracellular volume, including in the brain, and this will be exacerbated if ADH is preventing the normal excretion of free water and acting via aquaporin 4 receptors in the brain to increase cerebral water.

This physiological response has been clearly demonstrated in case series and reports and in clinical trials of perioperative and in-hospital fluid administration [39, 40]. A recent systematic review by Choong et al. [41] examined six randomized controlled trials of intravenous fluids, four surgical and two medical (gastroenteritis, cases of hospital-acquired hyponatremia). The conclusion of this systematic review was that patients receiving hypotonic maintenance fluids were 17.2 times more likely to develop hyponatremia than those who were given isotonic solutions.

The dangers of hyponatremia are well documented. By 2002 there were over 50 case reports in the literature of neurological morbidity including 26 deaths. The incidence of in-hospital hyponatremia in children with pneumonia is 45%, and in those with meningitis rises to 50% [42]. Babies with bronchiolitis have also been shown to be at risk [40]. Clinical researchers at the Hospital for Sick Children, Toronto, have demonstrated an alarmingly high incidence of hyponatremia in the in-hospital population, many of whom received intravenous fluids in greater than recommended volumes [43]. They were able to show in a further study that those who developed hyponatremia received significantly more electrolyte free water (dextrose solutions) and had more neurological sequelae [44].

In 2004 Ulster Television broadcast a programme "When Hospitals Kill" alleging that three children had died unnecessarily related to in-hospital fluid management, leading the government of the UK to announce an inquiry into these hyponatremia-related deaths. Prior to this, in the wake of these deaths, a Working Group in Northern Ireland had developed and published guidelines (Department of Health, Social Services and Public Safety 2002) [45, 46] on prevention of hyponatremia in children receiving prescribed fluids. However, a point survey of fluid prescribing practices in Northern Ireland carried out in 2003 found that implementation of these guidelines was incomplete [47]. It did not uncover any significant hyponatremia, although the numbers were small.

Holliday and Segar have recently published a modification of their original guidelines recommend firstly that any dehydration should be rapidly replaced with isotonic fluids at 20–40 ml/kg and that maintenance should then be continued with hypotonic fluids at 50% of the originally suggested rate [48]. The authors believe that this approach would prevent dehydration, with its effect of stimulating ADH, and would compensate for the low urine output seen in the immediate postoperative period due to nonosmotic stimuli to ADH secretion. They make a strong argument that hypovolemia at presentation is often inadequately treated and that infants with moderate to severe dehydration should be given 60–100 ml/kg of isotonic saline in the first 2–4 hours after presentation. Further correspondence has ensued with the proponents of isotonic fluid maintenance [49–51] with a heated debate concerning sodium load and lack of proof of safety and efficacy on both sides.

In 2007 Holliday et al. reported an extensive review of the development of fluid therapy guidelines from the administration of 0.8% saline by intraperitoneal injection for treatment of diarrheal dehydration in 1918 to the most recent literature, commenting further on the current isotonic/hypotonic debate [52]. They again called for trials of both intravenous and oral rehydration regimens and of how ADH levels change with rehydration. Many authors [53, 54] have already called for large, randomized controlled studies to evaluate the impact of changing the recommended solutions for perioperative and in-hospital maintenance from hypotonic to isotonic solutions.

Such trials are awaited, but until results are available it would appear prudent to adjust our policies since the case report and series evidence is difficult to ignore. Some authors [55, 56] have stated strongly that hypotonic fluids should no longer be administered in the perioperative situation while others [57] have argued equally forcefully against this position! Some hospitals have removed hypotonic fluids from their wards and units. However, situations remain when hypotonic solutions would be more appropriate, including for patients with cirrhosis and cardiac failure, when both sodium and water must be restricted.

However, reasonable suggestions made by several authorities include:

1. Careful monitoring of plasma sodium in all children receiving iv fluids
2. Avoidance of hypotonic solutions in children with an initial plasma sodium of <136 mmol/l
3. Measurement of plasma and urine sodium and osmolality in those in whom ADH secretion is suspected because of decreasing urine output or in all receiving intravenous fluids for more than 24 hours
4. Daily weight and fluid balance
5. Restriction of maintenance fluid volumes if the underlying condition suggests ADH secretion, e.g. bronchiolitis, spinal fusion postoperatively, and there are no ongoing fluid losses
6. Use of solutions containing dextrose/glucose only as needed, including for premature infants and some newborns, with intraoperative glucose monitoring.

Conclusion

Fluid management in children requires an understanding of pediatric physiology and an appreciation of the pathophysiology of the perioperative period. Careful monitoring of hemodynamics and laboratory values will avoid most problems if used to guide the fluids prescribed.

References

1. Friis-Hansen B (1961) Body water compartment changes in children: changes during growth and related changes in body composition. Pediatrics 28:169–181
2. Association of Paediatric Anaesthetists (2007) APA consensus guideline on perioperative fluid management in children. Association of Paediatric Anaesthetists, London
3. Splinter WM, Schaefer JD (1990) Unlimited clear fluid ingestion 2 hours before surgery in children does not affect volume or pH of stomach contents. Anaesth Intensive Care 18:522–526
4. Aehlert B (2006) Pediatric advanced life support study guide, 2nd edn. American Heart Association. Mosby, Philadelphia
5. Woloszczuk-Gebicka B (2005) How to limit allogenic blood transfusion in children. Paediatr Anaesth 15:913–924
6. Wales PW, Lau W, Kim PC (2001) Directed blood donation in paediatric general surgery: is it worth it? J Pediatr Surg 36(5):722–725
7. Chiavetta JA, Maki E, Gula CA, Newman A (2000) Estimated risk of transfusion transmitted infection in the Canadian blood supply (1987–1996). Vox Sang 78 [Suppl 1]; abstract P360
8. Desmet L, Lacroix J (2004) Transfusion in paediatrics. Crit Care Clin 20:299–311
9. Lacroix J, Hebert PC, Hutchison JS et al (2007) Transfusion strategies for patients in paediatric intensive care units. N Engl J Med 356:1609–1619
10. Winslow RM (2003) Alternative oxygen therapeutics: products, status of clinical trials, and future prospects. Curr Hematol Rep 2:503–510
11. Cochrane Injuries Group Albumin Reviewers (1998) Human albumin administration in critically ill patients: systematic review of randomized controlled trials. BMJ 317:235–240
12. Soni N (1998) Validity of review methods must be assessed. BMJ 317:883–884
13. Petros A, Schindler M, Pierce C et al (1998) Human albumin administration in critically ill patients. Evidence needs to be shown in paediatrics. BMJ 317:882
14. SAFE Study Investigators; Finfer S, Bellomo R, McEvoy S et al (2006) Effect of baseline serum albumin concentration on outcome of resuscitation with albumin or saline in patients in intensive care units: analysis of data from the saline versus albumin fluid evaluation (SAFE) study. BMJ 333(7577):1044
15. The Albumin Reviewers (Alderson P, Bunn F, Li Wan Po A et al) (2004) Human albumin solution for resuscitation and volume expansion in critically ill patients. Cochrane Database of Systematic Reviews, Issue 4. Article no. CD001208
16. Boluyt N, Bollen CW, Bos AP et al (2006) Fluid resuscitation in neonatal and paediatric hypovolemic shock: a Dutch Paediatric Society evidence-based clinical practice guideline. Intensive Care Med 32:995–1003
17. Gandhi SD, Weiskopf RB, Jungheinrich C et al (2007) Volume replacement therapy during major orthopedic surgery using Voluven (hydroxyethyl starch 130/0.4) or hetastarch. Anesthesiology 106:1120–1127
18. Vincent J-L (2007) The pros and cons of hydroxyethyl starch solutions (editorial). Anesth Analg 104:484–486
19. World Health Organization (2000) Management of the child with a serious infection or severe malnutrition. Guidelines for care at the first-referral level in developing countries. World Health Organization, Geneva, pp 57–73
20. Molyneux EM, Maitland K (2005) Intravenous fluids – getting the balance right. N Engl J Med 353:941–944
21. Winters RW (1973) The body fluids in paediatrics, 1st edn. Little, Brown and Company, Boston, p 113
22. Berry FA (1990) Anesthetic management of difficult and routine pediatric patients, 2 edn. Churchill Livingstone, New York
23. Holliday MA, Segar WE (1957) The maintenance need for water in parenteral fluid therapy. Paediatrics 19:823–832

24. Talbot NB (1938) Basal metabolism standards for children. Arch Dis Child 55:455–459

25. Crawford JD, Terry ME, Rourke GM (1950) Simplification of doing dosage calculation by application of the surface area principle. Pediatrics 5:783–790

26. Briassoulis G, Venkataraman S, Thompson A (2000) Energy expenditure in critically ill children. Crit Care Med 28:1166–1172

27. Verhoeven JJ, Hazelot JA, van der Voort E et al (1998) Comparison of measured and predicted energy expenditure in mechanically ventilated children. Crit Care Med 24:464–468

28. Coss-Bu JA, Klish WJ, Walding D et al (2001) Energy metabolism, nitrogen balance, and substrate utilization in critically ill children. Am J Clin Nutr 74:664–669

29. Theye RA, Michenfelder JD (1975) Whole-body and organ VO2 changes with enflurane, isoflurane, and halothane. Br J Anaesth 47:813–817

30. Lindahl SGE (1988) Energy expenditure and fluid and electrolyte requirements in anesthetized infants and children. Anesthesiology 69:377–382

31. Illner K, Brinkmann G, Heller M et al (2000) Metabolically active components of fat free mass and resting energy expenditure in nonobese adults. Am J Physiol Endocrinol Metab 278:E308–E315

32. Heeley AM, Talbot NB (1955) Insensible water losses per day by hospitalized infants and children. Am J Dis Child 90:251–255

33. Lamke LO, Nilsson GE, Reithner HL (1977) Insensible perspiration from the skin under standardized environmental conditions. Scand J Clin Lab Invest 37:325–331

34. Bluemle LW, Potter HP, Elkington JR (1956) Changes in body composition in acute renal failure. J Clin Invest 10:1094–1108

35. Pickering DE, Winters RW (1954) Fluid and electrolyte management in children. Pediatr Clin N Am 873–899

36. Al-Dahhan J, Jannoun L, Haycock GB (2002) Effect of salt supplementation of newborn premature infants on neurodevelopmental outcome at 10-13 years of age. Arch Dis Child Fetal Neonatal Ed 86:F120–F123

37. Dubois MC, Gouyet L, Murat I, Saint-Maurice C (1992) Lactated ringer with 1% dextrose: an appropriate solution for peri-operative fluid therapy in children. Paediatr Anaesth 2:99–104

38. Welborn LG, Norden JM, Seiden N et al (1993) Effect of minimizing preoperative fasting on perioperative blood glucose homeostasis in children. Paediatr Anaesth 3:167–171

39. Steele A, Gowrishankar M, Abrahamson S et al (1997) Postoperative hyponatremia despite near-isotonic saline infusion: a phenomenon of desalination. Ann Intern Med 126:20–25

40. Hanna S, Tibby SM, Durward A, Murdoch IA (2003) Incidence of hyponatraemia and hyponatraemic seizures in severe respiratory syncytial virus bronchiolitis. Acta Paediatr 92:430–434

41. Choong K, Kho ME, Bohn D (2007) Hypotonic versus isotonic saline in hospitalized children: a systematic review. Arch Dis Child 91:828–835

42. Shann F, Germer S (1985) Hyponatraemia associated with pneumonia or bacterial meningitis. Arch Dis Child 60:963–966

43. Halberthal M, Halperin ML, Bohn D (2001) Acute hyponatraemia in children admitted to hospital: retrospective analysis of factors contributing to its development and resolution. BMJ 322:780–782

44. Hoorn EJ, Geary D, Robb M et al (2004) Acute hyponatremia related to intravenous fluid administration in hospitalized children: an observational study. Paediatrics 113:1279–1284

45. Department of Health, Social Services and Public Safety (2002) Hyponatraemia wall chart. Department of Health, Social Services and Public Safety, Belfast. Available at: http://www.dhsspsni.gov.uk/hypno_wallchart.pdf

46. Jenkins JG, Taylor B, McCarthy M (2003) Prevention of hyponatraemia in children receiving fluid therapy (editorial). Ulster Med J 72:69–72

47. McAloon J, Kottyal R (2005) A study of current fluid prescribing practice and measures to prevent hyponatraemia in Northern Ireland's paediatric departments. Ulster Med J 74:93–97

48. Holliday MA, Segar WE, Friedman A (2003) Reducing errors in fluid therapy management. Paediatrics 111:424–425
49. Vajda Z, Sulyok E, Dóczi T, Nielsen S (2004) Intravenous fluids for seriously ill children (letter). Lancet 363:241
50. Holliday MA (2005) Isotonic saline expands extracellular fluid and is inappropriate for maintenance therapy (letter). Pediatrics 115:193
51. Hoorn EJ, Halperin ML, Bohn D (2005) Isotonic saline expands extracellular fluid and is inappropriate for maintenance therapy (reply). Pediatrics 115:194
52. Holliday MA, Ray PE, Friedman AL (2007) Fluid therapy for children: facts, fashions and questions. Arch Dis Child 92:546–550
53. Taylor D, Durward A (2004) Pouring salt on troubled waters. Arch Dis Child 89:411–414
54. Duke T, Molyneux EM (2003) Intravenous fluids for seriously ill children: time to reconsider. Lancet 362:1320–1323
55. Arieff AI (1998) Postoperative hyponatraemic encephalopathy following elective surgery in children. Paediatr Anaesth 8:1–4
56. Moritz ML, Ayus JC (2003) Prevention of hospital-acquired hyponatremia: a case for using isotonic saline. Paediatrics 111:227–230
57. Hatherill M (2004) Rubbing salt in the wound. Arch Dis Child 89:414–418

Chapter 12

Adrenal Insufficiency in Pediatric Critical Illness

Giuliana Rizzo, Kusum Menon

Introduction

The hormonal response to nonendocrine illness has a crucial importance in pediatric critical illness. Prompt recognition of hormonal deficiency or excess as a cause of critical illness leads to specify therapy for what often appears to be a nonspecific clinical syndrome. In recent years, we have become more aware of the physiological, possibly adaptive, alterations in endocrine function that occur in response to critical illness. The pediatric intensivist needs to interpret the hormonal studies properly and to treat the childhood endocrine disorders and the life-threatening complications that can occur in the course of a pediatric critical illness.

In this chapter we review the pathophysiology, physical and laboratory diagnosis and treatment of acute adrenal insufficiency in pediatric critical illness.

Anatomy of the Adrenal Gland

The adrenal glands, which are also called the suprarenal glands, are small, triangular glands located on the top of each kidney. The adrenal gland comprises two parts: the outer region called the adrenal cortex and the inner region called the adrenal medulla.

Physiology of the Hypothalamic Pituitary Adrenal Gland

The adrenal glands are part of the hypothalamic adrenal axis which is responsible for the production of cortisol. The hypothalamus produces corticotropin-releasing hormone (CRH), which stimulates the pituitary gland which in turn produces adrenocorticotropic hormone (ACTH). ACTH stimulates the adrenal cortex to produce cortisol which then provides feedback inhibition to the pituitary and hypothalamus. The adrenal cortex and medulla perform very separate

M. Astuto (ed), *Basics*, Anesthesia, Intensive Care and Pain in Neonates and Children.
ISBN 978-88-470-0654-6 © Springer-Verlag Italia 2009

functions. The adrenal cortex secretes hormones that have an effect on the body's metabolism, biochemistry, and certain physical characteristics. The adrenal cortex secretes corticosteroids and other hormones directly into the bloodstream. The hormones produced by the adrenal cortex include corticosteroids, androgens and aldosterone. The adrenal medulla is part of the neurosympathetic system and secretes epinephrine and norepinephrine.

Secretion, Physiological Actions and Metabolism of Cortisol

Cortisol is the major endogenous glucocorticoid secreted by the adrenal cortex. Over 90% of circulating cortisol is protein-bound with the majority being bound to corticosteroid-binding globulin (CBG) and the remainder bound to albumin and less than 10% in the free, biologically active form. Albumin has a high capacity and low affinity for binding cortisol and therefore cortisol bound to albumin is considered to be physiologically active. Normal serum cortisol concentrations range between 5 and 20 µg/dl. Cortisol exerts its effects by passing through cell membranes and binding to receptors in the cytosol of nucleated cells. The steroid-receptor complex migrates to the nucleus and influences gene transcription. Cortisol has several important physiological actions on metabolism, cardiovascular function and the immune system. The metabolic effects of cortisol include increasing blood glucose concentrations through activation of key enzymes involved in hepatogluconeogenesis and inhibiting glucose uptake in adipose tissue. In addition, lipolysis is activated resulting in the release of free fatty acids into the circulation.

Cortisol has permissive effects on other hormones including catecholamines and glucagons, with resultant development of insulin resistance and hyperglycemia. Glucocorticoids are required for normal cardiovascular reactivity to angiotensin II, epinephrine and norepinephrine, contributing to the maintenence of cardiac contractility, vascular tone and blood pressure. These effects are mediated partly by the increased transcription and expression of the receptors for these hormones. Glucocorticoids are required for the synthesis of Na^+,K^+-ATPase and catecholamines. The effects of glucocorticoid on synthesis of catecholamines and catecholamine receptors are partially responsible for the positive inotropic effects of these hormones. Cortisol has a profound effect on the inflammatory process as it inhibits the functions of almost every cell involved in inflammation. This inhibition is mediated by altering the transcription of cytokine genes (interleukins IL-1 and IL-6) and by inhibiting the production of proinflammatory substances (leukotrienes and prostaglandins). Cortisol is metabolized in the liver with subsequent renal excretion of the metabolites. Therefore, liver disease markedly impairs the metabolism of cortisol and renal disease reduces the excretion of the metabolites.

Responses of the Hypothalamic-pituitary-adrenal Axis to Acute and Prolonged Critical Illness

Critical illness, anesthesia, surgery, trauma, burns, hemorrhage, infection, pain, cold, fever and emotional disorders are stressors that activate the hypothalamic-pituitary-adrenal (HPA) axis [1]. The HPA axis is an essential component of the general adaptation to stress and plays a crucial role in cardiovascular, metabolic and immunological homeostasis. The hypothalamus releases CRH, which elicits a series of events. The initial event involves the stimulation of the sympathetic nervous system to release norepinephrine and epinephrine, which causes vascular smooth muscle vasoconstriction and enhances inotropic response. Secondly, the posterior pituitary is stimulated to release antidiuretic hormone (ADH) to promote intravascular fluid retention. Lastly, stimulation of the anterior pituitary leads to release of adrenocorticotropin hormone (ACTH), which stimulates the adrenal cortex to release the mineralocorticoid (aldosterone) to promote intravascular fluid retention and the glucocorticoid (cortisol) to increase availability of substrates for metabolism and modulate the immune/inflammatory response. These responses are beneficial as they augment cardiovascular function, reduce and redirect energy metabolism, and protect against the biological effects of the immune response (Fig. 12.1).

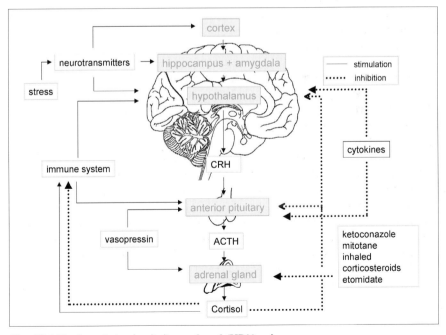

Fig. 12.1 The hypothalamic-pituitary-adrenal (HPA) axis

Pathophysiology

The mechanisms leading to dysfunction of the HPA axis during critical illness are complex and poorly understood and probably include decreased production of CRH, ACTH and cortisol as well as their receptors. In neonates, particularly preterm infants, immaturity of the HPA axis may limit the ability to increase cortisol production in response to stress [2]. Patients of any age may mount an inadequate cortisol response due to preexisting hypothalamic-pituitary or adrenocortical disease, exhaustion of secretory adrenocortical reserve, or suppression of cortisol and ACTH by inflammatory mediators [3]. In 1911 Waterhouse recognized, in the setting of meningococcemia, that adrenal hypoperfusion and hemorrhage may cause acute adrenal insufficiency in sepsis [4]. Drug-induced changes in steroid metabolism or production can also contribute to adrenal insufficiency; the use of etomidate, which inhibits enzymes involved in cortisol synthesis, in the pediatric intensive care unit has resulted in adrenal insufficiency that persists for 24 hours after administration and has been associated with increased mortality [5].

The pathophysiology of relative adrenal insufficiency and the effects of glucocorticoid therapy are not well understood. Inflammatory cytokines, released during sepsis, appear to promote corticosteroid resistance so that normal adrenal responses are suppressed [6]. The systemic inflammatory response syndrome results in the release of cytokines (tumor necrosis factor), which in vitro suppresses CRH [6]. In addition, patients treated with long-term corticosteroid are likely to have secondary adrenal insufficiency which may increase the risk of developing adrenal insufficiency [7].

Epidemiology of Adrenal Insufficiency in Critical Illness

The incidence of adrenal dysfunction in critically ill children reported in the literature varies considerably from 4% for to 52% [8, 9]. However, the available studies focused on adrenal insufficiency presenting in children with septic shock and after open-heart surgery [10, 11]. It is important to distinguish between patients presenting to hospital with evidence of chronic adrenal insufficiency (Addison's disease) and those with "acute adrenal insufficiency" [12]. The prevalence of adrenal insufficiency in the neonatal population is unclear, since the normal adrenal response to critical illness has not been fully defined for neonates at various gestational ages [3].

Acute Adrenal Insufficiency

Acute adrenal insufficiency is a clinical condition that in its extreme is characterized by tachycardia and hypotension which are resistant to fluids and vasopressor therapy, and must be distinguished from the underlying illness [9]. If unrecognized and not promptly treated with stress doses of replacement gluco-corticoids and mineralocorticoids, may be fatal. Treatment courses for as short a period as 2 weeks may result in transient suppression of endogenous cortisol production. There are few data regarding death or hospitalization in children without hypothalamic pituitary disease caused by withdrawal of pharmacological glucocorticoid therapy [13, 14]. Clinical signs and symptoms common to both primary and secondary adrenal insufficiency include: nausea, vomiting, diarrhea, fever, hypotension and tachycardia. Laboratory findings include hyponatremia, hypoglycemia, normocytic normochromic anemia and eosinophilia. Mineralocorticoid deficiency is present only in primary adrenal insufficiency [15]. Mineralocorticoid deficiency is responsible of urinary losses of water and electrolytes (Na, Cl, K). The result is hyponatremia associated with volume contraction, elevated blood urea nitrogen (BUN) and creatinine, and hyperkalemia and hypotension.

Hyperkalemia is not present and hyponatremia is dilutional because an increase in ADH [15].

These clinical signs and symptoms can be very difficult to detect in critically ill patients where tachycardia and hypotension are clinical findings common to various critical illness and electrolyte abnormalities are often masked by continuous exogenous electrolyte replacement.

Causes of Adrenal Insufficiency

The causes of adrenal insufficiency can be primary or secondary (Table 12.1).

To minimize morbidity and mortality, prompt recognition and treatment of adrenal crisis is critical.

Table 12.1 Causes of adrenal insufficiency

Primary adrenal insufficiency	Secondary adrenal insufficiency
Abnormal adrenal development (adrenal hypoplasia congenita, AHC)	Withdrawal from glucocorticoid therapy
Steroidogenesis disorders (congenital adrenal hyperplasia)	Familial glucocorticoid deficiency (unresponsiveness to adrenocorticotropin hormone)
Peroxisomal disorders (adrenoleukodystrophy, ALD)	Hypothalamic tumors
Adrenal damage (hemorrhage, infarction) Tuberculosis, fungal infection, AIDS	Irradiation of the central nervous system Drugs
Sepsis	Trauma, surgery
Autoimmune adrenalitis	Hypopituitarism

In the pediatric intensive care unit, adrenal insufficiency should be particularly considered in the following clinical settings: shock, head injury, and history of an antecedent precipitating stress (e.g. surgery or infection).

Adrenal crisis should be considered in all children with hypotension and shock unresponsive to fluid resuscitation and inotropic medications; other clinical manifestations are usually related to the cause of adrenal insufficiency, such as vomiting, diarrhea, hypovolemia, hyponatremia, hyperkalemia, hypoglycemia, and hypotension.

Adrenal Damage Bilateral destruction of the adrenal glands by factors extrinsic to the adrenal gland is a less-common cause of primary adrenal insufficiency in children than in adults. However, damage to normal adrenal glands still causes adrenal insufficiency in a significant number of children.

Adrenal Hemorrhage In the newborn, bilateral subcapsular bleeding into the adrenal glands results from injury during delivery to the fine subcapsular vascular plexus. This vascular supply is separated from the adrenal parenchyma, causing ischemic damage to the adrenal glands.

Bilateral Adrenal Hemorrhage or Infarction Bilateral adrenal hemorrhage or infarction because of bacterial endotoxin is a life-threatening complication in children with serious bacterial infection. Although *Neisseria meningitidis* meningitis usually is identified with adrenal crisis (known as Waterhouse-Friderichsen syndrome), other pathogens associated with adrenal hemorrhage include *Pseudomonas aeruginosa*, *Streptococcus pneumoniae*, *Staphylococcus aureus*, and group B streptococcus. Adrenal insufficiency also may result from anticoagulant therapy.

Infections Infections of the adrenal gland can lead to adrenal insufficiency in children.

Tuberculosis produces chronic adrenocortical insufficiency as a result of initial infiltration and subsequent bilateral destruction of the adrenal glands. In some cases, calcification of the adrenal glands can be seen on abdominal radiographs. Fungal infections, such as histoplasmosis, coccidiomycosis and blastomycosis, can cause adrenal insufficiency in a similar manner to tuberculosis.

Adrenal abnormalities in patients with human immunodeficiency virus (HIV) disease may be because of a direct pathogenic effect of HIV, damage from secondary infections (e.g. cytomegalovirus or *Mycobacterium avium-intracellulare*), medications (e.g. ketoconazole), and/or malnutrition. Abnormalities include the inability to produce adrenal hormones as a result of damage to adrenocortical cells, blunted cortisol response to ACTH stimulation, or a decrease in cortisol reserve as measured by serum cortisol response to prolonged ACTH stimulation. Some have limited cortisol reserve (possibly because of chronic stress), and are at increased risk of adrenal insufficiency during periods of acute stress.

Drugs Drugs that inhibit cortisol synthesis include aminoglutethimide, keto-conazole, and etomidate. Adrenal suppression also has been reported with the use of megestrol acetate, a progestational agent used as an appetite stimulant, in children with HIV disease or with malignancies. Prolonged use of high doses of megestrol acetate can cause Cushing syndrome.

Diagnosis of Acute Adrenal Insufficiency in Critical Illness

There is no consensus regarding the criteria used for the diagnosis of adrenal insufficiency in critical illness, especially in children. It is interesting to note that the potential criteria used by pediatric endocrinologists are different from the criteria used by pediatric intensivists [9].

A high index of suspicion of adrenal insufficiency should be considered in the presence of unexplained catecholamine-resistant hypotension, despite adequate fluid resuscitation and ongoing evidence of inflammation (without an obvious source) that does not respond to empirical treatment [2, 9].

HPA reactivity has been assessed using the corticotrophin stimulation test. To perform this test a low dose (1 µg) of synthetic corticotrophin is administered; a number of studies [2] have demonstrated that a low dose of corticotropin is more sensitive in the diagnosis of secondary adrenal insufficiency. The normal response to a low dose of corticotropin is an increase in cortisol level of 18 µg or more at baseline 30 to 60 minutes after infusion.

Traditionally a high-dose ACTH stimulation test using 250 µg of intravenous corticotropin has been used to diagnose adrenal insufficiency in critical illness with cortisol levels being obtained at baseline and 30 minutes and 60 minutes following ACTH administration. A basal cortisol level less than 5 µg/dl is generally accepted as being adrenally insufficient even in outpatients and after ACTH stimulation a serum cortisol level <18 µg/dl, or an increase in the cortisol concentration of <9 µg/dl in a hypotensive patient is highly suggestive of adrenal insufficiency [2].

Treatment

There are no randomized controlled trials on the treatment of adrenal insufficiency in pediatric critical illness. Despite this critically ill children are still empirically treated with glucocorticoids in the pediatric intensive care unit [9].

A meta-analysis of several prospective, randomized, controlled trials in adults demonstrated a reduction in time to shock reversal at 7 days, and decreased 28-day mortality, in patients with adrenal insufficiency treated with low-dose hydrocortisone (300 mg per day hydrocortisone or equivalent; 175 mg/m^2 per day) with no increase in adverse events [2]. This contrasts with previous studies of high-dose short-duration dexamethasone treatment that does not confer benefit in either adults or neonates [16, 17].

There are some studies demonstrating an increased mortality in pediatric patients who received steroids [18–20].

The focus of previous studies has been to examine the efficacy of both dexamethasone and hydrocortisone treatment for hypotension and prevention of chronic lung disease [2] in critically ill preterm infants. Studies in preterm infants with volume and pressor-resistant hypotension demonstrate that steroid treatment improves blood pressure and stabilizes cardiovascular status.

A study [21] of term critically ill neonates demonstrated improvement in hemodynamic parameters with hydrocortisone therapy only in those patients with initial low (<15 mg/dl) cortisol concentrations, with no improvement in those patients without evidence of relative adrenal insufficiency.

In another study [22] low-dose hydrocortisone therapy was adopted in preterm infants in the attempt to determine the utility of steroids in preventing bronchopulmonary dysplasia. However, this study did not base hydrocortisone therapy on biochemical evidence of adrenal insufficiency and during therapy some patients developed very high cortisol levels which appeared to be associated with an increased risk of complications. However, some evidence suggests that even short-term glucocorticoid use in pediatric critical illness may be associated with hyperglycemia, leukocytosis and polyneuropathy [9].

Taken together, the evidence suggests the need for careful assessment of which patients will benefit from replacement therapy and the use of hydrocortisone only in patients with demonstrated adrenal insufficiency.

Some experts [2] recommend keeping ACTH in the pediatric intensive care unit pharmacy, to allow quick access and prompt testing. Hydrocortisone can be started immediately after testing, but should be continued only if adrenal insufficiency is confirmed by laboratory testing. In the absence of any conclusive evidence on the treatment of suspected adrenal insufficiency in the pediatric critical care literature, it is reasonable to use (lower) stress doses of 50–100 mg/m^2 per day of hydrocortisone every 4 hours intravenously (or by infusion) during the acute phase of the child's illness followed by a wean over 3–4 days once stabilized.

Conclusion

There is no consensus on the incidence, diagnosis and treatment of adrenal insufficiency in pediatric critical illness which is supported by a recent survey involving 16 tertiary care pediatric intensive care units and all pediatric endocrinologists in Canada [9]. In light of this, large-scale epidemiological studies using adrenal function testing that correlate various definitions of adrenal insufficiency with clinically important outcomes are necessary to determine the optimum definition, diagnosis and ultimately management of adrenal insufficiency in pediatric critical illness.

References

1. Williams HW, Dluhy RG (1998) Diseases of the adrenal cortex. In: Fauci AS, Braunwald E, Isselbacher KJ et al (eds) Harrison's principles of internal medicine. McGraw-Hill, New York, pp 2035–2057
2. Langer M, Modi BP, Agus M (2006) Adrenal insufficiency in the critically ill neonate and child. Curr Opin Pediatr 18:448–453
3. Watterberg KL (2004) Adrenocortical function and dysfunction in the fetus and neonate. Semin Neonatol 9:13–21
4. Waterhouse R (1911) A case of suprarenal apoplexy. Lancet 1:577–578
5. Wagner RL, White PF, Kan PB et al (1984) Inhibition of adrenal steroidogenesis by the anesthetic etomidate. N Engl J Med 310:1415–1421
6. Papanicolaou DA, Tsigos C, Oldfield EH, Chrousos GP (1996) Acute glucocorticoid deficiency is associated with plasma elevations of interleukin-6: does the latter participate in the symptomatology of the steroid withdrawal syndrome and adrenal insufficiency? J Clin Endocrinol Metab 81:2303–2306
7. Cooper MS, Stewart PM (2003) Corticosteroid insufficiency in acutely ill patients. N Engl J Med 348:727–734
8. Menon K, Clarson C (2002) Adrenal function in pediatric critical illness. Pediatr Crit Care Med 3:112–116
9. Menon K, Lawson M (2007) Identification of adrenal insufficiency in pediatric critical illness. Pediatr Crit Care Med 8:276–278
10. Hildebrandt T, Mansour M, Al Samsam R (2005) The use of steroids in children with septicemia: review of the literature and assessment of current practice in PICUs in the UK. Paediatr Anaesth 15:358–365
11. Hatherill M, Tibby SM, Hilliard T et al (1999) Adrenal insufficiency in septic shock. Arch Dis Child 80:51–55
12. Pizarro CF, Troster EJ, Damiani D, Carcillo JA (2005) Absolute and relative adrenal insufficiency in children with septic shock. Crit Care Med 33:855–859
13. Shulman DI, Palmert MR, Kemp SF; Lawson Wilkins Drug and Therapeutics Committee (2007) Adrenal insufficiency: still a cause of morbidity and death in childhood. Pediatrics 119:e484–e494
14. White PC, Speiser PW (2000) Congenital adrenal hyperplasia due to 21-hydroxylase deficiency. Endocr Rev 21:245–291
15. Trimarchi T (2006) Endocrine problems in critically ill children: an overview. AACN Clinical Issues 17:66–78
16. Van den Berghe G (2003) Endocrine evaluation of patients with critical illness. Endocrinol Metab Clin N Am 32:385–410
17. Johnson KL, Rn CR (2006) The hypothalamic-pituitary-adrenal-axis in critical illness. AACN Clin Issues 17:39–49
18. Cronin L, Cook DJ, Carlet J et al (1995) Corticosteroid treatment for sepsis: a critical appraisal and meta-analysis of the literature. Crit Care Med 23:1430–1439
19. Fernandez E, Schrader R, Watterberg K (2005) Prevalence of low cortisol values in term and near-term infants with vasopressor-resistant hypotension. J Perinatol 25:114–118
20. Watterberg KL, Gerdes JS, Cole CH et al (2004) Prophylaxis of early adrenal insufficiency to prevent bronchopulmonary dysplasia: a multicenter trial. Pediatrics 114:1649–1657
21. Stoll BJ, Temprosa M, Tyson JE et al (1999) Dexamethasone therapy increases infection in very low birth weight infants. Pediatrics 104:e63
22. Markovitz BP, Goodman DM, Watson RS et al (2005) A retrospective cohort study of prognostic factors associated with outcome in pediatric severe sepsis: what is the role of steroids? Pediatr Crit Care Med 6:270–274

Chapter 13

Perioperative Care in Pediatric Cardiac Surgery

Joseé Lavoie

Introduction

Congenital heart disease (CHD) is the commonest form of congenital disease with an incidence of 11.6 per 1,000 live births [1]. The perioperative care of children with CHD undergoing cardiac surgery requires an integrated multidisciplinary team approach. The great strides achieved in the care of these children would not have been possible without dedicated teams of medical personnel working with a concerted and standardized approach. The achievements have been such that perioperative mortality rates have decreased significantly. In fact, overall perioperative mortality is currently on average 3.6% [2], with straightforward atrial septal defect (ASD) repair at close to 0% [3] and stage 1 palliation for hypoplastic left heart syndrome at 29% [4]. Expected lifetimes without treatment are 19.5 years for acyanotics and 1.4 years for cyanotics compared to 64.9 years and 46 years, respectively, in treated patients. Although efforts towards reduction of perioperative mortality are continuing, there has been increasing interest in improving perioperative morbidity. Perioperative morbidity may involve the hematological, respiratory, cardiac and nervous systems. In a one-year survival and neurological outcome study (single-center), the overall survival rate was 92% and the incidence of acute neurological events was 17% in survivors [5]. The risk factors were the presence of elevated red blood cell count, low Apgar score and abnormal preoperative brain imaging.

There has been growing interest in neurological outcome because of its impact on quality of life. Recent studies have focused on pre-existing neurological dysfunction, neurological monitoring and perioperative strategies to improve neurological outcome.

Preoperative Evaluation

History taking and physical examination are fundamental in the evaluation of the patient with CHD. There should be emphasis put on determining the presence of risk factors. The risk factors associated with the worst outcomes in CHD are listed

M. Astuto (ed), *Basics*, Anesthesia, Intensive Care and Pain in Neonates and Children.
ISBN 978-88-470-0654-6 © Springer-Verlag Italia 2009

in Table 13.1 [6, 7]. Odegard et al. have studied the frequency of anesthesia-related cardiac arrest in patients with CHD undergoing cardiac surgery [8]. The younger patients, neonates and infants were at higher risk as well as patients with altered coronary perfusion, i.e. lesions with run-off of blood flow from the systemic to pulmonary circulation and low aortic root diastolic pressure. Another study on the incidence of complications during cardiac catheterization has demonstrated an incidence of events of 9.3% with the highest incidence being in infants and in therapeutic interventions other than patent ductus arteriosus or ASD occlusion [9].

The nature of previous surgical procedures must be clarified, as these may impact on management. For example, a previous aortic coarctation repair using a subclavian flap involves sacrificing the right subclavian artery, which will render measurement of blood pressure, and possibly pulse oximetry, in the right upper limb unreliable. Similar issues may arise with aortopulmonary shunts. In patients who have undergone multiple cardiac catheterization procedures and/or central venous cannulations, it would be wise to establish patency of vessels preoperatively. In this regard, ultrasound technology may be quite useful.

Current medication, cardiac and otherwise, will not only give an indication of the patient's clinical status, but may also have repercussions on intraoperative management. For instance, angiotensin-converting enzyme (ACE) inhibitors have been associated with an increased risk of intraoperative hypotension, which may require the use of vasopressors to maintain blood pressure [10]. This phenomenon is caused by sympathetic blockade, a decreased response to α-adrenergic agonists, impaired degradation of bradykinin causing vasodilation and inhibition of the receptor binding of angiotensin ll. The hypotension is usually a result of a severely decreased cardiac index. Vasopressin may be a useful vasopressor in cases of severe refractory hypotension.

Table 13.1 Risk factors for noncardiac and cardiac surgery in patients with congenital heart disease

Risk factors	Noncardiac surgery[a]	Cardiac surgery[b]
Pulmonary hypertension	✔	–
Cyanosis	✔	–
Congestive heart failure	✔	–
Poor general health		–
Procedures on the respiratory or nervous systems	✔	–
Single ventricle physiology	–	✔
Re-do operation	–	✔

[a]Warner et al. [6]
[b]Andropoulos et al. [7]

Preoperative imaging now increasingly relies on breath-hold electrocardiographically gated cardiac magnetic resonance (MR) imaging and contrast material enhanced MR angiography (MRA) as a diagnostic tool in CHD. As such, heart catheterization is now mostly reserved for patients undergoing cardiac interventions. The advantages of MR imaging and angiography include its noninvasiveness, lack of ionizing radiation, and the accuracy and clarity of 3-D reconstruction programs for identification of vascular anatomy (Fig. 13.1). It is especially useful for deep structures that are difficult to image by echocardiography and may be difficult to access via standard catheterization. Its disadvantages are that it does not provide pressure readings in the cardiac cavities nor in vessels, although it does provide indices to function and functional impact of stenosis. Thus, pre-Fontan evaluations must still be performed by heart catheterization.

Interventions performed via cardiac catheterization are becoming more sophisticated. To the armamentarium of device closures, stenting and dilations, have been added percutaneous implantations of pulmonary valves and aortic valves [11, 12]. In a series of 59 consecutive patients with pulmonary regurgitation after repair of CHD, Khambadkone et al. successfully implanted percutaneous pulmonary valves in 58 of 59 consecutive patients [11]. The right ventricular pressure and grade of pulmonary regurgitation decreased significantly after the procedure. This procedure is reserved for older children due to equipment size. It may be of particular interest in patients with free pulmonary insufficiency following transannular repair of tetralogy of Fallot.

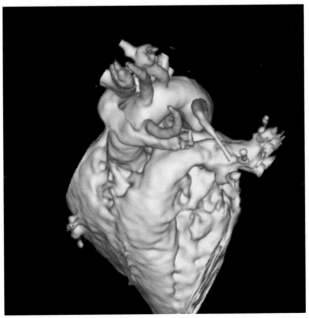

Fig. 13.1 Magnetic resonance angiography with 3-D reconstruction

Intraoperative Management

Endocarditis Prophylaxis

The major change in intraoperative management has undoubtedly been the introduction of new guidelines in the management of endocarditis [13]. The rationale
for revising the guidelines was to base these on evidence, and it is clear that
endocarditis is much more likely to result from frequent exposure to bacteremias
associated with daily activities than from bacteremia caused by procedures on
the teeth, the gastrointestinal tract or the genitourinary tract. The cardiac conditions considered at high risk of an adverse outcome from endocarditis are prosthetic cardiac valves, cardiac valvulopathy in cardiac transplantation recipients,
previous infectious endocarditis, and certain CHDs. Whereas most patients with
CHD used to require endocarditis prophylaxis, now only a small number of them
do, and these are patients with:
- Unrepaired cyanotic CHD, including palliative shunts and conduits
- Completely repaired congenital heart defect with prosthetic material or
  device, during the first 6 months after the procedure
- Repaired CHD with residual defects at the site or adjacent to the site of a
  prosthetic patch or prosthetic valve.

Procedures for which antibiotic prophylaxis is recommended are dental procedures that involve manipulation of gingival tissues or the periapical region of
the teeth or perforation of the oral mucosa. In addition, procedures on the respiratory tract that involve incision or biopsy of the respiratory mucosa, as well as
procedures on infected skin, skin structures or musculoskeletal tissue also
require prophylaxis. However, antibiotic prophylaxis is not recommended for
genitourinary or gastrointestinal procedures on the basis of endocarditis prophylaxis alone. Ampicillin remains the mainstay of the antibiotic regimen.

Anesthetic Agents

Induction of anesthesia may be performed safely in most patients using sevoflurane as it maintains cardiac index and heart rate. It causes less hypotensive and
negative inotropic effects than isoflurane or halothane [14]. Propofol may also
be used as an induction agent; it does, however, show significant hemodynamic
effects secondary to a decrease in systemic vascular resistance [15].
Consideration should be given to using a reduced dosage or avoiding the agent
altogether in patients with compromised cardiac function. In those patients with
hemodynamic compromise, etomidate at a dose of 0.3 mg/kg produces minimal
cardiovascular effects [16]. Ketamine may also be used in these patients.
However, although it indirectly releases catecholamines, it is a direct myocardial
depressant. Thus, it should be used with care in catecholamine-depleted patients
or not at all. Narcotics such as fentanyl or sufentanil provide stable hemodynamics on induction and during maintenance by preserving ventricular function.

Furthermore, the combination of fentanyl and midazolam used in conjunction with pancuronium in patients with single-ventricle physiology has been shown to preserve myocardial function [17].

Patients with increased pulmonary vascular pressures pose a particular challenge. In children aged less than 3 years, ketamine and nitrous oxide have not been shown to increase pulmonary pressures [18, 19]. Options for the treatment of elevated pulmonary vascular resistance are summarized in Table 13.2. In an observational study of 294 patients with severe postoperative pulmonary hypertension undergoing atrioventricular defect repair, the authors found that there was a high

Table 13.2 Treatment options for pulmonary hypertension

Drug	Dose range
Inhaled nitric oxide	5–80 ppm
Intravenous milrinone	0.1–0.7 µg/kg per min
Oral sildenafil	0.5 mg/kg every 4 h
Inhaled prostacyclin	50 ng/kg per min for 15 min
Inhaled milrinone	0.07 mg/kg
Combined nitric oxide and intravenous milrinone	

probability of postoperative mortality reduction in patients treated with inhaled nitric oxide (NO) at 25 ppm [20]. The combined effects of a continuous infusion of milrinone and inhaled NO produce a greater decrease in pulmonary artery pressure in children after cardiopulmonary bypass (CPB) surgery [21]. In postoperative patients who presented with pulmonary hypertension preoperatively, inhaled prostacyclin administered at a rate of 50 ng/kg per minute for a 15-minute period, has been shown to reduce the mean pulmonary artery pressure and improve the PaO_2/FiO_2 ratio without associated decreases in systemic blood pressure, heart rate or cardiac index [22]. Sildenafil, a highly selective phophodiesterase type 5 inhibitor, is being used increasingly in the treatment of pulmonary hypertension in children with congenital heart defects. In a small study of postoperative CHD patients who were on NO for pulmonary hypertension, the addition of 0.5 mg/kg of sildenafil orally every 4 hours resulted in a significant reduction in pulmonary artery pressure without an associated decrease in systemic arterial pressure [23]. Finally, there are emerging studies in adults using inhaled milrinone to treat postoperative pulmonary hypertension. This mode of administration seems to be effective in decreasing positive airway pressure (PAP) without causing systemic hypotension [24].

Monitoring

Monitoring of the patient undergoing cardiac surgery has become increasingly sophisticated. Transesophageal echocardiography (TEE), near infrared spectroscopy (NIRS) and transcranial Doppler ultrasonographic (TCD) monitoring have been added to the basic armamentarium of pulse oximetry, end-tidal capnometry, ECG and noninvasive blood pressure monitoring.

Pulse oximetry readings may be altered in the presence of CHD. At low levels of saturation, it overestimates the true value [25]. However, high hematocrit levels have not been shown to be responsible for impaired accuracy [25]. End-tidal CO_2 monitoring will be influenced by the presence of shunts. In patients with Qp/Qs ratios above 2:1, there will be an increased end-tidal to arterial CO_2 gradient [26].

The internal jugular vein (IJV) is the preferred site for central venous monitoring. The use of real-time ultrasound guidance is slowly becoming the standard of care [27]. It is one of the safety practices with the greatest strength of supporting evidence [28]. In fact, ultrasound guidance for central venous line placement has been demonstrated to be cost effective, to reduce the rate of complications, and increase the success rate of cannulations [29, 30].

Another monitor that has become a fixture in the cardiac operating room is TEE. It is used in most patients with CHD undergoing cardiac surgery with CPB and in selected non-CPB congenital heart surgery.

Monitoring of the nervous system is the most rapidly evolving area with the introduction of new monitors that are portable and compatible with the operating room environment. The neuromonitors currently available are NIRS, TCD and processed EEG. They may be used alone or in combination. They are best used in a standardized approach with predetermined interventional algorithms. Figure 13.2 illustrates one of the neuromonitoring algorithms that is used at the Montreal Children's Hospital. NIRS is a noninvasive monitor of brain tissue oxygenation. The Somanetics Invos NIRS monitor is currently the only monitor with FDA approval. The values of the Somanetics Invos monitor range from 15% to 95%. Studies seem to indicate a correlation between low cerebral saturations and adverse neurological outcome. Austin et al. studied 250 pediatric patients undergoing cardiac surgery with CPB. They found that amongst the 41% of patients with NIRS values 20% below baseline, 25% had postoperative adverse neurological events [31]. There exists a controversy as to whether or not bilateral monitoring should be used in surgery for CHD. There are isolated case reports of unilateral changes in NIRS from aortic cannula malposition and differences in measurements during regional low-flow cerebral perfusion [32, 33]. NIRS has also been used to guide low-flow cerebral perfusion during hypoplastic aortic arch repair [34]. Furthermore, NIRS may be useful to monitor splanchnic oxygenation after a Norwood repair or during aortic coarctation repair [35, 36]. However, these uses have not been validated.

TCD applied to the temporal region provides a window to the middle cerebral arteries. TCD is used to assess cerebral blood flow velocity and detect emboli. It may be useful in determining appropriate CPB flows during regional low-flow perfusion and in avoiding excessive flows. It has also helped in detecting acute decreases in cerebral blood flow from aortic cannula malposition, in conjunction with NIRS.

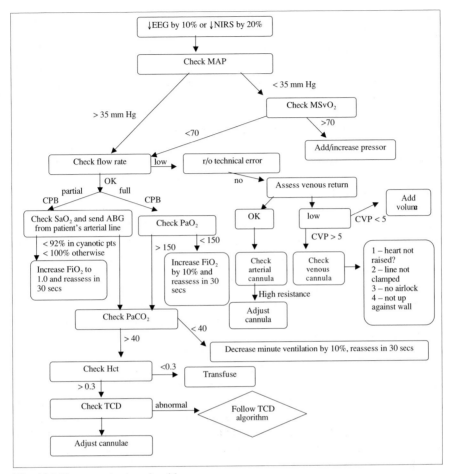

Fig. 13.2 Neuromonitoring algorithm

The processed EEG monitors have not been studied extensively. There is currently a paucity of pediatric studies. It has mostly been used in combination with the previously described monitors. It may be used to establish the presence of an isoelectric EEG prior to initiating total circulatory arrest. In the study by Austin et al., abnormal EEG findings alone did not correlate with adverse postoperative outcomes [31].

Hemostasis

One of the many challenges in pediatric cardiac anesthesia is achieving adequate hemostasis perioperatively. Hemostasis depends on preoperative patient characteristics, good surgical technique, short CPB times, control of the inflammatory reaction and the nature of the surgical procedure. In addition, it is essential to maintain adequate calcium levels and normothermia. The addition of antifibrinolytics such as E-amino-caproic acid, Tranexamic acid or Aprotinin may also contribute to decreasing perioperative blood loss and transfusions [37, 38]. Aprotinin has, according to certain authors, both antifibrinolytic and antiinflammatory properties [39]. In the context of CPB, this latter property may seem advantageous. Aprotinin is, however, associated with an anaphylaxis rate of 4.1% upon reexposure within 6 months [40]. Some animal studies have hinted towards a neuroprotective role [41]. Mossinger et al. found that in 60 infants weighing less than 10 kg and treated with aprotinin, there was a decrease in postoperative bleeding and in the amount of blood transfused, and a shortened duration of ventilation [42]. On 5 November 2007, Bayer temporarily halted marketing of the drug. This has followed the early termination of a Canadian multicenter trial on high-risk adult cardiac surgical patients, the BART study, because interim analysis of the data found increased mortality rates (all causes) in the study patients. The findings also demonstrated decreased bleeding. The marketing has been stopped temporarily until the complete data have been analyzed.

Another method of decreasing blood loss during pediatric cardiac surgery is to use whole blood less than 48 hours old in the bypass prime [43]. Manno et al. studied over 150 patients randomized to one of three groups: very fresh whole blood, fresh whole blood <48 hours, and reconstituted whole blood. The mean age of the children was 2.8, 3.9 and 3.8 years, respectively. The blood loss was 50.9, 44.8 and 74.2 ml/kg, respectively. However, a more recent study performed in infants has found different results [44]. Patients were randomized to receive either fresh whole blood (96 patients) or reconstituted blood (104 patients) for bypass circuit priming. The length of stay in the intensive care unit was shorter in the group receiving reconstituted blood. This group also had a smaller cumulative fluid balance at 48 hours. There were no differences between the groups with regard to postoperative chest-tube output and blood product transfusion requirements.

In patients with postoperative bleeding, coagulation testing should be performed, using thromboelastography as well as a laboratory coagulation profile that includes prothrombin time (PT), partial thromboplastin time (PTT), international normalized ratio (INR), fibrinogen and fibrin split products. Platelets should be administered initially, as it has been shown that the trauma of CPB affects platelet function most. Cryoprecipitate concentrates should be administered next followed by fresh frozen plasma. Recombinant factor VIIa has been used as a rescue drug. However, there are no large randomized controlled trials validating its safety and efficacy in pediatric cardiac surgery, and there are concerns regarding its potential for thrombosis [45].

Postoperative Period

The most significant single contribution to postoperative care has been the refinement of mechanical circulatory support. Although extracorporeal membrane oxygenation (ECMO) has been in use for some time, the bulk of the experience has been in patients with respiratory distress. During recent decades, the indications for ECMO have expanded to include patients with CHD [46]. These indications include bridge to recovery and bridge to transplantation in patients with postoperative ventricular dysfunction, or complex, lethal or chronic end-stage CHD. The bridge to transplantation option is particularly useful considering the paucity of pediatric hearts available for transplantation, and this may decrease the mortality rate during the waiting period. Devices available for circulatory support are listed in Table 13.3. The choice of apparatus will depend on the indication, the estimated duration of support required and the size of the patient. The options available for support in infants and neonates are limited due to size restrictions. ECMO does not have any size restrictions. Its ease and rapidity of implantation as well as the cannulation site options and its potential for full cardiopulmonary support make it an attractive choice. However, it remains a short-term option and there is a disadvantage with regard to its higher anticoagulation requirements and the risk of hemorrhage.

Ventricular assist devices (VAD) such as the Berlin Heart and the Medos-HIA system may be used in patients as small as 2 kg. These VADs offer circulatory support only but have the advantage of requiring less anticoagulation. There is an increasing amount of literature on the long-term use of these devices for left, right or biventricular circulatory support [47, 48]. Furthermore, patients with these VADs may be discharged from the intensive care unit and ambulate freely.

Table 13.3 Mechanical devices for circulatory support

Device	Short-term	Long-term	Weight	Right ventricular assist device	Left ventricular assist device	Biventricular assist device	Cardio-pulmonary support
Extracorporeal membrane oxygenation	✔	–	No restrictions	–	–	–	✔
Centrifugal ventricular assist device	✔	–	No restrictions	✔	✔	✔	–
Thoratec	–	✔	>17 kg	✔	✔	✔	–
Berlin Heart, Medos VAD	–	✔	>2 kg	✔	✔	✔	–
DeBakey Child VAD	–	✔	>0.7 m^2	✔	✔	✔	–
Intraaortic balloon pump	✔	–	–	–	✔	–	–

VAD, ventricular assist device

Conclusion

Anesthesia for patients with CHD is becoming an increasingly complex endeavor. The great strides achieved in the fields of anesthesia, cardiology, cardiac surgery and intensive care have resulted in higher survival rates of patients, even those with the most complex forms of CHD. It follows that pediatric cardiac anesthesia is becoming a subspecialty requiring specific training. The anesthetic considerations for the patient with CHD are multiple and include the choice of appropriate anesthetics, the need for neuromonitoring and neuroprotection, the identification of risk factors, the maintenance of hemostasis, treatment of coagulation anomalies after bypass and treatment of postoperative ventricular dysfunction.

It is a challenge to maintain an evidence-based practice in CHD because there are fewer randomized controlled trials in children and the number of patients is often too low to reach significant conclusions. Thus, it becomes essential that anesthesiologists taking care of patients with CHD unite into a network to promote exchange of information, participate in multicenter trials and share expertise. This would best serve the interest of the patients and help anesthesiologists provide the best care for this patient population by fostering evidence-based decisions.

References

1. Meberg A, Hals J, Thaulow E (2007) Congenital heart defects – chromosomal anomalies, syndromes and extracardiac malformations. Acta Pediatr 96:1142–1145
2. Bazzani LG, Marcin JP (2007) Case volume and mortality in pediatric cardiac surgery patients in California, 1998–2003. Circulation 115:2652–2659
3. Butera G, Carminati M, Chessa M et al (2006) Percutaneous versus surgical closure of secundum atrial septal defect: comparison of early results and complications. Am Heart J 151:228–234
4. Nilsson B, Mellander M, Sudow G, Berggren H (2006) Results of staged palliation for hypoplastic left heart syndrome: a complete population-based series. Acta Paediatr 95:1594–1600
5. Chock VY, Reddy VM, Bernstein D, Madan A (2006) Neurologic events in neonates treated surgically for congenital heart disease. J Perinatol 26:237–242
6. Warner MA, Lunn RJ, O'Leary PW, Schroeder DR (1998) Outcomes of noncardiac surgical procedures in children and adults with congenital heart disease. Mayo Clin Proc 73:728–734
7. Andropoulos DB, Stayer SA, Skjonsby BS et al (2002) Anesthetic and perioperative outcome of teenagers and adults with congenital heart disease. J Cardiothorac Vasc Anesth 16:731–736
8. Odegard KC, DiNardo JA, Kussman BD et al (2007) The frequency of anesthesia-related cardiac arrests in patients with congenital heart disease undergoing cardiac surgery. Anesth Analg 105:335–343
9. Bennett D, Marcus R, Stokes M (2005) Incidents and complications during pediatric cardiac catheterization. Paediatr Anaesth 15:1083–1088
10. Behnia R, Molteni A, Igic R (2003) Angiotensin-converting enzyme inhibitors: mechanisms of action and implications in anesthesia practice. Curr Pharm Des 9:763–776

11. Khambadkone S, Coats L, Taylor A et al (2005) Percutaneous pulmonary valve implantation in humans: results in 59 consecutive patients. Circulation 112:1189–1197
12. Block PC, Bonhoeffer P (2005) Percutaneous approaches to valvular heart disease. Curr Cardiol Rep 7:108–113
13. Wilson W, Taubert KA, Gewits M et al (2007) Prevention of infective endocarditis. Guidelines from the American Heart Association. Circulation 116:1736–1754
14. Rivenes SM, Lewin MB, Stayer SA et al (2001) Cardiovascular effects of sevoflurane, isoflurane, halothane, and fentanyl-midazolam in children with congenital heart disease. Anesthesiology 94:223–229
15. Oklü E, Bulutcu FS, Yalçin Y et al (2003) Which anesthetic agent alters the hemodynamic status during pediatric catheterization? Comparison of propofol versus ketamine. J Cardiothorac Vasc Anesth 17:686–690
16. Sarkar M, Laussen PC, Zurakowski D et al (2005) Hemodynamic responses to etomidate on induction of anesthesia in pediatric patients. Anesth Analg 101:645–650
17. Ikemba CM, Su JT, Stayer et al (2004) Myocardial performance index with sevoflurane-pancuronium versus fentanyl-midazolam-pancuronium in infants with a functional single ventricle. Anesthesiology 101:1298–1305
18. Hickey PR, Hansen DD, Cramolini GM et al (1985) Pulmonary and systemic hemodynamic responses to ketamine in infants with normal and elevated pulmonary vascular resistance. Anesthesiology 62:287–293
19. Hickey PR, Hansen DD, Strafford M et al (1986) Pulmonary and systemic hemodynamic effects of nitrous oxide in infants with normal and elevated pulmonary vascular resistance. Anesthesiology 65:374–378
20. Journois D, Baufreton C, Mauriat P et al (2005) Effects of inhaled nitric oxide administration on early postoperative mortality in patients operated for correction of atrioventricular canal defects. Chest 128:3537–3544
21. Khazin V, Kaufman Y, Zabeeda D et al (2004) Milrinone and nitric oxide: combined effect on pulmonary artery pressures after cardiopulmonary bypass in children. J Cardiothorac Vasc Anesth 18:156–159
22. Carroll CL, Backer CL, Mavroudis C et al (2005) Inhaled prostacyclin following surgical repair of congenital heart disease – a pilot study. J Card Surg 20:436–439
23. Raja SG, Danton MD, MacArthur KJ, Pollock JC (2007) Effects of escalating doses of sildenafil on hemodynamics and gas exchange in children with pulmonary hypertension and congenital cardiac defects. J Cardiothorac Vasc Anesth 21:203–207
24. Lamarche Y, Perrault LP, Maltais S et al (2007) Preliminary experience with inhaled milrinone in cardiac surgery. Eur J Cardiothorac Surg 31:1081–1087
25. Schmitt HJ, Shuetz WH, Proeschel PA, Jaklin C (1993) Accuracy of pulse oxymetry in children with cyanotic congenital heart disease. J Cardiothorac Vasc Anesth 7:61–65
26. Burrows FA (1989) Physiologic dead space, venous admixture, and the arterial to end-tidal carbon dioxide difference in infants and children undergoing cardiac surgery. Anesthesiology 70:219–225
27. Feller-Kopman D (2005) Ultrasound-guided central venous catheter placement: the new standard of care? Crit Care Med 33:1875–1877
28. Rothschild JM (2001) Ultrasound guidance of central vein catheterization. In: Rothschild JM (ed) Evidence report/technology assessment no. 43. Making health care safer: a critical analysis of patient safety practices. Agency for Healthcare Research and Quality, Rockville, pp 245–253
29. Wigmore TJ, Smythe JF, Hacking MB et al (2007) Effect of the implementation of NICE guidelines for ultrasound guidance on the complication rates associated with central venous catheter placement in patients presenting for routine surgery in a tertiary referral centre. Br J Anaesth 99:662–665
30. Milling TJ, Rose J, Briggs WM et al (2005) Randomized, controlled clinical trial of point-of-care limited ultrasonography assistance of central venous cannulation: the third sonography outcomes assessment program (SOAP-3) trial. Crit Care Med 33:1764–1769

31. Austin EH, Edmonds HL, Auden SM et al (1997) Benefit of neurophysiologic monitoring for pediatric cardiac surgery. J Thorac Cardiovasc Surg 114:707–717
32. Gottlieb EA, Fraser CD Jr, Andropoulos DB, Diaz LK (2006) Bilateral monitoring of cerebral oxygen saturation results in recognition of aortic cannula malposition during pediatric congenital heart surgery. Paediatr Anaesth 16:787–789
33. Andropoulos DB, Diaz LK, Fraser CD Jr et al (2004) Is bilateral monitoring of cerebral oxygen saturation necessary during neonatal arch reconstruction? Anesth Analg 98:1267–1272
34. Andropoulos DB, Stayer SA, McKenzie ED, Fraser CD Jr (2003) Novel cerebral physiologic monitoring to guide low-flow cerebral perfusion during neonatal aortic arch reconstruction. J Thorac Cardiovasc Surg 125:491–499
35. Li J, Van Arsdell GS, Zhang G et al (2006) Assessment of the relationship between cerebral and splanchnic oxygen saturations measured by near-infrared spectroscopy and direct measurements of systemic haemodynamic variables and oxygen transport after the Norwood procedure. Heart 92:1678–1685
36. Berens RJ, Stuth EA, Robertson FA et al (2006) Near infrared spectroscopy monitoring during pediatric aortic coarctation repair. Paediatr Anaesth 16:777–781
37. Bulutcu FS, Ozbek U, Polat B et al (2005) Which may be effective to reduce blood loss after cardiac operations in cyanotic children: tranexamic acid, aprotinin or a combination? Paediatr Anaesth 15:41–46
38. Chauhan S, Das SN, Bisoi A et al (2004) comparison of epsilon aminocaproic acid and tranexamic acid in pediatric cardiac surgery. J Cardiothorac Vasc Anesth 18:141–143
39. Day JR, Taylor KM, Lidington EA et al (2006) Aprotinin inhibits proinflammatory activation of endothelial cells by thrombin through the protease-activated receptor 1. J Thorac Cardiovasc Surg 131:21–27
40. Dietrich W, Ebell A, Busley R, Boulesteix AL (2007) Aprotinin and anaphylaxis: analysis of 12,403 exposures to aprotinin in cardiac surgery. Ann Thorac Surg 84:1144–1150
41. Grocott HP, Sheng H, Miura Y et al (1999) The effects of aprotinin on outcome from cerebral ischemia in the rat. Anesth Analg 88:1–7
42. Mossinger H, Dietrich W, Braun SL et al (2003) High-dose aprotinin reduces activation of hemostasis, allogeneic blood requirement, and duration of postoperative ventilation in pediatric cardiac surgery. Ann Thorac Surg 75:430–437
43. Manno CS, Hedberg KW, Kim HC et al (1991) Comparison of the hemostatic effects of fresh whole blood, stored whole blood and components after open heart surgery in children. Blood 77:930–936
44. Mou SS, Giroir BP, Molitor-Kirsch EA et al (2004) Fresh whole blood versus reconstituted blood for pump priming in heart surgery in infants. N Engl J Med 351:1635–1644
45. Agarwal HS, Bennett JE, Churchwell KB et al (2007) Recombinant factor seven therapy for postoperative bleeding in neonatal and pediatric cardiac surgery. Ann Thorac Surg 84:161–168
46. Delmo Walter EM, Stiller B, Hetzer R et al (2007) Extracorporeal membrane oxygenation for perioperative cardiac support in children I: Experience at the Deutsches Herzzentrum Berlin (1987–2005). ASAIO J 53:246–254
47. Potapov EV, Stiller B, Hetzer R (2007) Ventricular assist devices in children: current achievements and future perspectives. Pediatr Transplant 11:241–255
48. Laliberté E, Cecere R, Tchervenkov C et al (2004) The combined use of extracorporeal life support and the Berlin Heart pulsatile pediatric ventricular assist device as a bridge to transplant in a toddler. J Extra Corpor Technol 36:158–161

Chapter 14

Acute Pain Service: Clinical Assessment and Standard of Care

Joëlle Desparmet

Introduction

Acute pain has long been underestimated and undertreated in children and this is still true in some medical centres. The implementation of acute pain services in pediatric settings has lead to increased understanding and better management of pain in this group of patients. The role of an acute pain service (APS) is to assess pain, provide adequate and safe analgesia by monitoring the effects and treating the side effects of analgesic therapy, to provide information and education about pain, and to perform research in the field of pain and its management. An APS identifies patients at risk of complications, establishes monitoring and treatment guidelines and is available around the clock to intervene. Additionally an APS improves pain management by assessing and treating pain in a timely manner and by raising awareness of the need for adequate analgesia for all patients throughout the hospital. Pain should be considered as the fifth vital sign along with heart rate, respiratory rate, blood pressure and temperature. Pain relief is a basic human right and no one should be left to suffer.

Acute pain is most often nociceptive and results from injury, surgery or an internal disease. Specialized nerve endings called nociceptors attached to nerve fibers (A-delta and C fibers) collect the pain message at the site of injury and forward it to spinal targets and eventually to cortical structures resulting in conscious pain perception and conscious and subconscious responses to the pain. Different receptors and neurochemicals are involved in the transmission of the pain message along the pain pathways. This is why the treatment of acute pain should be multimodal and involve medications which target these different receptors. For example, opioids target μ and κ receptors in the spinal cord, ketamine, NMDA receptors, and nonsteroidal antiinflammatory drugs (NSAIDs) act at the level of cyclooxygenase and prostaglandins. Each potentiates the analgesic potency of the other, thereby reducing the required dose of each medication and the incidence of side effects due to each drug.

It was long thought that infants could not feel pain and that older children did not remember it. Fear of overdosing or complications also prevented adequate pain relief in children. We now know that a fetus has pain systems that are

M. Astuto (ed), *Basics*, Anesthesia, Intensive Care and Pain in Neonates and Children.
ISBN 978-88-470-0654-6 © Springer-Verlag Italia 2009

mature enough to process pain as early as 24 weeks of gestation, and that children who experience pain in early life may develop higher sensitivity to pain and may be more susceptible to chronic pain in their adult years [1–3]. In addition, pharmacokinetic and pharmacodynamic studies of pain medications in children have demonstrated their safety and reliability.

Hence, there is little justification for withholding adequate analgesia from a patient for the sole reason that he is "too young".

Definitions

While the general term of nociception is the perception of a painful sensation, pain can be divided into different categories:
- Somatic pain refers to pain of the musculoskeletal system such as that felt after a bone fracture
- Visceral pain is the pain originating in the internal organs. Pancreatitis is a good example of visceral pain
- Neuropathic pain is initiated or caused by a lesion or dysfunction of the nervous system. Diabetes and drugs used in oncology can cause neuropathic pain.

History of Pain Management

Until the mid-1970s, little was known about pain in children. In 1968, a survey about the use of analgesics in pediatric intensive care departments showed that the proportion of children who received analgesics after general surgery was as low as 3%. Some of the reasons given included, for example, "pediatric patients seldom need relief of pain after general surgery. They tolerate discomfort well". The International Association for the Study of Pain (IASP), founded in 1973–75, became a home base for many pediatric specialists around 1985, and the first international conference on pediatric pain did not take place until 1988 in Seattle, USA. The first books on pain in children were written in the late 1980s.

Development of Nociception in Children

Dorsal horn cells in the spinal cord form synapses with developing sensory neurons by 6 weeks of gestation. Peripheral nerves migrate to the skin of the limbs by 11 weeks and by birth, the density of nociceptive nerve endings is similar to that in adults. Neonates have considerable maturation of peripheral, spinal, and supraspinal afferent pain transmission by 24–26 weeks of gestation and myelination starts at 30 weeks. However, while the nociceptive system is still immature at birth, neonates respond to tissue injury by demonstrating specific behaviors, with hormonal, and metabolic signs of stress and distress.

There are potential long-term consequences for neonates who experience pain. Peripheral nerve injury in neonates can cause rapid and extensive death of the dorsal root ganglion cells which results in major changes within the spinal cord. Repeated painful procedures can affect sensory processing in infants who will exhibit hypersensitivity to touch and to pain following surgery and repeated heel lancing. Taddio et al. [4] demonstrated a stronger pain response to routine immunizations at 4 and 6 months in infants who had been circumcized at birth without EMLA cream.

Developmental Pharmacology

The pharmacokinetics and dynamics of analgesics change during development of the child. Different hepatic enzymes mature at different rates so there is a lower clearance of drugs at birth. The composition of the body compartments changes, and renal and hepatic functions develop so that at birth there is an increased duration of action of drugs due to an increased volume of distribution and slow elimination. The concentration of plasma proteins changes after birth: α1-glycoproteins, the main proteins to which local anesthetics bind, are low at birth and do not reach normal levels until 1 to 2 months of age. Thus, dosing intervals should be increased to avoid accumulation. Due to decreased ventilatory reflexes, there is an increased potential for respiratory pauses and apnoea and an increased risk of hypoventilation, hypoxemia and atelectasis. This should always be taken into consideration when prescribing analgesics to small children.

A new field of research, pharmacogenetics, explores the role of genetics in the pharmacology of drugs. Patients have genetically different forms of cytochromes, which can influence the metabolism of drugs and their interaction with other drugs. This would explain why, for instance, some patients do not have pain relief after receiving large doses of codeine.

Clinical Assessment of Pain

It is likely that pain will be undertreated if it is not assessed appropriately and regularly. Pain should be considered as the fifth vital sign and as such be measured as often and as thoroughly as temperature, blood pressure, heart rate and respiratory rate. Assessment of pain must be age-appropriate, easy and quick to implement at the bedside, and result in a reasoned and prompt adjustment of the analgesic dose.

Children often do not have the means to express pain as an adult patient would, and scales to measure pain in this group of patients must take into account their age and their cognitive development. Toddlers at age 2 years can say if they have pain or not and say that they have a little, some or a lot of pain. Children as young as 4 years can report pain. Most can understand that they have pain, but the quantification of the pain is more difficult for them. For instance, when given an equal number of chips to represent units of pain, some children thought that when the chips were placed in a line the number of chips was greater than when the chips were placed in a pile, while others thought the opposite. This difference in visual evaluation is an example of the impact of the choice of scale used to quantify pain in children. By the age of 5 years, children can understand simple ratios and use interval pain scales like the visual analogue scales (VAS), faces scales and numerical scales.

Assessment of pain relies on two groups of measures: physiological parameters and behavioral factors. Physiological parameters such as increases in heart rate, respiratory rate and blood pressure and the presence of sweating, high cortisol and cortisone levels, and endorphin concentrations are all responses to pain, but they are nonspecific. Thus behavioral scales are the primary pain scoring methods for neonates, infants, children under 4 years of age or children who cannot communicate verbally. These scales rely on facial expressions (crying, grimacing), motor responses, guarding, and verbal responses. An example of such a scale is shown in Table 14.1.

Self-report scales and VAS are available to measure pain in children. Typically, self-report will be used in older children. VAS, the faces pain scale (Fig. 14.1), and the Oucher (colored pictures of one child's face arranged vertically to show increasing levels of discomfort) are self-report measures of pain that are commonly used following surgery in children. With the faces scale, the child chooses the face that corresponds to how he feels. On the other side of the scale, there is the pain score for that face. Children older than 6 or 7 years can

Table 14.1 FLACC (face, legs, activity, cry, consolability) scale. The highest score is 10, but a score above 5 signifies pain that needs to be treated

	0	1	2
Face	No particular expression or smile	Occasional grimace or frown, withdrawn, disinterested	Frequent to constant quivering chin, clenched jaw
Legs	Normal position or relaxed	Uneasy, restless, tense	Kicking, or legs drawn up
Activity	Lying quietly, normal position, moves easily	Squirming, shifting back and forth, tense	Arched, rigid or jerking
Cry	No cry (awake or asleep)	Moans or whimpers; few complaints	Crying steadily, screams or sobs, frequent complaints
Consolability	Content, relaxed	Reassured by touching, hugging, or being talked to, distractable	Difficult to console or comfort

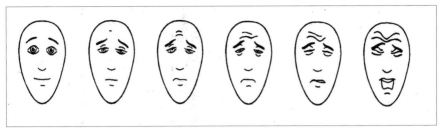

Fig. 14.1 Faces pain scale. On the other side of the scale there is the score corresponding to each face

understand VAS. Faces scales and the Oucher are better for younger children.

The FLACC (face, legs, activity, cry, consolability) and CHEOPS (Children's Hospital of Eastern Ontario pain scale) are behavioral scales that are used for infants and very young children. Unfortunately, there is a disparity between these scales and self-report scales. In fact, behavioral scales tend to underestimate severe pain.

Scales are important tools for the measurement of pain, but do not provide absolute pain scores. For instance, a score of 5/10 in one child could be equivalent to 9/10 in another. What is more important is the score as it evolves during the day, before and after the administration of an analgesic, or with movement and at rest. Based on these changes in pain scores, the dose of analgesic will be increased or modified. This explains the importance of establishing an APS that is able to manage pain within a continuum of care.

Management of Pain

The management of pain should provide maximum pain relief with minimum side effects. Multimodal analgesia is an approach that uses the synergistic effect of analgesics from different families of drugs, resulting in a decreased need for each drug and thus a decreased incidence of side effects from each. It can also apply to drugs given by different routes such as a regional block and rectal or oral medication.

Nociception is the result of four processes: transduction is the conversion of a noxious stimulus into an electrical signal, transmission is the propagation of this signal along the pain pathways, modulation describes the process by which the pain signal is modified by various nerve endings, and perception is the subjective experience of pain that is influenced by cognitive, emotional and cultural factors. Most analgesics exercise their effect on one of the first three of these processes and associating one or more of these drugs will result in all of these processes being affected.

The best example of the synergistic effect of drugs is the morphine-sparing effect of certain drugs. Korpela et al. [5] studied the effect of three target doses of acetaminophen on the need for morphine postoperatively in children. With the addition of rectal acetaminophen, the percentage of children who did not need morphine two hours after surgery went from 10% with no acetaminophen to a significant 60% with 40 mg/kg and 80% with 60 mg/kg.

Analgesics

Analgesic drugs can be divided into minor, moderately active or major analgesics.

Acetaminophen is in the first category, but given with moderate or major analgesics it can enhance analgesia [5].

Acetaminophen is the most commonly prescribed analgesic in children. Its mechanism of action is primarily through the inhibition of cyclooxygenase. It can be given orally or rectally. Birmingham et al. [6] studied the pharmacokinetics of rectal acetaminophen and found that an initial dose of 30 mg/kg is needed to achieve therapeutic serum concentrations of 10–20 µg/ml. Although the optimum dose of acetaminophen in children has not been determined, the commonly recommended dose range is 10 to 15 mg/kg orally. In another study, Birmingham et al. found that a loading dose of 40 mg/kg rectally followed by 20 mg/kg every 4 to 6 hours depending on the child's age provides blood levels of acetaminophen that are well below toxic concentrations with no accumulation during 24 hours [7]. Hepatic failure has rarely been reported with high doses of acetaminophen in children who had severe infections, and it is wise to administer acetaminophen for short periods in these patients.

Opioids are indicated for moderate to severe pain. Pain relief occurs when a minimum effective analgesic concentration (MEAC) is achieved in the serum. In order to reach the MEAC, intermittent boluses, continuous infusions or both can be delivered via a patient-controlled analgesia (PCA) pump. The MEAC of opioids differs from one patient to another and varies from day to day in the same patient. Lynn et al. found that the MEAC of morphine in children following cardiac surgery is between 12 and 25 ng/ml. Below this range there may not be adequate pain relief and above side effects such as respiratory depression may occur. This concentration requires a loading dose of 0.05–0.1 mg/kg and an infusion rate 0.01–0.03 mg/kg per hour. In fact, in the study of Lynn et al., a serum level of 30 ng/ml did not affect baseline respiration [8].

The elimination of morphine is dependent on the age of the child. The elimination half-life is an average of 9 hours in preterm neonates, 6.5 hours in term neonates and 2 hours in infants and children. This shows that intervals between doses compared to those in children should be increased fourfold in premature babies and two to three fold in newborns.

Particular care should be given when prescribing opioids to newborns as they have a number of reasons to have complications. They have a decreased metabolism of opioids due to immature liver conjugation and renal filtration. Thus there is a risk of accumulation of drug in the blood after repeated administration of opioids or excessive infusion rates. Because they have low protein-binding capacity due to low α1-glycoprotein levels and low albumin levels until 1 month of age, they have an increased free drug fraction. This unbound drug crosses the blood–brain barrier more easily and exposes newborns to opioid-induced seizures. Newborns also have a decreased ventilatory response to hypoxia and hypercarbia. In fact, newborns respond to hypercarbia by apnoea rather than an increase in respiratory rate. For all these reasons doses of opioids should be decreased and given at longer intervals, and infusion of morphine should not exceed 10 µg/kg per hour. The doses of morphine for PCA are shown in Table 14.2.

The risk factors for respiratory depression in children receiving morphine are age below 12 months, renal or hepatic insufficiency, pulmonary disease, obstructive sleep apnoea such as seen in children with chronic enlarged tonsils, neuromuscular and neurological disorders, obesity and interactions with sedative medication. These patients are at an increased risk of respiratory depression and should be particularly monitored.

NSAIDs inhibit the biosynthesis of prostaglandins by inactivation of cyclooxygenase, which is necessary for the conversion of arachidonic acid to prostaglandin endoperoxides. This process reduces the prostaglandins mediating inflammation as well as those involved with homeostatic functions such as platelet aggregation, renal blood flow, protection of the gastric mucosa and osteoblastic activity.

Ketorolac, one of the few intravenous forms of NSAIDs with diclofenac, has been studied in children. It was shown that a dose between 0.3 and 0.5 mg/kg is as effective for analgesia as higher doses and is associated with fewer side effects. Watcha et al. showed that ketorolac used alone for minor surgery (myringotomy) decreased pain scores, decreased the need for supplemental analgesics and was superior to 10 mg/kg acetaminophen and placebo [9]. Munro et al. studied nausea and vomiting after strabismus surgery and found that the administration of 0.75 mg/kg of ketorolac resulted in less nausea and vomiting than 0.1 mg/kg morphine with metoclopramide [10]. When given with opioids

Table 14.2 Dose and interval of administration of opioids used for patient-controlled analgesia

Drug	Dose	Interval (min)	Basal rate	Break-through pain
Morphine	0.02 mg/kg	6–10	0.004 mg/kg/h	0.04 mg/kg every 10 min up to three doses every 2 h
Hydromorphone	0.004 mg/kg	6–10	0.001 mg/kg/h	0.008 mg/kg
Fentanyl	0.5 µg/kg	6–8	0.1 µg/kg/h	0.4 µg/kg
Nalbuphine	0.02 mg/kg	6–10	0.004 mg/kg/h	0.04 mg/kg

after major surgery, NSAIDs improve postoperative pain, reduce the need for additional opioids by 30% and reduce opioid-related side effects [11, 12]. Splinter et al. compared the local infiltration of the wound with ketorolac (1 mg/kg) to a caudal block for analgesia after inguinal hernia repair. They found that the pain scores, the incidence of nausea and vomiting and the time to ambulation were lower in the ketorolac group [13]. In a study of the efficacy of ketorolac in suppressing bladder spasms after ureteral reimplantation, 25% of patients receiving ketorolac experienced bladder spasms compared with 83% of those receiving placebo [14].

NSAIDs should not be used in patients with a history of peptic ulceration or gastrointestinal hemorrhage, in those with hemorrhagic diathesis, a reaction to aspirin or NSAIDs, renal impairment or hypovolemia, or in those on anticoagulants, or after an operation associated with a high risk of postoperative bleeding.

Adjuvants

Some medications, while not used alone for analgesia, are used to potentiate other analgesics. Ketamine and clonidine are such drugs.

Ketamine is a noncompetitive antagonist at NMDA receptors sites. It has analgesic properties at subanesthetic doses and reduces central sensitization to a painful stimulus. A single bolus dose of 0.15 mg/kg of ketamine decreases morphine requirements after arthroscopic knee ligament repair. There are few studies on the use of ketamine in children, but they all show the benefit of adding ketamine to an analgesic regimen after surgery. Marcus et al. found that children who received ketamine had greater pain scores at 30 minutes after surgery compared to those who received morphine, but the same pain scores after 4 hours. Side effects were the same in both groups and the incidence of bad dreams was low in both groups [15].

Clonidine is a partial agonist of alpha-2 adrenergic receptors that are found at the presynaptic site of nerve endings and noradrenergic neurons in the central nervous system and postsynaptically in the liver, pancreas, kidneys and platelets. Its mean half-life of elimination is 12 hours, and it has no active metabolites. It can be administered via the rectal, oral, transdermal, neuraxial or parenteral route. Its bioavailability is 100% orally and 95% rectally. Clonidine given as a premedication in children at a dose of 3–4 µg/kg, provides preoperative sedation and enhances postoperative analgesia [16, 17], reduces the hemodynamic response to intubation [18] and reduces the MAC of halothane and sevoflurane [19, 20]. It decreases the incidence of vomiting [21] and reduces the response to atropine and the hyperglycemic response to stress [22, 23].

Given as an adjuvant to caudal anesthesia, clonidine increases the duration of postoperative analgesia by 50–114% and decreases analgesic requirements. It has no effect on the incidence of vomiting or urinary retention, but does increase the level of sedation [24–26].

Regional Techniques

Regional anesthesia is a well-established technique for postoperative analgesia in children. An APS is essential to evaluate and optimize its efficacy and to monitor and treat side effects. The most common regional blocks followed by a pediatric APS are continuous epidural or caudal blocks, and continuous peripheral blocks, usually femoral or brachial plexus blocks.

The doses of local anesthetics are shown on Table 14.3. A low concentration of local anesthetic (0.1–0.125%) provides the same duration and quality of postoperative analgesia as bupivacaine 0.25% with less motor blockade. The pharmacokinetic parameters of local anesthetics are different in infants compared to older children. Infants up to 1 month of age have low levels of $\alpha 1$-glycoproteins, the main protein that binds to local anesthetics. Unbound, free molecules of local anesthetic enter cardiac and nerve cells more easily leading to greater toxicity. The volume of distribution of local anesthetics is greater in children and the half-life of elimination is longer so that there is a risk of accumulation in newborns, infants and small children. Infusion rates should be halved in this age group.

Berde and Sethna [27] conducted a survey of toxicity of local anesthetics in children and infants with the Anesthesia Patient Safety Foundation. They found reports of convulsions in ten patients. Three infants had independent risk factors but the other seven received bupivacaine at infusion rates above 0.5 mg/kg per hour.

A mixture of a low concentration local anesthetic and an opioid (morphine or fentanyl) provides adequate analgesia with few side effects. The most frequent side effects of epidural opioids are pruritus, nausea and vomiting, sedation and urinary retention. Pruritus is frequent, and an infusion of low-dose naloxone (1 µg/kg per hour) is sufficient to eliminate this side effect. Because urinary retention occurs in 50–80% of children, a urinary catheter should be placed systematically as long as the epidural infusion is administered. The incidence of these side effects increases with the concentration of opioid. Glensky et al. [28] showed that an increase in epidural morphine does not improve analgesia but increases the incidence of side effects (Table 14.4).

Table 14.3 Maximum recommended doses for regional blockade

Drug	Dose		Infusion rate (mg/kg/h)
	Plain (mg/kg)	With epinephrine (mg/kg)	
Lidocaine	5	7	0.8–1.6
Bupivacaine	2–2.5	2.5–3.0	0.2–0.40
Ropivacaine	0.5–2.5		0.1–0.6

Table 14.4 Increase in side effects with dose of epidural morphine. From [28]

Dose of morphine (µg/kg)	Duration of analgesia (h)	Frequency of side effects (%)
<100	12.1	0
100–150	10.1	2.9
>150	11.2	5.4

The incidence of respiratory depression is low and varies according to its definition. In pediatric studies, respiratory depression has been defined as respiratory rate of less than eight per minute, the need for naloxone, or a reduction in the ventilation/end-tidal CO2 (Ve/PetCO2) slope. The risk of respiratory depression increases with intrathecal administration of opioids, especially with greater dose, and with administration of intravenous opioids as well as intrathecal or epidural opioids.

Adjuvants may be added to prolong the duration of analgesia. Clonidine increases the duration and quality of analgesia but can lead to over-sedation. Ketamine has been studied in adult patients, but not in children.

Monitoring

Monitoring of children receiving analgesia is an essential role of an APS. Guidelines for the management of these patients should be developed with the nursing staff in order to ensure safe conditions. A prescription for an analgesic regimen, whether a PCA or a continuous block, should always include a prescription for the treatment of possible side effects. Patients should be evaluated throughout the day and night to detect and treat side effects in a timely manner. Someone should be available 24 hours a day to attend to changes in the need for medication or to adapt a treatment.

Infants and patients at risk of respiratory depression should be particularly monitored for apnoea and signs of toxicity. Oxygen saturation, heart rate, respiratory rate via an apnoea monitor, and blood pressure should be monitored continuously. A fidgety baby could be experiencing local anesthetic toxicity rather than increased pain, and particular attention should be given to maximum doses of medications in this age group.

A pediatric APS should be composed of physicians and one or more nurses specializing in the management of acute pain in children. The service should be available at all times and ensure continuity of care. Children should be evaluated by the members of the APS at least two to three times a day or more if needed. Pain scores, sedation scores side effects and vital signs should be recorded hourly. Modifications are brought to the analgesic regimen based on those data. Precise guidelines indicating medications, dosing, treatment of side effects and troubleshooting interventions should be developed with the collaboration of nursing staff on the wards, the hospital pharmacy and the surgical and medical staff responsible for the patients. Education and quality assurance are essential duties of the APS so that pain management can be improved at all levels.

Conclusion

Efficient and safe postoperative analgesia is available to children of all ages providing repeated evaluations, precise dosing according to weight and age and strict safety precautions are followed. An APS provides 24-hour coverage and ensures safe conditions. It also provides education and support to the nursing staff and physicians in training concerning the management of pain. Pain is the fifth vital sign and as such is evaluated, recorded regularly and treated just as a decrease in blood pressure would be treated. An APS provides the most efficient means to manage pain successfully.

References

1. Anand KJ, Aynsley-Green A (1985) Metabolic and endocrine effects of surgical ligation of patent ductus arteriosus in the human preterm neonate: are there implications for further improvement of postoperative outcome? Mod Probl Paediatr 23:143–157
2. Anand KJ (1998) Clinical importance of pain and stress in preterm neonates. Biol Neonate 73:1–9
3. Anand KJ, Hickey PR (1987) Pain and its effects in the human neonate and fetus. N Engl J Med 317:1321–1329
4. Taddio A, Katz J, Ilersich AL et al (1997) Effect of neonatal circumcision on pain response during subsequent routine vaccination. Lancet 349:599–603
5. Korpela R, Korvenoja P, Meretoja OA et al (1999) Morphine-sparing effect of acetaminophen in pediatric day-case surgery. Anesthesiology 91:442–447
6. Birmingham PK, Tobin MJ, Henthorn TK et al (1997) Twenty-four-hour pharmacokinetics of rectal acetaminophen in children: an old drug with new recommendations. Anesthesiology 87:244–252
7. Birmingham PK, Tobin MJ, Fisher DM et al (1997) Initial and subsequent dosing of rectal acetaminophen in children. Anesthesiology 94:385–389
8. Lynn AM, Opheim KE, Tyler DC (1984) Morphine infusion after pediatric cardiac surgery. Crit Care Med 12:863–866
9. Watcha MF, Ramirez-Ruiz M, White PF et al (1992) Perioperative effects of oral ketorolac and acetaminophen in children undergoing bilateral myringotomy. Can J Anaesth 39:649–654
10. Munro HM, Riegger LQ, Reynolds PI et al (1994) Comparison of the analgesic and emetic properties of ketorolac and morphine for paediatric outpatient strabismus surgery. Br J Anaesth 72:624–628
11. Vetter TR, Heiner EJ (1994) Intravenous ketorolac as an adjuvant to pediatric patient-controlled analgesia with morphine. J Clin Anesth 6:110–113
12. Gillies GW, Kenny GN, Bullingham RE et al (1987) The morphine sparing effect of ketorolac tromethamine. A study of a new, parenteral non-steroidal anti-inflammatory agent after abdominal surgery. Anaesthesia 42:727–731

13.   Splinter WM, Reid CW, Roberts DJ et al (1997) Reducing pain after inguinal hernia repair in children: caudal anesthesia versus ketorolac tromethamine. Anesthesiology 87:542–546

14.   Park JM, Houck CS, Sethna NF et al (2000) Ketorolac suppresses postoperative bladder spasms after pediatric ureteral reimplantation. Anesth Analg 91:11–15

15.   Marcus RJ, Victoria BA, Rushman SC et al (2000) Comparison of ketamine and morphine for analgesia after tonsillectomy in children. Br J Anaesth 84:739–742

16.   Ramesh VJ, Bhardwaj N, Batra YK et al (1997) Comparative study of oral clonidine and diazepam as premedicants in children. Int J Clin Pharmacol Ther 35:218–221

17.   Lavrich PS, Hermann D, Pang LM et al (1996) Clonidine as a premedicant in children. Anesthesiology 85:A1085

18.   Mikawa K, Maekawa N, Azano M (1995) Attenuation of the catecholamine response to tracheal intubation with oral clonidine in children. Can J Anaesth 42:869–874

19. Nishina K, Mikawa K, Maekawa N et al (1996) The efficacy of clonidine for reducing perioperative haemodynamic changes and volatile anaesthetic requirements in children. Acta Anaesthesiol Scand 40:746–751

20.   Nishina K, Mikawa K, Shiga M et al (1997) Oral clonidine premedication reduces minimum alveolar concentration of sevoflurane for tracheal intubation in children. Anesthesiology 87:1324–1327

21.   Mikawa K, Nishina K, Maekawa N et al (1995) Oral clonidine premedication reduces vomiting in children after strabismus surgery. Can J Anaesth 42:977–981

22.   Nishina K, Mikawa K, Maekawa N et al (1995) Oral clonidine premedication blunts the heart rate response to intravenous atropine in awake children. Anesthesiology 82:1126–1130

23.   Nishina K, Mikawa K, Maekawa N et al (1998) Effects of oral clonidine premedication on plasma glucose and lipid homeostasis associated with exogenous glucose infusion in children. Anesthesiology 88:922–927

24.   Jamali S, Monin S, Begon C et al (1994) Clonidine in pediatric caudal anesthesia. Anesth Analg 78:663–666

25.   Lee JJ, Rubin AP (1994) Comparison of a bupivacaine-clonidine mixture with plain bupivacaine for caudal analgesia in children. Br J Anaesth 72:258–262

26.   Klimscha W, Chiari A, Michalek-Sauberer A et al (1998) The efficacy and safety of a clonidine/bupivacaine combination in caudal blockade for pediatric hernia repair. Anesth Analg 86:54–61

27.   Berde CB, Sethna NF (2002) Analgesics for the treatment of pain in children. N Engl J Med 347:1094–1103

28.   Glenski JA, Warner MA, Dawson B, Kaufman B (1984) Postoperative use of epidurally administered morphine in children and adolescents. Mayo Clinic Proc 59:530–533

Chapter 15

Anesthesia Outside the Operating Room

Teresa Valois

Scope of the Problem

Sedation for children outside the operating room has been the subject of numerous discussions in the last 20 years, especially for pediatric anesthesiologists. Among the reasons why this was and continues to be an important topic (Fig. 15.1) for us are:

- An increase in the number and type of procedures outside and inside the operating room (OR), versus a decreased or equal number of anesthesiologists available, all scheduled as day surgery
- An increase in the demand for special conditions to produce better images/results (e.g. MRI, dentistry)
- An Increase in the complexity of cases due to an increase in survival rates of children with complex pathology.

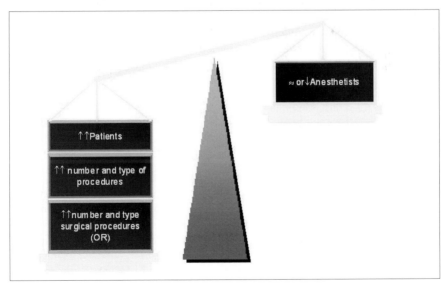

Fig. 15.1 The scope of off-site sedation problems

M. Astuto (ed), *Basics*, Anesthesia, Intensive Care and Pain in Neonates and Children.
ISBN 978-88-470-0654-6 © Springer-Verlag Italia 2009

Nonanesthesiologists face the challenge of performing procedures in children that generally require sedation, and they need to guarantee optimal conditions in the face of the unavailability of enough anesthesiologists to provide sedation services.

Some of the solutions suggested [1] include: sedation services [2], trained nursing personnel, sedation rooms, sedation team (combining provider types). Sedation recipes have not been successful, and are not recommended, as careful evaluation and patient selection is required before administering sedation or anesthetic drugs, to avoid adverse outcomes.

This chapter is addressed to anesthesiologists and discusses current definitions of sedation, techniques and complications.

Historical Background

Following reports of several sedation mishaps (including death) associated with sedation procedures provided by nonanesthesiologists in the early 1980s [3–7], the first sedation guidelines were developed by Coté et al. [1, 6]. Three definitions were included: conscious sedation, deep sedation, and general anesthesia. Later in 1992 [7], the Committee on Drugs of the American Association of Pediatrics (AAP), published revised guidelines in which pulse oximetry was recommended for all patients undergoing sedation and no sedation was to given by parents at home [5]. In 2002 an addendum eliminated the term "conscious sedation" [8] and it was suggested that the guidelines apply to any location (including hospitals). Also, the concept of patient rescue was introduced.

Finally, in 2006 the AAP and American Association of Dentists joined forces and published guidelines for monitoring and management of pediatric patients during and after sedation and therapeutic procedures [9]. Around the same time (2004), the Scottish Intercollegiate Guidelines Network published guidelines [10] aimed at improving sedation practices. Both guidelines reiterate the importance of proper preparation, proper evaluation, appropriate skills to rescue the patient, and proper recovery.

Current Definitions

Four criteria are used to determine the level of sedation [11]:
1. *Responsiveness*: normal response, purposeful response to verbal or tactile stimulation, purposeful response following repeated or painful stimulation, and unarousable.
2. *Airway*: unaffected, no intervention required, intervention may be required, and intervention often required.
3. *Spontaneous ventilation*: unaffected, adequate, may be adequate, and frequently inadequate.
4. *Cardiovascular function*: unaffected, usually maintained, usually maintained, and may be impaired.

Based on these criteria, there are four levels of sedation depth [11]:

1. *Minimal sedation* [5, 12] (anxiolysis): a drug-induced state in which patients respond normally to verbal commands. Although cognitive function and coordination may be impaired, ventilatory and cardiovascular functions are unaffected.

2. *Moderate sedation/analgesia* [11]: a drug-induced depression of consciousness in which patients respond purposefully to verbal commands, either alone or accompanied by light tactile sensation. No interventions are required to maintain a patent airway and spontaneous ventilation is adequate. Cardiovascular function is usually maintained.

3. *Deep sedation/analgesia* [5, 11]: a drug-induced depression of consciousness in which patients cannot be easily aroused but respond purposefully following repeated or painful stimulation. The ability to independently maintain ventilatory function may be impaired. Patients may require assistance in maintaining a patent airway, and spontaneous ventilation may be inadequate. Cardiovascular function is usually maintained.

4. *General anesthesia*: a drug-induced loss of consciousness during which patients are not arousable, even by painful stimulation. The ability to independently maintain ventilatory function is often impaired. Patients often require assistance in maintaining a patent airway, and positive pressure ventilation may be required because of depressed spontaneous ventilation or drug-induced depression of neuromuscular function. Cardiovascular function may be impaired.

These definitions are summarized in Table 15.1.

Table 15.1 Continuum of the depth of sedation: definition of general anesthesia and levels of sedation/analgesia [11]

	Minimal sedation (anxiolysis)	Moderate sedation/analgesia (conscious sedation)	Deep sedation/analgesia	General anesthesia
Responsiveness	Normal response to verbal stimulation	Purposeful[a] response to verbal or tactile stimulation	Purposeful[a] response after repeated or painful stimulation	Unarousable, even with painful stimuli
Airway	Unaffected	No intervention required	Intervention may be required	Intervention of ten required
Spontaneous ventilation	Unaffected	Adequate	May be inadequate	
Cardiovascular function	Unaffected	Usually maintained	Usually maintained	May be impaired

[a]Reflex withdrawal from a painful stimulus is not considered a purposeful response

The provider of the sedation should be capable of rescuing the patient from the next depth level. For example, when providing moderate sedation, the person should be able to recognize, manage and rescue the patient from deep sedation analgesia. As stated in the ASA document:

"Because sedation is a continuum, it is not always possible to predict how an individual patient will respond. Hence, practitioners intending to produce a given level of sedation should be able to rescue[1] patients whose level of sedation becomes deeper than initially intended. Individuals administering Moderate Sedation/Analgesia ("Conscious Sedation") should be able to rescue patients who enter a state of Deep Sedation/Analgesia, while those administering Deep Sedation/Analgesia should be able to rescue patients who enter a state of General Anesthesia." [11]

Anesthesia Considerations

A stepwise approach will ensure that shortcuts are not taken, and safety is not compromised. The general goals of a sedation service are outline in Figure 15.2. The major goals [1] of the sedation procedure itself are:

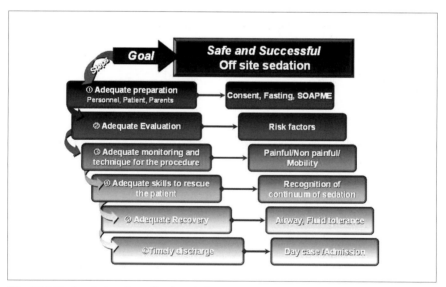

Fig. 15.2 Goal and steps in pediatric sedation

---

[1] "Rescue of a patient from a deeper level of sedation than intended is an intervention by a practitioner proficient in airway management and advanced life support. The qualified practitioner corrects adverse physiologic consequences of the deeper-than-intended level of sedation (such as hypoventilation, hypoxia and hypotension) and returns the patient to the originally intended level of sedation." [9]

- Anxiety relief
- Pain control
- Control of excessive movement.

Consent for sedation/anesthesia should be obtained prior to any procedure, diagnostic or therapeutic. The risks and possible complications are discussed and any questions from the parents or patient are addressed in detail. When assessing the patient a thorough medical and sedation history should be obtained.

Patients with an ASA physical status (PS) [13] of I and II can be sedated on an outpatient basis. Patients with an ASA PS III and higher should be hospitalized and sedation provided by anesthesia as these patients are at higher risk of respiratory adverse events [14–16]. Despite the fact that ASA PS is not the best tool for classifying patients (high interobserver variability), it gives an estimate of the risk related to sedation.

Patients with the following risk factors are not good candidates for sedation by a nonanesthesiologist, and when appropriate should be assessed before the procedure by an anesthesiologist (preanesthetic consultation):

- Craniofacial malformations
- Known difficult airway
- Cervical spine instability
- Trisomy 21 (Down syndrome): these patients are difficult to sedate and are at higher risk of paradoxical reactions [17]
- Ex-premature children
- Children younger than 1 year
- Syndromes
- Respiratory tract infections
- Respiratory and/or cardiac failure [10]
- Increased intracranial pressure [10]
- Neuromuscular disease [10]
- Bowel obstruction
- Known allergy to sedative [10]
- Previous adverse reactions [10]
- Obstructive sleep apnea [18]
- Anticonvulsants or opioid therapy [10]
- Emergency cases [10].

Patient fasting guidelines (Table 15.2) [19] are the same as for general anesthesia.

The acronym SOAPME underscores the proper preparation procedure [20]:

Suction
Oxygen
Airway equipment
Pharmaceutical (medications)
Monitors
Equipment (special)

Table 15.2 Fasting guidelines

Ingested material	Minimum fasting period (h)
Clear fluids[a]	2
Breast milk	4
Infant formula	6
Nonhuman milk	6
Light meal[b]	6

[a]For example, water, fruit juices without pulp, carbonated beverages, clear tea, black coffee.
[b]A light meal typically consists of toast and clear liquids. Meals that include fried or fatty foods or meat may prolong gastric emptying time. Both the amount and type of foods ingested must be considered when determining an appropriate fasting period.

Whenever a general anesthesia is planned, standard monitors should be applied. Pulse oximetry is mandatory and capnography is highly recommended [20].

Medications

Multiple approaches have been described in the literature for sedation, especially for nonpainful procedures, such us MRI or CT scan. The options include: propofol, propofol/remifentanil, midazolam/ketamine, ketamine, pentobarbital, chloral hydrate, dexmedetomidine, midazolam/fentanyl. In a recent phone survey in Canada, Usher and Kearney [21] found that total intravenous anesthesia (TIVA) is used predominantly and airway instrumentation was less likely in these circumstances. In institutions in which a volatile technique was used, a laryngeal mask airway (LMA) was more commonly inserted. The dose of propofol ranges from 2 to 6 mg/kg and 100 to 250 µg/kg/min. Safety is still a concern with the use of nasal prongs with TIVA or propofol boluses [21]. At the Montreal Children's Hospital, for MRI and CT scans, TIVA and inhalational techniques are used according to the preference of the anesthesiologist. For hematology procedures (bone marrow biopsies and lumbar punctures), intravenous induction with propofol and maintenance with sevoflurane is the most common practice. Radiotherapy and PET scans are done solely with TIVA.

There are many reports mainly in the United States literature of the use of dexmedetomidine, an α-2 agonist more potent than clonidine and of shorter half life. Among its advantages are: short duration of action, preservation of spontaneous ventilation and analgesic properties [22–24]. However, severe bradycardia has been reported following bolus administration [25–27]. Midazolam, although a useful drug, particularly when combined with opioids (fentanyl, morphine, meperidine), is associated with an increased risk of hypoxemia and hypotension

[28, 29]. Paradoxical reactions are also of concern [30–36]. The use of mela-tonin as a sedative has been reported, but with no success for MRI procedures [37]. Atropine is highly recommended as, as well as its antisialagogic effect, it may enhance the upper airway dilator muscles [38].

Nonpharmacological techniques are also part of the armamentarium of the anesthesiologist. Parental presence seems to decrease sedative requirements [10], although it is not always helpful and evidence of its benefits is still scarce [39–42]. Preparation for the procedure has been shown to be helpful [43, 44], as it provides both parents and the child with coping tools. Hypnosis and virtual reality might be used in older children [45–47]. Some of these techniques may become popular, especially in view of reports that as many as 54% of patients may have maladaptive behaviors postoperatively [40].

Adverse Events

Life-threatening adverse events such as respiratory depression and hypoxemia may have long-term consequences. The incidence varies in the literature, depending on the sedation provider (anesthesiologist, sedation nurse, emergency physician), location (radiology department, emergency department, gastroen-terologist's office, dentist's office, etc), and procedure performed (endoscopy, scan, fracture reduction, etc). The real incidence is difficult to determine. The overwhelming majority of critical events are preventable and are caused by oper-ator error or lack of robust rescue systems when incidents do occur [1, 4]

Blike et al. [48] reported, from a database of adverse events created in 2005, one adverse event per 29 patients (Table 15.3). The expected incidence of a seda-tion-induced crisis should be in the order of one in tens of thousands [49]. The most common adverse event in this database was prolonged sedation and recov-ery. Laryngospasm was in third place. Although not the most common adverse event, when looked at with the number of unplanned treatments (see Table 15.4), is clear that appropriate airway skills and ability to recognize airway obstruction are necessary for sedation providers.

Hypoxemia during sedation has been reported to occur in 2.9% of procedures [15] and is more common in patients with ASA PS III and IV. Failed sedation occurs in approximately 7% of procedures and inadequate sedation ranges from 0.29 (1 in 338 patients) [1] to 16% [15]. Older children, ASA PS III and IV, and the use of benzodiazepines as sole agent have been associated with failed seda-tion [15].

Future

Sedation procedures will continue to increase, and the training of nonanesthesi-ologists to provide safe sedation seems to be one possible approach. This should be guided and supervised by anesthesiologists, as we possess the expertise in air-

Table 15.3 Sedation adverse events (1 per 29 patients [49])

Event	Per 10,000 patients
Cardiac arrest	0.3
Aspiration	0.3
Hypothermia	1.3
Laryngospasm	4.3
Prolonged sedation	13.6
Prolonged recovery	22.3

Table 15.4 Unplanned treatments (1 per 89 patients [49])

	Per 10,000 patients
Reversal agent	1.7
Emergency anesthesia consultation	2
Admission to hospital	7
Intubation required	9.7
Bag mask ventilation	63.9

way management, pharmacology, integrated physiology and crisis management, and such procedures are part of our daily routine. Also, anesthesia has been a pioneer specialty in the medical field in working with a systems approach, and integrating critical events analysis, taken mostly from the aviation industry, and this has made anesthesia one the safest specialties. Simulation, as has been used for many years in aviation, is a very useful tool in training and preparing personnel for critical incident recognition and management, as well as for developing good communication skills that are needed when working in a team [48, 50].

Multicenter and/or international registries for documentation of critical events are needed to provide a better picture of current practices and sedation pitfalls [48].

New drug developments, such as dexmedetomidine, are encouraging, although better powered studies are needed. Recent reports of the effects of anesthetics on brain development may influence current sedation practices, although it is not possible currently to predict how they will be influenced.

In summary, anesthesiology departments are strongly encouraged to participate actively in the creation of sedation guidelines for their own hospitals. Having a clear mission (see Fig. 15.2), steps to achieve it, and continuous quality assurance evaluations will improve current sedation practices and help us face the challenging increase not only in the number of patients but also in the locations and procedures where our services are required.

References

1. Cravero JP, Blike GT (2004) Review of pediatric sedation. Anesth Analg 99:1355–1364
2. Litman RS (2005) Sedation by non-anesthesiologists. Curr Opin Anaesthesiol 18:263–264
3. Coté CJ, Karl HW, Notterman DA et al (2000) Adverse sedation events in pediatrics: analysis of medications used for sedation. Pediatrics 106:633–644
4. Coté CJ, Notterman DA, Karl HW et al (2000) Adverse sedation events in pediatrics: a critical incident analysis of contributing factors. Pediatrics 105:805–814
5. American Society of Anesthesiologists Task Force on Sedation and Analgesia by Non-Anesthesiologists (2002) Practice guidelines for sedation and analgesia by non-anesthesiologists. Anesthesiology 96:1004–1017
6. Committee on Drugs and Section on Anesthesiology (1985) Guidelines for the elective use of conscious sedation, deep sedation, and general anesthesia in pediatric patients. Pediatrics 76:317–321
7. American Academy of Pediatrics Committee on Drugs (1992) Guidelines for monitoring and management of pediatric patients during and after sedation for diagnostic and therapeutic procedures. Pediatrics 89:1110–1115
8. Coté CJ (2001) "Conscious sedation": time for this oxymoron to go away! J Pediatr 139:15–17
9. Coté CJ, Wilson S (2006) Guidelines for monitoring and management of pediatric patients during and after sedation for diagnostic and therapeutic procedures: an update. Pediatrics 118:2587–2602
10. Scottish Intercollegiate Guidelines Network (2004) Safe sedation of children undergoing diagnostic and therapeutic procedures. A national clinical guideline. Scottish Intercollegiate Guidelines Network, Edinburgh. http://www.sign.ac.uk/pdf/sign58.pdf
11. American Society of Anesthesiologists (2004) Continuum of depth of sedation definition of general anesthesia and levels of sedation/analgesia. American Society of Anesthesiologists, Park Ridge, IL. http://www.asahq.org/publicationsAndServices/standards/20.pdf
12. American Society of Anesthesiologists Task Force on Sedation and Analgesis by Non-Anesthesiologists (1996) Practice guidelines for sedation and analgesia by non-anesthesiologists. Anesthesiology 84:459–471
13. Aplin S, Baines D, De Lima J (2007) Use of the ASA Physical Status Grading System in pediatric practice. Paediatr Anaesth 17:216–222
14. Malviya S, Voepel-Lewis T, Tait AR (1997) Adverse events and risk factors associated with the sedation of children by nonanesthesiologists. Anesth Analg 85:1207–1213
15. Malviya S, Voepel-Lewis T, Eldevik OP et al (2000) Sedation and general anaesthesia in children undergoing MRI and CT: adverse events and outcomes. Br J Anaesth 84:743–748
16. Maxwell LG, Tobias JD, Cravero JP, Malviya S (2003) Adverse effects of sedatives in children. Expert Opin Drug Saf 2:167–194
17. Baum VC, O'Flaherty JE (2006) Anesthesia for genetic metabolic and dysmorphic syndromes of childhood. Lippincott, Williams & Williams, Philadelphia
18. American Society of Anesthesiologists Task Force on Perioperative Management of Patients with Obstructive Sleep Apnea (2006) Practice guidelines for the perioperative management of patients with obstructive sleep apnea. http://www.asahq.org/publicationsAndServices/sleepapnea103105.pdf
19. American Society of Anesthesiologist Task Force on Preoperative Fasting (1999) Practice guidelines for preoperative fasting and the use of pharmacologic agents to reduce the risk of pulmonary aspiration: application to healthy patients undergoing elective procedures. http://www.asahq.org/publicationsAndServices/NPO.pdf
20. Coté CJ (2007) Pediatric sedation and adverse events (How we got from there to here). Department of Anesthesia, Harvard University, Boston. Conference Proceedings
21. Usher A, Kearney R (2003) Anesthesia for magnetic resonance imaging in children: a survey of Canadian pediatric centres. Can J Anaesth 50:425
22. Koroglu A, Demirbilek S, Teksan H et al (2005) Sedative, haemodynamic and respiratory

effects of dexmedetomidine in children undergoing magnetic resonance imaging examination: preliminary results. Br J Anaesth 94:821–824

23. Rosen DA, Daume JT (2006) Short duration large dose dexmedetomidine in a pediatric patient during procedural sedation. Anesth Analg 103:68–69

24. Heard CM, Joshi P, Johnson K (2007) Dexmedetomidine for pediatric MRI sedation: a review of a series of cases. Paediatr Anaesth 17:888–892

25. Berkenbosch JW, Tobias JD (2003) Development of bradycardia during sedation with dexmedetomidine in an infant concurrently receiving digoxin. Pediatr Crit Care Med 4:203–205

26. Finkel JC, Quezado ZM (2007) Hypothermia-induced bradycardia in a neonate receiving dexmedetomidine. J Clin Anesth 19:290–292

27. Hammer GB, Drover DR, Cao H et al (2008) The effects of dexmedetomidine on cardiac electrophysiology in children. Anesth Analg 106:79–83

28. Pitetti R, Davis PJ, Redlinger R et al (2006) Effect on hospital-wide sedation practices after implementation of the 2001 JCAHO procedural sedation and analgesia guidelines. Arch Pediatr Adolesc Med 160:211–216

29. Litman RS (1996) Airway obstruction after oral midazolam. Anesthesiology 85:1217–1218

30. Massanari M, Novitsky J, Reinstein LJ (1997) Paradoxical reactions in children associated with midazolam use during endoscopy. Clin Pediatr (Phila) 36:681–684

31. McGraw T, Kendrick A (1998) Oral midazolam premedication and postoperative behaviour in children. Paediatr Anaesth 8:117–121

32. Kumar SS (2000) Premedication with midazolam in pediatric anesthesia. Anesth Analg 90:498

33. Kain ZN, Mayes LC, Wang SM, Hofstadter MB (1999) Postoperative behavioral outcomes in children: effects of sedative premedication. Anesthesiology 90:758–765

34. Malviya S, Voepel-Lewis T, Prochaska G, Tait AR (2000) Prolonged recovery and delayed side effects of sedation for diagnostic imaging studies in children. Pediatrics 105:E42

35. Finley GA, Stewart SH, Buffett-Jerrott S et al (2006) High levels of impulsivity may contraindicate midazolam premedication in children. Can J Anaesth 53:73–78

36. Stewart SH, Buffett-Jerrott SE, Finley GA et al (2006) Effects of midazolam on explicit vs implicit memory in a pediatric surgery setting. Psychopharmacology (Berl) 188:489–497

37. Sury MR, Fairweather K (2006) The effect of melatonin on sedation of children undergoing magnetic resonance imaging. Br J Anaesth 97:220–225

38. Brown K (2007) Pediatric considerations in sedation for patients with the obstructive sleep apnea syndrome. Semin Anesth 26:94–102

39. Kain ZN, Caldwell-Andrews AA, Krivutza DM et al (2004) Trends in the practice of parental presence during induction of anesthesia and the use of preoperative sedative premedication in the United States, 1995–2002: results of a follow-up national survey. Anesth Analg 98:1252–1259

40. Kain ZN, Mayes LC, Wang SM et al (1998) Parental presence during induction of anesthesia versus sedative premedication: which intervention is more effective? Anesthesiology 89:1147–1156

41. Kain ZN, Caldwell-Andrews AA, Wang SM et al (2003) Parental intervention choices for children undergoing repeated surgeries. Anesth Analg 96:970–975

42. Kain ZN, Caldwell-Andrews AA, Mayes LC et al (2003) Parental presence during induction of anesthesia: physiological effects on parents. Anesthesiology 98:58–64

43. Bellew M, Atkinson KR, Dixon G, Yates A (2002) The introduction of a paediatric anaesthesia information leaflet: an audit of its impact on parental anxiety and satisfaction. Paediatr Anaesth 12:124–130

44. Kain ZN, Caldwell-Andrews AA, Mayes LC et al (2007) Family-centered preparation for surgery improves perioperative outcomes in children: a randomized controlled trial. Anesthesiology 106:65–74

45. Boswinkel JP, Litman RS (2005) Sedating patients for radiologic studies. Pediatr Ann 34:650–654, 656

46. Dexter F, Yue JC, Dow AJ (2006) Predicting anesthesia times for diagnostic and interventional radiological procedures. Anesth Analg 102:1491–1500
47. Kazak AE, Penati B, Brophy P, Himelstein B (1998) Pharmacologic and psychologic interventions for procedural pain. Pediatrics 102:59–66
48. Blike GT, Christoffersen K, Cravero JP et al (2005) A method for measuring system safety and latent errors associated with pediatric procedural sedation. Anesth Analg 101:48–58
49. Cravero JP, Blike GT, Beach M et al (2006) Incidence and nature of adverse events during pediatric sedation/anesthesia for procedures outside the operating room: report from the Pediatric Sedation Research Consortium. Pediatrics 118:1087–1096
50. Farnsworth ST, Egan TD, Johnson SE, Westenskow D (2000) Teaching sedation and analgesia with simulation. J Clin Monit Comput 16:273–285

Chapter 16

Tracheotomy in Children

Giuliana Rizzo, Paolo Murabito, Francesca Rubulotta, Carmela Cutuli,
Massimiliano Sorbello, Marinella Astuto

Introduction

Tracheotomy in children is a relatively uncommon and high-skill procedure,
which is generally performed if ventilator support is required for months to
years [1, 2]. Although the procedure is difficult and challenging to perform, it is
truly rewarding to access a safe and protected airway. However, the issue
remains complex from the psychosocial point of view, for both the growing child
and the caregivers and family members [3].

Definition and Anatomy

Tracheotomy is a surgical procedure that opens up the windpipe (trachea). It is
performed in an emergency situation, in the operating room, or at the bedside of
a critically ill patient. The term tracheostomy is sometimes used interchange-
ably with tracheotomy. Strictly speaking, however, tracheostomy refers to the
opening itself, while a tracheotomy is the actual operation. Compared with the
anatomy of the adult trachea, pediatric anatomy is different and rapidly changing, bearing in mind that tracheotomy is performed in patients over the whole
pediatric age range from preterm babies to children in the late teenage years [4].

Anatomy is the most intricate problem from the surgical point of view because
of both the small dimensions of the pediatric trachea and interindividual variations. Compared with adult patients, the hyoid bone, and the thyroid and cricoid
cartilages lie higher in the neck, and are particularly difficult to palpate and to distinguish in the small neck of a child, and this may be even more complicated by
the quite common presence of a fat pad in the anterior neck region [5–7].

In contrast to the anatomy in adults, different structures might lie in the lower
neck region of pediatric patients, such as the innominate artery, the left brachio-
cephalic veins, the apices of the lungs and thymus residuals. Therefore, particularly
if neck hyperextension is requested, a low tracheotomy is rarely formed in a child.
Furthermore, recurrent laryngeal nerves lie lateral to the trachea, and so they might
be damaged accidentally especially in patients with deviation from the midline.

Last but not least, it must be underlined that in pediatric patients the trachea
is a developing structure, so whatever the procedure it should be treated as gen-

M. Astuto (ed), *Basics*, Anesthesia, Intensive Care and Pain in Neonates and Children.
ISBN 978-88-470-0654-6 © Springer-Verlag Italia 2009

tly as possible, with the main aim of minimizing long-term damage. The optimal tracheal incision for tracheotomy in children is therefore a vertical incision through the second to fourth tracheal cartilages, as a "higher" tracheotomy might damage either the first tracheal or the cricoid cartilage, with an increased risk of formation of an anterior flap, resulting in a higher risk of post-tracheotomy stenosis [8]. In fact a horizontal incision or a vertical incision that is too short might result in tracheal stricture due to posterior dislocation of the cartilages, and similarly in the percutaneous technique, postprocedural stenosis could be due to fracture or rupture of the cartilages which might occur during the dilational phase [9].

Surgical Technique

The child is placed supine, the head fixed and the neck moderately hyperextended by the use of a small pillow under the shoulders. A lidocaine-adrenaline solution is then infiltrated above the sternal notch to provide anesthesia and vasoconstriction. Mechanical ventilation is maintained through the existing tracheal tube.

A small horizontal incision is created to provide the future stoma. The subcutaneous fat pad is removed and underlying muscles are picked up and dissected in layers in the midline. Once reached, the thyroid gland can be either retracted superiorly or incised in the midline and ligated or electrically cauterized. As soon as the trachea is exposed, one monofilament stay suture is placed on each side of the intended vertical tracheotomy. They should be fixed with tape and clearly indexed (i.e. "left" and "right") and clearly labeled with a "do not remove" warning [10]. The trachea is then incised vertically in the midline between the second and fourth ring, with an extension of at least two rings, and the tracheotomy cannula is positioned while withdrawing the endotracheal tube. Other alternatives are to make a horizontal incision, to excise a part of the anterior tracheal wall, or to create an inferiorly-based tracheal flap [3–6].

Starplasty tracheotomy is a new technique based on the geometry of a three-dimensional Z-plasty [11]: an "X"-shaped incision is made half way between the sternal notch and the cricoid cartilage, the triangular skin flaps are undermined and subcutaneous fat removed. After careful tracheal dissection a "+"-shaped incision is formed in the anterior tracheal wall, while suturing the tips of the tracheal flaps to the troughs of the skin flaps and, in turn, the troughs of the tracheal flaps to the tips of the skin flaps. The tracheotomy cannula is then inserted and fixed securely with a cotton tape tied around the neck and, differently from the standard surgical technique, the cannula is not sutured to the skin. Recent reports [12] suggest that this technique is better than the standard technique in preventing serious complications in pediatric tracheotomy, particularly pneumothorax and death from accidental decannulation, and in reducing the incidence of tracheal stenosis after tracheotomy. Because of the design of the procedure, patients who undergo decannulation will have a persistent tracheocutaneous fistula that may require secondary reconstruction after decannulation [13].

The main concern when performing a pediatric tracheotomy is the choice of the correct tube size [14]. The tube should be small enough to allow the child to speak and yet not so small that a large insufflation leak causes hypoventilation, especially during sleep. Unlike adults, children need to have their tracheotomy tube size increased as they grow. A comprehensive paper by Behl and Watt [14] concludes that the classic Cole's formula [15] can be adapted to choose the right cannula diameter: ID = (age in years/3) + 3.5; OD = (age in years/3) + 5.5 (*ID*, inner diameter; *OD*, outer diameter). An interesting alternative might be preoperative ultrasound assessment of the airway diameters [16].

Although representing a far away problem to be solved [17], the surgical vs percutaneous question is also relevant for pediatric tracheotomy [18]. The percutaneous technique, described as an alternative to the surgical approach, was first described by Sheldon et al. [19], whereas the first percutaneous technique was described by Ciaglia et al. [20], whose method, which is based on progressive dilatation with blunt-tipped dilators, is the most frequently used. In 1997 Fantoni and Ripamonti [21] described the so-called translaryngeal technique, in which an armored tracheal cannula is pulled outwards through the oral cavity, larynx and trachea. The procedure is performed under direct endoscopy, via a rigid or flexible bronchoscope. Although both percutaneous and translaryngeal techniques have been used in children, the latter is probably more suitable for use in children, especially in those below 10 years of age, because of the high pliability of the cartilaginous frame. Lack of external compression of the trachea minimizes the possibility of collapse of the tracheal walls [13].

As an alternative in children less than 4 years old, a Melker cricothyrotomy set (COOK), either cuffed or uncuffed, might be used, while in children more than 10–11 years old with normal anthropometric features, regular small size adult sets can be used. In younger children, despite endoscopic control, anatomical landmarks are more difficult to define with precision, and the trachea is smaller and consequently more difficult to fix and puncture. Moreover, the smallest currently available commercial sets include a 5.5-mm outer diameter tube, therefore limiting the age of patient in whom the percutaneous approach can be performed to 4–5 years. The PercuTwist (Teleflex Medical) for the Frova percutaneous technique is actually available in sizes 7, 8 and 9, but it should be readily available in a pediatric version to be used in small children ranging from 4 years of age.

Whatever the chosen technique, endoscopic control (either rigid or flexible) is mandatory before, during and after the procedure, in order to assess the risks, evaluate intraoperative complications and maneuvers and assess follow-up, respectively [8, 13, 22, 23].

In experienced hands, the percutaneous approach is a safe and effective alternative to standard tracheotomy, so that it has almost replaced this technique in adult ICUs [24]. Undoubtedly, some advantages of the percutaneous technique (such as safety, shorter performance time, bedside feasibility without patient transport, lower periprocedural bleeding, need for less dissection and consequently lower stomal infection rate and less severe aesthetic consequences) [25] might encourage its use in the pediatric population.

On the other hand the main concerns still limiting its use are the risk of posterior tracheal wall lesions (depending on the technique) and difficult to control bleeding, the easily collapsible nature of pediatric tracheal structures (thus limiting the application of excessive external pressure), the limited percutaneous sets availability, the suggested high incidence of postprocedural stenosis, fistulas, granuloma and cartilage necrosis [8], and finally the risks due to accidental decannulation and difficult/impossible cannula reinsertion [26].

Experience with percutaneous pediatric tracheostomy is limited to a few reports, and it is highly characterized by descriptions of complications. Toursarkissian et al. [22] used a nonendoscopic guided procedure with three complications over 11 procedures (patient ages 10–20 years). Scott et al. report two cases of tracheal stenosis after the use of the Ciaglia multiple dilator technique [8], while Silvia Bárbara et al. [23] report the safe use of the Ciaglia Blue Rhino method with endoscopic guidance in adolescents, concluding that this technique can be considered safe in expert hands and using endoscopic control. Fantoni and Ripamonti [21] report a series of translaryngeal tracheotomy done in very young patients, including infants of only a few months of age. They found the technique to have a high level of intrinsic safety and to be perfectly suitable to the anatomy of the child.

In conclusion, the percutaneous technique is still rarely used in children, either because tracheotomy is less often performed in children than in adults or because of the lack of appropriate methods and/or equipment. It seems to be a safe, quick and simple bed-side procedure, and associated with a low rate of complications and stoma infections.

No percutaneous technique should be attempted in an emergency if the diameter of the larynx is too small in relation to the size of the available tracheotomy tube, if there was a previous direct trauma to the larynx, and in cases of active papillomatosis or hemangioma. Surgical tracheostomy remains fully justified in critical situations [13].

Postprocedural Chest Radiography

Postoperative radiography after tracheotomy is generally indicated for two purposes: the first is for detection of complications (such as pneumothorax, pneumomediastinum) and the second is control of the cannula tip position. The second issue has clearly been resolved by perioperative and follow-up endoscopic control [7], while the first still remains a matter of debate.

Published rates of pneumothorax in children vary, but were low in a recent large series: 1.3% for pneumothorax, 0.8% for pneumomediastinum, and 0.5% for subcutaneous emphysema, although in some series higher values have been reported (10–17% vs. 0–4% in adults) [7]. For these reasons, while it is generally accepted that periprocedural complications are higher in children than in adults, some authors do suggest routine use of postoperative chest radiography [7], while others do not recommend its routine use considering it unnecessary and expensive, and to have a low sensitivity [27, 28], while highlighting the importance of a careful and complete clinical examination.

Probably, considering the risky nature of pediatric tracheotomy, all kinds of controls, including clinical, endoscopic and radiographic, should be performed routinely, particularly in emergency, difficult and high-risk cases.

Complications

Tracheotomy-related complication can be divided into early (intraoperative up to 1 week) and late (after 1 week) complications [9, 26, 29–31]. Tracheotomy-related mortality was very high in the 1940s and 1950s (5–10%) [2], while it actually ranges from 5% to 39% if considered globally (including underlying conditions and diseases) and from 0 to 3% for the procedure itself [29, 32–35].

Morbidity and periprocedural complications (see Table 16.1) occur in 20% to 90% of patients [3, 5, 8, 32, 35–37], especially in emergency situations and in infants, and might occur in up to 70% of premature and very low birth weight patients [34–41]. Complications and morbidity are lower in adults with both the percutaneous and the standard open technique than in children [7, 42].

Table 16.1 Complications of pediatric tracheotomy [30] (multiple complications occur in 35.9% of patients [29])

Early (13.6%)	Late (15.5%)
Intraoperative death	Innominate artery erosion
False passage	Stomal cellulitis
Tube plugging[a]	Suture abscess
Decannulation	Stomal granuloma
Bleeding	Keloid formation
Subcutaneous emphysema	Cartilage necrosis
Pneumomediastinum[a]	Tracheitis
Pneumothorax[a]	Tracheal stenosis
Aspiration pneumonia	Tracheocutaneous fistula
	Tracheoesophageal fistula

[a]More frequently reported complications [21]

Early Complications

- *Obstruction*: Mucus and crusts might easily obstruct the inner lumen of the cannula, especially in small children requiring a small diameter cannula [43]. Obstruction remains one of the most frequent complications, and prompt suctioning and adequate hydration and inhaled gas humidification result in a lower incidence of this potentially fatal complication.
- *Apnea*: Apnea may occur due to the sudden reduction of dead space (loss of upper airway anatomical dead space) especially in children with chronic airway obstruction or central breathing control impairment.
- *Accidental decannulation*: Accidental decannulation can be extremely dangerous in the first days after tracheostomy, as the stoma is not yet formed and stable. The stay suture is therefore the optimal solution to increase safety and allow prompt recannulation, as if left in place and easily accessible, it allows immediate identification and access to the stoma.
- *Air leak*: This complication might occur if the stoma is not tightly adherent to the cannula, in cases of wide neck dissection and fat pad removal, or after sudden unexpected traction on the cannula. The consequence is typically subcutaneous emphysema, generally easily treated by correcting the source of the leak. However, in some cases air leak can lead further to the development of pneumomediastinum or pneumothorax which can be life-threatening complications requiring immediate surgical treatment.
- *Pneumothorax/pneumomediastinum*: These complications are possible consequences of air leak or of a defective surgical approach, especially for low tracheotomies.
- *False passage*: This complication is typically a consequence of a (difficult) cannula exchange in the first days after tracheotomy. It might result in airway loss, obstruction, hemodynamic consequences and death if not recognized and promptly treated.
- *Hemorrhage*: Early hemorrhage is typically due to a defective surgical approach, to an undetected vascular abnormality, or to insufficient care in cauterization. Treatment might be either topical or surgical, with emergent access to the operating theatre.

Late Complications

- *Obstruction*: In the later phase, obstruction might be due to granuloma formation or to mucus plugs. Granulomas might occur at the site of the stoma or above it, within the tracheal lumen, resulting in either obstruction or dangerous bleeding during tube exchange maneuvers, requiring emergency surgical treatment [8].
- *Acquired tracheoesophageal/tracheocutaneous fistula*: This is a rare compli-

cation in the pediatric population generally occurring in less than 1% of cases. It is due to the cuff being overdistended, prolonged use, and use in combination with a stiff nasogastric tube. The high metabolic state of patients along with associated injuries and infection, hypotension and steroid administration also increase the likelihood of developing this complication [35, 44].

- *Hemorrhage*: Late hemorrhage is generally due to friction against and continuous erosion of close blood vessels, particularly an abnormal innominate artery. The consequences are generally catastrophic, as this rare complication generally occurs late after tracheotomy, when the child is no longer in a safe and protected environment such as a hospital ward.
- *Infections*: Different infections might affect either the lungs or the tracheostomy. As observed in adults [24], local infections are generally more frequent with the open technique than with the percutaneous technique due to the tighter adhesion of the stoma with the latter. Severe forms might include suture abscess, stomal cellulitis, and deep chest infections.

One of the most challenging factors regarding late complications is that they can occur long after hospital discharge in the domiciliary setting, thus exposing the child to a higher risk of unskilled help far from the safe hospital environment [32, 45].

Postprocedural tracheal stenosis seems to occur, according to Walz, in up to 30% of patients, but is clinically relevant in 1–5% of patients [24]. Unfortunately, although in most case series postprocedural stenosis has been reported to occur in less than 1% of children [8], even minimal stenosis which would have been undetected and asymptomatic in an adult may produce clinical symptoms in a child because of the smaller tracheal diameter.

Cannula Exchange

In the first week, tube exchange or accidental decannulation might be quite easily managed thanks to the stay sutures. They allow safe tube exchange which is generally performed once a week in the first period after tracheotomy. However, tube exchange might be required more frequently.

After the stay sutures are removed, cannula exchange could be dangerous and difficult, and reintroduction might be difficult even weeks after the tracheotomy [8]. For this purpose a smaller internal diameter tracheal tube, a small suction catheter or dedicated airway exchange catheters should be used for any preplanned exchange [46], remembering that the stoma route is almost vertical due to the anatomical features of pediatric patients [10]. A light hyperextension obtained with a small pillow under the shoulders might be helpful. The stoma should be inspected at any tube exchange, and the procedure should always be performed in a fasted child.

Early Decannulation

After a tracheotomy has been performed, the opening must be kept patent with a tube. The size and style of the tube chosen will vary according to the size of the trachea and the needs of the individual patient. The most common materials used for tracheotomy tubes are polyvinyl chloride (PVC) or PVC-based (siliconized PVC), silver and silicone. Silver is expensive, but durable because it withstands repeated cleaning and sterilizing procedures. PVC and silicone tubes are disposable, although the inner cannula can be cleaned and some can be reused several times in the same patient. These tubes are lighter than the silver tubes and some soften at body temperature, which can make them more comfortable to wear. PVC or silicone tubes are always used when radiotherapy is given to an area that includes the tracheotomy, because the presence of metal in the treated area can result in tissue necrosis. These tubes have an enormous range of features, from decannulation plugs through to speaking attachments for cuffed tubes.

Tracheotomy suctioning is carried out by nurses and is supervised by the Pediatric Tracheostomy Team. It is needed to maintain a clear airway and normal breathing sounds and pattern, without exaggerated effort or awareness of the sensation of breathing and without causing trauma or hypoxia. Suctioning needs to be carried out when the patient is unable to clear his or her own secretions, or is only able to clear them into the tracheotomy tube with cough-like mechanisms.

The removal of the tube is called decannulation and can take place from days to months after surgery, but never until the patient breathes with the tube occluded for 24 hours continuously. If the tube has been in place for any significant length of time, occlusion is carried out gradually to determine the patient's ability to breathe with the tracheotomy closed and to help him or her become accustomed, psychologically and physically, to breathing without the tube. Strategies used to work toward decannulation include reducing the size of the tube at each tube change, use of a fenestrated tube (allowing the patient to breathe through the larynx, whereas the external tube opening can be blocked by a speaking valve or decannulation plug), and blocking the tube with a 'cork' or capping device, or a decannulation plug, for varying and increasing lengths of time [29, 34, 37, 38, 41–43, 47].

Irrespective of the method used, close observation for respiratory distress is necessary. The tube should not be removed until a full and continuous 24-hour period has passed without the tube being used for respiration. Once the tube is removed, a firm, airtight dressing should be applied to prevent air entering and escaping the tracheostomy site and to promote healing. A small tube and tracheal dilators should be available at the bedside for a minimum of 48 hours after removal in case respiratory distress occurs.

Speaking Valve

Children of all ages, including infants, may be candidates for the use of a speaking valve. A tracheostomy speaking valve offers another option for voice production with a tracheostomy tube. A speaking valve is a one-way removable valve that is attached to the open end of the tracheostomy tube. Speaking valves that are used in children include: the Passy-Muir speaking valve (Passy-Muir, Irvine, CA), the Shiley Phonate speaking valve (Nellcor Puritan Bennett, Pleasanton, CA), and the Montgomery tracheostomy speaking valve (Boston Medical Products, Westborough, MA) [4].

There are some contraindications to the use of a speaking valve; these include:
- the presence of severe tracheal or laryngeal obstruction
- a laryngectomy
- the use of an inflated cuffed tracheotomy tube
- the presence of excessive secretions that cannot be managed adequately
- gross aspiration
- bilateral adductor vocal cord paralysis
- serious illness
- an unconscious state.

Indications for Tracheotomy in Children

Over the years, indications for tracheotomy in children have changed. During the period 1960 to 1970, the primary indication was acute inflammatory upper airway obstruction (diphtheria, epiglottitis and laryngotracheobronchitis) [47]. With improvement in neonatal and pediatric intensive care services and survival of critically sick children after prolonged intubation and ventilation, subglottic stenosis is now becoming a major indication for tracheotomy with neurological impairment and prolonged ventilation [2–4, 10, 35]. In the late 1960s and early 1970s, patients intubated for ventilation often had tracheotomies within 48 hours of intubation. Over the years however, the duration of intubation, especially in neonates and infants, has increased to several weeks before tracheotomy is done [3, 47. 48]. Arcand and Granger reported 19 tracheotomized patients who were intubated for an average of 29 days prior to tracheotomy. Of these patients, seven developed subglottic stenosis after a mean intubation period of 40 days [48].

Other important factors which contribute to the development of postintubation subglottic stenosis include:
- movement of the tube
- number of reintubations required
- trauma at the time of intubation
- size and material of the tube
- prematurity
- the presence of upper airway infection
- gastroesophageal reflux disease.

There is also a definite reduction in the number of tracheotomies required in pediatric patients [49]; Wetmore et al. found no difference in the number of tracheotomies performed in their center between the period 1971–1980 (37.5 cases per year) and the period 1981–1992 (42 cases per year), but found a declining incidence of tracheotomy in relation to the number of hospital admissions [50]. Symptoms of airway obstruction often do not appear until several weeks after the primary insult and extubation. The symptom-free interval between extubation and appearance of obstructive symptoms may vary. Even the opinion as to the (expected) intubation period after which a child is tracheotomized has changed fundamentally within the last 30 years. In the 1970s it was recommended that a patient receive a prophylactic tracheotomy if it was foreseeable that the patient would have to be ventilated for more than 8 days. Today, the period after which a patient is tracheotomized is increasingly determined individually [4].

More recent studies recommend that the indication for pediatric tracheotomy should also be decided individually according to clinical and endoscopic findings [4]. The intubation periods in these studies ranged from 2 to 134 days (average 31 days). However, this remains a matter of controversy, and many pediatric intensive care departments still have the rule to do tracheotomy in case of prolonged intubation. Other conditions requiring tracheotomy, which have been seen with increasing frequency, are tracheal stenosis and microtrachea, respiratory papillomatosis, caustic alkali ingestion, and craniofacial syndromes. The incidence of tracheotomy in some conditions has fallen: subglottic hemangioma is now often treated by endoscopic intralesional injection of steroids or submucosal excision via an external approach, avoiding the need for tracheotomy. Similarly, short laryngeal clefts can be repaired endoscopically [4].

How to Approach the Indication for Tracheotomy

With the increasing complexity of the underlying medical problems, the decision to tracheotomize a child has become an interdisciplinary process involving intensive care and pulmonology specialists, pediatric otorhinolaryngologists, pediatric surgeons, social care workers, and respiratory nurses. The attitudes of patients and care-givers influence the choice of treatment just as much as socioeconomic factors, funding, and the availability of professional support at home.

Pediatric Tracheotomy Management

Training for Care-givers

A structured training protocol, tailored to the needs of the individual child and equipment, has proved to be useful. The achievements of the trainee care-givers are monitored step by step in an appropriate record book.

Education is started preferably before elective tracheotomy. Topics include indications for tracheotomy, the relevant anatomy and physiology, and differences from 'normal' breathing. Models, drawings and videos provide support for understanding the often complex situation. During the postoperative period, parents are encouraged to spend as much time as possible with their child in order to gain confidence in mastering the expected challenge of having a child with a tracheotomy at home.

Feeding, bathing, lifting the child out of bed, cuddling and carrying are demonstrated and gradually taken over by the parents. Once they feel confident with handling their child, teaching progresses to stoma and tube care as well as to monitoring vital signs. Special emphasis is directed towards a correct suction technique, and mock emergency situations and the appropriate resuscitation measures are discussed and practiced over and over again. The equipment purchased for domiciliary care should already be used on the ward to practice correct handling, cleaning, maintenance and troubleshooting.

Once all necessary knowledge and skills have been obtained and the child is ready to go home, the care-givers are admitted together with their child onto a side ward, where they can practice the home situation day and night and see for themselves whether they are competent and confident enough. An emergency package should be kept with the child at all times. This must contain spare tubes one the same size and the other one size smaller, scissors, ties, suction catheters, normal saline, gloves and an Ambubag with appropriate mask, together with an information card to quickly identify brand, size and length of the tube, catheter insertion depth, the reason for the tracheotomy, potential individual risks, and the names and telephone numbers of physicians, therapists, nurses, and service and maintenance companies [51–53].

Preparing the Home Environment

The home into which a child with a tracheotomy is to be discharged often needs adaptation that has to be planned with the help of the health-care team well in advance [54]. Additional electricity sockets around the bed and in the child's living area, as well as extra space for storing disposable utensils, are needed. Bath/shower facilities must be adapted to provide safety and to suit both child and care-givers. Occasionally, a clever rearrangement of rooms will substantially facilitate care-giving and monitoring. In case of room-sharing by siblings, consideration must be given to the disturbance of the other child by alarms and the various care measures. Transporting the child together with all necessary equipment often calls for adaptation of stairs, car seats, prams, etc.

Well before discharge, communication with the family doctor, pediatrician, pharmacist, nurse specialist, and when applicable also the speech pathologist and physiotherapist as well as the equipment supplier should be established. A telephone connection and power supply must be secured [51, 55].

Instructions to Parents

Parents should be instructed to avoid all dust, smoke, lint, pet hair, powder, sprays, small toys, and objects. The child should not be in contact with furry toys, clothes, or bedding. Contact sports and water sports are not permitted. The child may be bathed in 1–2 inches (2–5 cm) of water with a trained care-giver in attendance. Showers may be permissible for older children. Be aware of and participate in goals and planning of the feeding program, occupational therapy, physical therapy, and speech therapy.

Parents should be aware of and participate in the planning for return to school/classes and any out-of-home arrangements, e.g. day-care. Children who are at most risk of a serious episode of tracheotomy obstruction are younger patients who do not yet attend school; in older, school-aged children who have a critical airway in which the risk of obstruction is high, a trained care-giver should be in attendance throughout transport to and from school and at school, and should be aware of monitoring needs, if prescribed, and able to operate the monitor correctly and act on the information in accordance with the decannulation plan [51, 52].

Family Environment

Home tracheotomy care is a considerable burden and challenge for any family [54, 55]. A commitment to provide optimal care in the home and a conviction that home care is best for the child's social, communication and motor development helps care-givers cope with this challenge and strive for a family life as near normal as possible. As a prerequisite for tracheotomy home care, care-givers have to acquire the necessary knowledge and become competent in a spectrum of practical skills [53].

Once the child is at home, parental responsibility is massive; anxiety and preparedness for an emergency may cause substantial stress. Increased attention to the child and insecurity concerning disciplinary measures can cause jealousy and resentment in the rest of the family; social isolation as well as physical and emotional overload may follow. To prevent burn-out, additional care-givers have to be recruited and trained, and community resources made available. It often helps care-givers to consult with support groups and establish links with other families who have successfully cared for a child with a tracheotomy [56]. Provision needs to be made well in advance for accommodating the child in play group, kindergarten and school. When, due to the underlying pathology, voice generation fails, other ways of communication, such as an electrolarynx, sign language or a letter board, need to be considered in order prevent isolation of the child and family.

In summary, caring for a child with a chronic tracheotomy in the home provides a challenge that can be met by optimal medical management, motivated care-givers, adequate training and education, a well-prepared and equipped home environment, support from the extended family and community, and well-established communication with the health-care team. With these prerequisites, domiciliary tracheotomy care is as safe as, and in many other aspects superior to, long-term hospitalization.

Focus on Pediatric Tracheostomy Teams

The number of pediatric tracheostomy teams (PTT) is increasing. Initiatives from the Australian and New Zealand Intensive Care Society, organizations in the US including the Institute for Healthcare Improvement, the American Medical Association, the Joint Commission on the Accreditation of Healthcare Organizations, the Association of American Medical Colleges, and the Robert Wood Johnson Foundation, and other national and international groups, highlight the role of the tracheostomy team as conceptually related to rapid response systems (RRS). The intent of a RRS is to prevent harm and death in patients deteriorating in hospitals. The RRS, and therefore the PTT, were a relatively unknown concept several years ago, while they are now an expected standard of care in many health-care organizations [57].

The PTT should ideally focus on triggers to rescue the very sick child or the child at risk in a timely manner, and on in-hospital and at-home tracheotomy patients. In 2005, during the First International Conference on RRS, experts established that the RRS should include four components: event recognition and response trigger (afferent arm), provision of personnel and equipment resources (efferent arm), initiation of improvement activities post hoc, and administration of infrastructure to support the entire system [58]. Over the last decade several teams have been identified and improved such as: the medical emergency team, the outreach team, the sepsis team, the tracheostomy team, etc. [58]. The ideal PTT is composed of a trained group of health-care practitioners (doctors, nurses, psychologists and social workers) who respond to crises outside the emergency room or the intensive care unit. The purpose of the PTT is to improve patient outcome, considering that hospital safety has been clearly recognized to represent a leading element in the improvement of hospital quality [59].

In particular, children who have a tracheotomy tube require specialist care and education from a number of disciplines during their hospital stay. Most patients will have the tracheotomy tube removed before going home, but some will need the tube long term. Those living in the community with a tracheotomy tube require ongoing assistance and support. The Tracheostomy Review and Management Service (TRAMS) is a specialist service introduced at Austin Health, Victoria, Australia, in 2002. A team of doctors, nurses, physiotherapists and speech pathologists coordinate and direct the care of patients with a tracheotomy tube across three campuses and into the community. The team has improved the quality and safety of care of patients who have a tracheotomy tube. TRAMS has developed an extensive teaching and training program and the model is one which other centers have instituted. This expert team is recognized as a national and international leader in the area of tracheotomy care. TRAMS is a service working with both adults and children, and unfortunately data collected are not specific for pediatric patients. However, the mission pursued by the team reflects the needs of an ideal PTT (Table 16.2) [59].

According to Price [60], body image is concerned with control and function, as well as with physical appearance. The presence of a hole on the neck that is kept open by a tube, and through which sputum is expectorated, is likely to cause anxiety and affect self-esteem. Children may express their fears and distress by refusing to look at the tracheotomy or become involved in their own care. Dropkin [61] considered that acceptance of the stoma could be demonstrated through self-care tasks and that these normally preceded resocialization behaviors. Part of the nurses' and team role in caring for patients with a tracheotomy is to provide support when patients feel ready to look at their altered neck and become involved in their own care. The first sight of a stoma can be equally distressing for family and friends. An enormous range of defense and coping mechanisms, such as denial, anger, regression, passivity and projection, can be brought into play during this time and PTT members need to be aware of these reactions, and such awareness should be an important aspect of both in-hospital and at-home tracheotomy patient care [62].

In conclusion, pediatric airway management is a delicate field requiring expertise, dedicated skills, competencies and guidelines [63]. Pediatric tracheotomy is a highly specialized field in pediatric airway management, and it has been reported to be a surgical procedure with significant morbidity and mortality. The indications for a tracheotomy in airway management and tracheotomy outcome have changed over time, and more neonates and infants are undergoing tracheotomy and surviving. Pediatric tracheotomy is a safe procedure if the PTT is established in the hospital in conjunction with home care by well-trained parents.

Table 16.2 The ideal pediatric tracheotomy team

To ensure safety and quality of tracheotomy care
To provide ongoing education to patients, families and care-givers
To assist with equipment, education and support of patients in the community
To contribute to the knowledge base for tracheotomy care
To diffuse instrumental and device evolution
To encourage updating and multidisciplinary cooperation
To support education, training and simulation
To seek consensus on indications, timing, techniques and decannulation
To promote care-giver and family meetings
To create center-wide interdisciplinary policy and procedures
To monitor and audit quality and safety

References

1. Lewis CH, Carron JD, Perkins JA et al (2003) Tracheotomy in pediatric patients. A national perspective. Arch Otolaryngol Head Neck Surg 129:523–529
2. Bigler J, Holinger P, Johnson K (1954) Tracheotomy in infancy. Pediatrics 13:5
3. Trachsel D, Hammer J (2006) Indications for tracheotomy in children. Paediatr Respir Rev 7:162–168
4. Davis GM (2006) Tracheostomy in children. Paediatr Respir Rev 7 [Suppl 1]:S206–S209
5. Cochrane LA, Bailey CM (2006) Surgical aspects of tracheotomy in children. Paediatr Respir Rev 7:169–174
6. Hotaling AJ, Robbins WK, Madgy DN et al (1992) Pediatric tracheotomy: a review of technique. Am J Otolaryngol 13:115–119
7. Greenberg JS, Sulek M, de Jong A et al (2001) The role of postoperative chest radiography in pediatric tracheotomy. Int J Pediatr Otorhinolaryngol 60:41–47
8. Scott CJ, Darowski M, Crabbe DC (1998) Complications of percutaneous dilatational tracheostomy in children. Anaesthesia 53:477–480
9. Van Heurn LW, Theunissen PH, Ramsay G et al (1996) Pathological changes of the trachea after percutaneous dilational tracheotomy. Chest 109:1466–1469
10. Russel C, Matta B (eds) (2004) Tracheotomy. A multiprofessional handbook. Greenwich Medical Media, London
11. Koltai PJ (1998) Starplasty, a new technique of pediatric tracheotomy. Arch Otolaryngol Head Neck Surg 124:1105–1111
12. Eliashar R, Gross M, Attal P et al (2004) "Starplasty" prevents tracheotomy complications in infants. Int J Pediatr Otorhinolaryngol 68:325–329
13. Solares CA, Krakovitz P, Hirose K (2004) Starplasty: revisiting a pediatric tracheotomy technique. Otolaryngol Head Neck Surg 131:717–722
14. Behl S, Watt JWH (2005) Prediction of tracheotomy tube size for paediatric long-term ventilation: an audit of children with spinal cord injury. Br J Anaesth 94:88–91
15. Penlington GN (1974) Endotracheal tube sizes for children. Anaesthesia 29:494–495
16. Hardee PS, Cashman M (2003) Ultrasound imaging in the preoperative estimation of the size of tracheotomy tube required in specialised operations in children. Br J Oral Maxillofac Surg 41:312–316
17. Gullo A, Sorbello M, Frova G (2007) Percutaneous versus surgical tracheotomy: an unfinished symphony. Crit Care Med 35:682–683
18. Zawadzka-Glosa L, Rawiczb M, Chmielik M et al (2004) Percutaneous tracheotomy in children. Int J Pediatr Otorhinolaryngol 68:1387–1390
19. Sheldon CH, Pudenz RH, Freshwater DB et al (1955) A new method for tracheotomy. J Neurosurg 12:428–431
20. Ciaglia P, Firsching R, Syniec C (1985) Elective percutaneous dilatational tracheotomy: a new simple bedside procedure; preliminary report. Chest 87:715–719
21. Fantoni A, Ripamonti D (2002) Tracheotomy in pediatrics patients. Minerva Anestesiol 68:433–442
22. Toursarkissian B, Fowler CL, Zweng TN et al (1994) Percutaneous dilatational tracheotomy in children and teenagers. J Pediatr Surg 29:1421–1424
23. Silvia Bárbara C, Rodríguez Núñez A, López Franco M et al (2005) Traqueostomía percutánea bajo control endoscópico en adolescentes. An Pediatr (Barc) 63:160–163
24. Walz MK (1997) Percutaneous dilational tracheotomy: method indications, contraindications and results. Curr Opin Anesthesiol 10:101–105
25. Polderman KH, Spijkstra JJ, De Bree R et al (2003) Percutaneous dilatational tracheotomy in the ICU. Optimal organization, low complication rates, and description of a new complication. Chest 123:1595–1602
26. Kremer B, Botos-Kremer AI, Eckel HE (2002) Indications, complications, and surgical techniques for pediatric tracheotomies: an update. J Pediatr Surg 37:1556–1562

27. Pinto JM, Ansley J, Baroody FM (2001) Lack of utility of postoperative chest radiograph in pediatric tracheotomy. Otolaryngol Head Neck Surg 125:241–244
28. Hamburger MD, Wold JS, Berry JA et al (2000) Appropriateness of routine postoperative chest radiography after tracheotomy. Arch Otolaryngol Head Neck Surg 126:649–651
29. Ward RF, Jones J, Carew JF (1995) Current trends in pediatric tracheotomy. Int J Pediatr Otorhinolaryngol 33:233–239
30. Goldenberg D, Ari EG, Golz A et al (2000) Tracheotomy complications: a retrospective study of 1130 cases. Otolaryngol Head Neck Surg 123:495–500
31. Alladi A, Rao S, Das K et al (2004) Pediatric tracheotomy: a 13-year experience. Pediatr Surg Int 20:695–698
32. Carr MM, Poje CP, Kingston L et al (2001) Complications in pediatric tracheotomies. Laryngoscope 111:1925–1928
33. Lee W, Koltai P, Harrison M et al (2002) Indications for tracheotomy in the pediatric intensive care unit population. A pilot study. Arch Otolaryngol Head Neck Surg 128:1249–1252
34. Wetmore RF, Marsh RR, Thompson ME et al (1999) Pediatric tracheotomy: a changing procedure? Arch Otolaryngol Head Neck Surg 108:695–699
35. Carron JD, Derkay CS, Strope GL et al (2000) Pediatric tracheotomies: changing indications and outcomes. Laryngoscope 110:1099–1104
36. Gaudet PT, Peerless A, Sasaki CT et al (1978) Pediatric tracheotomy and associated complications. Laryngoscope 88:1633–1641
37. Citta-Pietrolungo TJ, Alexander MA, Cook SP et al (1993) Complications of tracheotomy and decannulation in pediatric and young patients with traumatic brain injury. Arch Phys Med Rehabil 74:905–909
38. Gianoli JG, Miller RH, Guarisco JL (1999) Tracheotomy in the first year of life. Ann Otol Rhinol Laryngol 99:896–901
39. Pereira KD, MacGregor AR, McDuffie CM et al (2003) Tracheotomy in preterm infants. Current trends. Arch Otolaryngol Head Neck Surg 129:1268–1271
40. Kenna MA, Reilly JS, Stool SE (1987) Tracheotomy in the preterm infant. Ann Otol Rhinol Laryngol 96:68–71
41. Rocha EP, Dias MD, Szajmbok FE et al (2000) Tracheostomy in children: there is a place for acceptable risk. J Trauma 49:483–485
42. Simma B, Spehler D, Burger R (1994) Tracheotomy in children. Eur J Pediatr 153:291–296
43. Gianoli G, Miller R, Guarisco J (1990) Tracheotomy in the first year of life. Ann Otol Rhinol 92:398–400
44. Birman C, Beckenham E (1998) Acquired tracheo-esophageal fistula in the pediatric population. Int J Pediatr Otorhinolaryngol 44:109–113
45. Duncan BW, Howell LJ, deLorimier AA et al (1992) Tracheotomy in children with emphasis on home care. J Pediatr Surg 27:432–435
46. Sorbello M, Guarino A, Morello G (2007) Practical aspects for managing extubation of the difficult airway. In: Gullo A (ed) Anaesthesia Pain Intensive Care and Emergency Medicine – A.P.I.C.E. Proceedings of the 22nd Postgraduate Course in Critical Care Medicine, Venice-Mestre, 9–11 November 2007. Springer Verlag Italia, pp 81–92
47. Prescott CA, Vanlierde MJ (1989) Tracheotomy in children – The Red Cross War Memorial Children's Hospital experience 1980-1985. Int J Pediatr Otorhinolaryngol 17:97–107
48. Arcand P, Granger J (1988) Pediatric tracheotomies: changing trends. J Otolaryngol 17:121–125
49. Line WS, Hawkins DB, Kahlstrom EJ et al (1986) Tracheotomy in infants and young children: the changing perspective 1970-1985. Laryngoscope 96:510–515
50. Wetmore RF, Handler SD, Potsic WP (1982) Pediatric tracheotomy. Experience during the past decade. Ann Otol Rhinol Laryngol 91:628–632
51. Oberwaldner B, Eber E (2006) Tracheotomy care in the home. Paediatr Respir Rev 7:185–190
52. Messineo A, Giusti F, Narne S et al (1995) The safety of home tracheotomy care for children. J Pediatr Surg 30:1246–1248

53. Buzz-Kelly L, Gordin P (1993) Teaching CPR to parents of children with tracheotomies. MCN Am J Matern Child Nurs 18:158–163

54. Bryant K, Davis C, Lagrone C (1997) Streamline discharge planning for the child with a new tracheotomy. J Pediatr Nurs 12:191–192

55. Carnevale FA, Alexander E, Davis M et al (2006) Daily living with distress and enrichment: the moral experience of families with ventilator assisted children at home. Pediatrics 117:e48–e60

56. Lewarski JS (2005) Long-term care of the patient with a tracheotomy. Respir Care 50:534–537

57. Rubulotta F, Pinsky MR (2006) Second International Conference on Rapid Response System and Medical Emergency Team, 28-30 June 2006, Pittsburgh, PA, USA. Crit Care 10:319

58. De Vita MA, Bellomo R, Hillman K et al (2006) Findings of the first consensus conference on medical emergency teams. Crit Care Med 34:2463–2478

59. Tobin AE, Santamaria JD (2008) An intensivist-led tracheotomy review team is associated with shorter decannulation time and length of stay: a prospective cohort study. Crit Care 12:R48

60. Price B (1992) Living with altered body image: the cancer experience. Br J Nurs 1:641–645

61. Dropkin MJ (1989) Coping with disfigurement and dysfunction after head and neck cancer surgery: a conceptual framework. Semin Oncol Nurs 5:213–219

62. Seay SJ, Gay SL (1997) Problem in tracheostomy patient care: recognizing the patient with a displaced tracheostomy tube. ORL Head Neck Nurs 15:10–11

63. Frova G, Guarino A, Sorbello M et al (2006) Recommendations for airway control and difficult airway management in paediatric patients. Minerva Anestesiol 72:723–748

Chapter 17

Infection Control in Neonates and Children

Richard E. Sarginson, Hendrick K.F. van Saene, Antonino Gullo

Introduction

Many patients are admitted to the pediatric intensive care unit (PICU) with infection as the primary problem, for example with viral pneumonitis or meningococcal disease. Other patients are admitted free of infection but are at risk of acquisition, particularly if their stay in the PICU is prolonged with invasive devices in situ. A further group are admitted with exacerbations of chronic conditions, where infection may be a contributing factor, for example, pulmonary aspiration in a child with cerebral palsy.

A high proportion of patients have already received systemic antimicrobial drugs, either as treatment or as surgical prophylaxis. Infections which develop on the PICU after admission are usually termed "nosocomial".

We have argued elsewhere that terminology based on the origin of the infections is more informative (Table 17.1) [1]. "Infection control" includes effective

Table 17.1 Origin of infections according to the carrier state. Primary endogenous infections are due to organisms carried in the throat and/or rectum at the time of admission. Secondary endogenous infections are due to organisms acquired in the ICU and carried in the throat and/or rectum prior to infection. The rates of this type of infection depend on the use of selective decontamination of the digestive tract (SDD). Exogenous infections are due to organisms never carried by the patient

Infection type	Potential pathogen	Timing	Frequency (%)	Preventative or therapeutic intervention
Primary endogenous	Six "normal", nine "abnormal" + high and low level pathogens	Mostly <1 week	55–60	Parenteral antimicrobials
Secondary endogenous	Mostly nine "abnormal"+ S. aureus and Candida spp	Mostly >1 week	5–30	Enteral antimicrobials
Exogenous	Mostly nine "abnormal" + low-level pathogens	Any time during ICU treatment	15–35	Hygiene measures

M. Astuto (ed), *Basics*, Anesthesia, Intensive Care and Pain in Neonates and Children.
ISBN 978-88-470-0654-6 © Springer-Verlag Italia 2009

diagnosis and treatment of existing infection and prevention of new infections, particularly bloodstream infections, ventilator-associated pneumonias, wound infections, and urinary tract infections.

Literature on this subject is extensive [2], although studies on the origin of infections are few. We focus mainly on prevention, based on our system of twice-weekly surveillance cultures and microbiology meetings.

Normal Flora

Humans have evolved with microorganisms and carry a complex "ecosystem" of bacteria and yeasts in the alimentary canal and on the skin and mucosal surfaces. The definition of normal flora depends on detailed longitudinal studies on healthy populations. These are scarce in infants and children. Carriage of species such as *Streptococcus pneumoniae* or *Haemophilus influenzae* is common in healthy individuals, whereas prolonged carriage of methicillin-resistant *Staphylococcus aureus* (MRSA) or *Pseudomonas aeruginosa* is rare and considered abnormal (Table 17.2).

Table 17.2 Potentially pathogenic microorganisms. "Normal" (or "community") microorganisms are frequently carried by normal healthy people. "Abnormal" (or "hospital") microorganisms are rarely carried by healthy individuals, but are often acquired during critical illness. However, patients with chronic illnesses may carry "abnormal" organisms in the community

	Species
"Normal" ("community")	*Streptococcus pneumoniae*
	Haemophilus influenzae
	Moraxella catarrhalis
	Staphylococcus aureus
	Escherichia coli
	Candida albicans
"Abnormal" ("hospital")	*Klebsiella* species
	Proteus species
	Morganella species
	Enterobacter species
	Citrobacter species
	Serratia species
	Acinetobacter species
	Pseudomonas species
	MRSA

Abnormal Carrier States

Abnormal carrier states develop over time in previously healthy patients on the PICU. Overgrowth of abnormal potential pathogenic microorganisms (PPMs) in the throat or gut is very likely to occur in patients undergoing prolonged therapy in the PICU. Overgrowth is defined as 10^5 PPM per milliliter of saliva or gram of faeces. For example, infants with a severe respiratory syncytial virus (RSV) infection frequently acquire overgrowth with PPM species, typically aerobic gram-negative bacteria (AGNB), during the first few days of ventilation. Some patients, typically with chronic illness, have abnormal flora in throat or rectal surveillance swabs on admission, for example, patients undergoing cardiac surgery for congenital heart disease. Unfortunately, the carrier state of individual patients is rarely known on the day of surgery.

Patients with severe chronic or degenerative neurological conditions, such as cerebral palsy and spinal muscular atrophy, can have very high rates of abnormal carriage at the time of PICU admission [3].

The natural history of untreated abnormal carrier states in the PICU is largely unknown. Most studies of abnormal carriage have been done in the context of using selective decontamination of the digestive tract (SDD) to control AGNB and yeasts. Institutions in which SDD is not used employ routine surveillance cultures rarely. We are not aware of any studies investigating the incidence rates of infection in patients with evolving abnormal carrier states.

Two important questions emerge. What is the cumulative risk of acquiring an infection due to abnormal carriage? Secondly, what is the risk of transmission of the carried pathogens?

Surveillance and Diagnostic Cultures

We use a system of surveillance cultures of the throat and rectum. These are taken on admission and then twice weekly, on Monday and Thursday mornings. Results are discussed at microbiology meetings on Tuesday and Friday afternoons. Standard diagnostic cultures are done on clinical indication. If the same strain of a microorganism is present in surveillance cultures, typically in overgrowth concentrations, and subsequently grows from a diagnostic culture, the presumption is that the origin of the infection is endogenous. Clearly, hygiene or isolation measures will be ineffective to control this type of infection. This is a neglected point in most articles and policies on infection control in ICUs, even though a major proportion of "nosocomial" ICU infections are "endogenous" (Fig. 17.1).

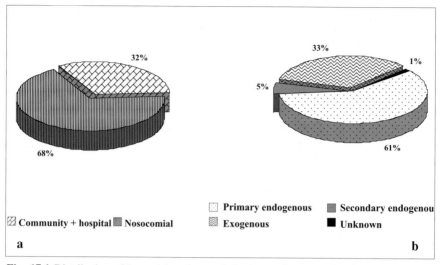

Fig. 17.1 Distribution of bacterial and yeast infections using two classification schemes. **a** The CDC 48-h cut-off scheme classifies infections as "nosocomial" if diagnosed 48 h or more after admission. **b** The microbial carrier state scheme shows infections identified by surveillance [1]

Classification of Infections

Infections can be classified by a number of schemes, including by the intrinsic pathogenicity of the causative organisms and the site, severity and origin of the infection. Knowledge of the origin of an infection is a crucial factor for establishing techniques of control.

In a 4-year study of patients staying four or more days in PICU, we found that approximately 60% of infections were due to organisms carried by the patient at the time of admission, primary endogenous infections (Fig. 17.1) [1]. Infections were classified as endogenous or exogenous, depending on the whether the causative microorganisms were present in surveillance cultures prior to the diagnosis of infection. Endogenous infections were classified as primary if the organism was present on surveillance at the time of admission and secondary if subsequently acquired on the PICU before the onset of infection. We used SDD selectively to control abnormal carriage, SDD "a la carte". The main aims of SDD are to control abnormal carrier states and to prevent secondary endogenous infection.

Tables 17.3, 17.4 and 17.5 illustrate the pattern of infections in a subgroup of longer stay patients on the PICU in Liverpool during the years 1999 through 2003 [1]. Figure 17.2 illustrates the day of onset for the same data.

Table 17.3 Classification of 803 bacterial and yeast infections using the criterion of carriage [1]. This pattern of infection is from a mixed regional cardiac/general PICU over a 4-year period. The population is the subgroup staying 4 or more days. SDD is used to control abnormal carrier states identified by surveillance cultures

Pathogens		Infection			
		Primary endogenous	Secondary endogenous	Exogenous	Not evaluable
High-level pathogens	*Neisseria meningitidis*	33			
	Streptococcus pyogenes	4			
	Streptococcus agalactiae	5			
	Bordetella pertussis	3			
	Mycobacterium tuberculosis	1			
"Community"	*Streptococcus pneumoniae*	20			
	Haemophilus influenzae	38			
	Moraxella catarrhalis	5			
	Escherichia coli	14		5	
	Staphylococcus aureus	62	19	38	1
	Candida species	49	2	5	1
"Hospital"	*Klebsiella* species	9	3	7	
	Proteus species	2	1	2	
	Citrobacter species			1	
	Enterobacter species	5		16	
	Serratia species	4	3		
	Acinetobacter species			22	
	Pseudomonas aeruginosa	33	12	56	1
	Pseudomonas non-aeruginosa	1	3	9	
	MRSA	6	16		1
Low-level pathogens	Coagulase-negative staphylococci	140		86	7
	Streptococcus viridans	5			
	Enterococci	27		2	
	Bacillus species			1	
	Anaerobes	5			
	Anaerobes/aerobes	6			
Miscellaneous	*Pneumocystis carinii*	2			
	Aspergillus fumigatus			3	
	Mycoplasma	1			
Total		480	59	253	11

Table 17.4 Sites of infection and microbial distribution in 803 infections (same data as in Table 17.3). A significant proportion of the wound infections were in patients with burns

Pathogen		Infection site				
		Blood	Lower airway	Wound	Urinary tract	Miscellaneous
High-level pathogens	*Neisseria meningitidis*	33				
	Streptococcus pyogenes		2	1		Bone 1
	Streptococcus agalactiae	2				Meninges 3
	Bordetella pertussis		3			3
	Mycobacterium tuberculosis		1			1
"Community"	*Streptococcus pneumoniae*	5	9			Meninges 1, eye 5
	Haemophilus influenzae	3	28			Eye 7
	Moraxella catarrhalis	1	4			
	Escherichia coli	5	3	1	7	Eye 1, peritoneum 2
	Staphylococcus aureus	13	66	32		Eye 7, bone 1, peritoneum 1
	Candida species	12		20	9	Peritoneum 4, vagina 10, bone 1, subphrenic 1
"Hospital"	*Klebsiella* species	9	1	2	6	Eye 1
	Proteus species				5	
	Citrobacter species				1	
	Enterobacter species	2	2	16		Peritoneum 1
	Serratia species	5	1	1		
	Acinetobacter species	4		17		Eye 1

↑ cont.

continue **Table 17.4**

Pseudomonas aeruginosa	13	30	43	10	Eye 10
Pseudomonas non-aeruginosa	1	7	3		Eye 2
MRSA	3	3	15		Eye 1, endocardium 1
Coagulase-negative staphylococci	230				V-P shunt 1, peritoneum 2
Streptococcus viridans	4				Pleura 1
Enterococci	18		2	4	V-P shunt 1, pleura 2, endocardium 1, gut 1
Bacillus species	1				
Anaerobes	2				Abscess 2, gut 1
Anaerobes/aerobes	1				Abdominal abscess 5
Pneumocystis carinii		2			
Aspergillus fumigatus		2	1		
Mycoplasma		1			
Total	367	165	159	37	75

Low-level pathogens (Coagulase-negative staphylococci through Anaerobes/aerobes); Miscellaneous (Pneumocystis carinii through Mycoplasma)

Table 17.5 Sites of infection and viral distribution in 193 infections (patients staying 4 or more days). These cannot be classified in the same way as bacterial and yeast infections. If the patient had the infection diagnosed within 5 days of admission, this was considered to be community-acquired, i.e. incubating at the time of admission. Otherwise the infection was considered to be ICU-acquired. Most infections were due to respiratory syncytial virus, followed by adenovirus and rotavirus

Virus	Infection site			Time of diagnosis	
	Lower airway	Wound	Miscellaneous	≤5 days (imported)	≥5 days (acquired)
Respiratory syncytial virus	143			123	20
Cytomegalovirus	5			5	
Adenovirus	4		Gut 6	5	5
Parainfluenza 3 virus	5			4	1
Influenza A virus	4			3	1
Herpes simplex virus	1	2	Brain 1, mouth 1	5	
Rotavirus			Gut 12	5	7
Astrovirus			Gut 1		1
Calicivirus			Gut 1		1
Small round structured virus			Gut 3		3
Echovirus	3			2	1
Rhinovirus			Upper airway 1		1
Total				155	38

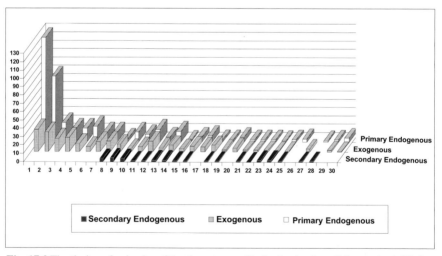

Fig. 17.2 The timing of episodes of the three types of infection by day of diagnosis. A 30-day cut-off point was used because sporadic infections occurred in a few patients with PICU stays of up to 6 months. Secondary endogenous infections did not occur before 8 days. Primary endogenous infections mostly occurred in the first week, but exogenous infections occurred throughout PICU stays. No time cut-off reliably distinguishes the epidemiological source of infection

Hand Washing and General Hygiene

The importance of reducing transmission of pathogens between patients or from contaminated environments by hospital staff has been advocated since the time of Semmelweis. Infection control campaigns typically place the main emphasis on hand washing, disposable items and rigorous cleaning of the environment [2]. In particular, peripatetic medical and nursing staff are seen as potential vectors of transmission of microorganisms by hand. There is also some evidence that bacteria, as well as viruses, can be transmitted by aerosol droplets by staff and relatives with symptomatic upper respiratory tract infections [4]. The potential roles of shared-use technological devices such as phones, computer keyboards and ultrasound devices for transmitting viral particles, bacteria and yeasts are largely unknown.

Some assessment of the effectiveness of general hygiene measures can be made by regular assessment of the prevalence of exogenous infections. This is illustrated in Figure 17.3 [1]. The monthly rate of exogenous infections is recorded (per 100 patient days) and is related to a threshold (calculated from the 95% confidence interval for 24 months of data). A period of a higher rate of exogenous infection is seen in the winter months of 2002. Adherence to hygiene standards is more likely to be compromised during periods of intense activity. Abnormally high rates of exogenous infections detected in this way can alert infection control teams.

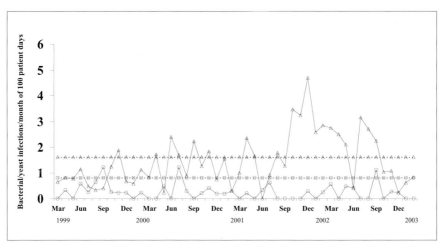

Fig. 17.3 Incidence density of secondary endogenous (○) and exogenous infections (Δ) over time. Two thresholds (—○—, —Δ—) were used for secondary endogenous and exogenous infections, respectively. These thresholds were calculated at the 95% confidence interval for the first 24 months of data, assuming the infection rates conformed to a Poisson distribution. A major prolonged rise above the thresholds would alert staff to potential breaches of hygiene

Admission Policies, Cohorting and Isolation

Many PICUs admit all patients from the local region requiring intensive care. Indeed, they may have to admit patients from adjacent regions during peak demand, typically during the winter respiratory virus epidemics. In most parts of the world there will typically be only one PICU facility per region except in very large cities. Consequently, all types of patient, ranging from those with acute respiratory illness to those scheduled for elective cardiac surgery and immuno-suppressed oncology patients will be admitted to the same unit.

Isolation serves two purposes: to protect vulnerable patients from acquiring infection and to prevent patients, infected with or carrying transmissible organisms, becoming sources for exogenous infections or abnormal carrier states. It is very difficult to study the effectiveness of such measures, particularly with regard to carrier states. Surveillance cultures are an essential tool for evaluation of these measures.

Patients with some infections, typically RSV, are managed in room cohorts in many PICUs where individual isolation facilities are limited, particularly during epidemic periods. Despite such measures, transmission may still occur [5].

Selective Decontamination of the Digestive Tract

SDD has been used for over two decades now [6–17]. The main principle is to control overgrowth of AGNB and yeasts in the alimentary canal of sick and vulnerable patients. Despite a large body of evidence supporting its use in reducing infections and mortality in adult ICUs, SDD has not gained universal approval. The full SDD protocol includes systemic cefotaxime to control primary endogenous infections and surveillance cultures (Table 17.6).

No large-scale randomized controlled trials (RCTs) to assess the effect of SDD have been done in PICUs. Four small-scale RCTs have been carried out [18–21]. Mortality rates in PICUs are considerably lower than in adult ICUs. Studies of the impact of infection prevention interventions on mortality are consequently difficult. The rationale for the use of SDD in PICUs comes from the recognition of similar patterns of abnormal carrier states in critically ill children as in critically ill adults. The rate of secondary endogenous infections is the cardinal indicator of the effectiveness of SDD. In our studies, secondary endogenous infections were limited to 5% of infections and no episode occurred before day 8 of admission (Fig. 17.2). This contrasts with secondary endogenous infection rates of 30% or more in the control arm of SDD RCTs in adults. Where secondary endogenous infection occurred, one or more of the factors described below under "Limitations of SDD" was usually present.

Table 17.6 The full four-component SDD protocol. This is administered on the basis of surveillance swabs and likely bacterial etiology for primary endogenous infections. If a patient has a high risk of an infection due to a *Pseudomonas* or a multiresistant AGNB, other parenteral agents will be used, e.g. ceftazidime, gentamicin or meropenem. In the presence of MRSA, vancomycin is added—enterally for the carrier state and parenterally for infection. Therapy is adjusted according to subsequent surveillance and diagnostic cultures

		Target pathogen	Antimicrobial	Total daily dose (four times daily)		
				<5 years	5–12 years	>12 years
1. Enteral antimicrobials ("abnormal pathogens")	Oropharynx	AGNB	Colistin with tobramycin	2 g 2% paste or gel		
		Yeasts	Amphotericin B or nystatin	2 g 2% paste or gel		
		MRSA	Vancomycin	2 g 4% paste or gel		
	Gut	AGNB	Colistin (mg)	100	200	400
			Tobramycin (mg)	80	160	320
		Yeasts	Amphotericin B (mg)	500	1,000	2,000
			Nystatin (Ux10^6)	2	4	8
		MRSA	Vancomycin (mg/kg)	20–40	20–40	500–2,000
2. Parenteral antimicrobials ("normal pathogens")			Cefotaxime (mg/kg)	150	200	4,000–8,000
3. Hygiene						
4. Surveillance cultures	Throat and rectum rectum		On admission, Monday, Thursday			

Limitations of SDD

SDD may fail for a number of reasons. The original regimen was designed to control infections due to aerobic gram-negative organisms (Table 17.2). Carriage of microorganisms, such as MRSA or low-grade pathogens such as coagulase-negative staphylococci, will not be eliminated by SDD. Also, there may be lapses in the administration of SDD, particularly the oral preparation. Occasional patients refuse the treatment.

Some patients have conditions which preclude enteral drug administration, for example necrotizing enterocolitis or following extensive gastrointestinal surgery. Other patients have problems with gut motility, where enteral antibiotics fail to penetrate the lower gastrointestinal tract despite administration. There is an argument for starting SDD prior to elective surgery where abnormal carrier states are demonstrated by preoperative surveillance swabs. In practice, this can be difficult to arrange and study due to the logistical complexities.

Carriage of AGNB with extended beta-lactamase (ESBL) genes is a significant problem, particularly where tobramycin resistance is present. Although most multiresistant AGNB are sensitive to colistin, it has proved difficult to control carriage of ESBL producing AGNB, including tobramycin resistance, with the standard SDD regimen [22].

SDD in the Context of Endemic MRSA

MRSA is a problem in most ICUs. However, the magnitude of the problem varies enormously between countries and specialist ICUs. Amongst RCTs designed to assess the impact of SDD, MRSA which is intrinsically resistant to the parenteral and enteral antimicrobial drugs used in the SDD protocol, was endemic in seven ICUs at the time the RCT was conducted [15, 23–28]. These RCTs report a trend towards higher MRSA carriage and infection rates in patients receiving SDD. Practically all were secondary endogenous infections, i.e. the patients did not import MRSA in their admission flora but acquired MRSA during treatment on the ICU. The MRSA was acquired first in the oropharynx, followed by gastric and intestinal carriage and overgrowth.

The addition of enteral vancomycin to the classical SDD regimen is required to control MRSA in ICUs with endemic MRSA (Table 17.6) [29–39].

Outbreaks

Many episodes of ICU infection outbreaks are exogenous infections due to breaches of hygiene. Exogenous infections may occur at any time during a patient's ICU stay (Fig. 17.1). The causative bacteria are acquired on the unit but were not present in the throat and/or gut flora of the patient at the time of ICU admission. For example, long-stay patients, particularly those with a tracheostomy, are at high risk of exogenous lower airway infections. Purulent lower airway secretions may yield a microorganism never previously carried by the patient in the digestive tract flora or, indeed, in their oropharynx. Although both the tracheostomy and the oropharynx are equally accessible for bacterial entry, the entry site for bacteria that colonize and infect the lower airways tends to be the tracheostomy [40].

Amongst the 56 reports of RCTs evaluating SDD, there is one describing an outbreak of exogenous lower airway infections due to *Acinetobacter* [15]. The policy of early tracheostomy was in place on the Respiratory Unit in Cape Town, South Africa, when a multiresistant *Acinetobacter* became endemic. The aim of the SDD trial was to eradicate the outbreak strain, using enteral polymyxin E and tobramycin. The investigators found that enteral application of polymyxin E and tobramycin successfully cleared *Acinetobacter* from the throat and gut, controlling endogenous lower airway colonization and infections with the outbreak strain in the test group. Fewer SDD-treated than placebo-treated patients had *Acinetobacter* infection, although the difference was not statistically significant. Since enteral antimicrobial drugs prevent only endogenous infection, the exogenous problem became more apparent. The main source of the outbreak strain was the long-term tracheotomized patients in the control group who were still carriers. In the Cape Town RCT, the *Acinetobacter* problem returned to former levels once SDD was discontinued.

The Problem of Resistance

The rising problem of antimicrobial drug-resistant bacteria is a subject of much discussion, both in the scientific literature [41] and political journalism. After 20 years of clinical research on SDD, an intriguing finding has emerged. Antibiotic resistance amongst AGNB is more likely to be controlled than increased in patients receiving SDD [16].

Two adult RCTs evaluated the impact of SDD on antimicrobial drug resistance amongst AGNB [17, 42]. The largest trial included 1,000 patients and showed that the rate of carriage of AGNB, resistant to imipenem, ceftazidime, ciprofloxacin, tobramycin and polymyxins, was lower among patients receiving SDD (16%) than among those receiving parenteral antibiotics alone (25%) [17]. This is in line with an earlier RCT which showed that the addition of enteral to parenteral antimicrobial drugs controls carriage and infections due to extended beta-lactamase producing *Klebsiella* [42].

Gut overgrowth of potential pathogens increases the frequency of spontaneous mutations or plasmid transmission of resistance genes, leading to polyclonality and antimicrobial resistance [43, 44]. As parenteral antimicrobial drugs generally fail to eradicate the overgrowth concentrations of abnormal carrier states, the enteral agents of SDD are required to clear carriage and overgrowth of resistant organisms. The essential point is that gut concentrations of excreted or metabolized parenteral antimicrobial agents are likely to be sublethal to overgrowth concentrations of PPMs.

Open Questions and Future Research

Infection control on the PICU is an evolving field, beset by many uncertainties and unanswered questions. The natural history of oropharyngeal and intestinal bacterial and yeast overgrowth carrier states in children, in the absence of enteral antibiotic use, is largely unknown. Consequently the risk of occurrence of secondary endogenous infections in the presence of abnormal carriage is also unknown. Although the control group in SDD trials can give an estimate of this type of infection, such trials in children are few and mainly restricted to small groups of patients with specific disorders such as liver disease and burns

[18, 20]. Furthermore, where a trial is conducted with a unit, SDD can be expected to have an impact on the endogenous flora acquired by patients not receiving the therapy.

The basic SDD formulation was designed when resistant organisms such as MRSA and multiresistant AGNB were less prevalent than today. Several commentators argue that SDD should not be used where the prevalence of such organisms is high. However, we and others have argued that enteral antimicrobial drugs can be used to control gastrointestinal tract overgrowth of resistant bacteria. However, as indicated above, changes in enteral antimicrobial formulation are needed to achieve this; for example, enteral vancomycin to control MRSA overgrowth and the substitution of paromomycin for tobramycin in the case of tobramycin-resistant ESBL producing AGNB. Further empirical tests of such policies are needed.

A further area of uncertainty concerns antimicrobial prophylaxis for surgical operations requiring ICU admission and postoperative ventilation. Few institutions assess the presence of abnormal carriage preoperatively in patients undergoing elective surgery. Is there a role for preoperative SDD as part of surgical prophylaxis for major cardiac or gastrointestinal surgery when the patients are shown to have abnormal carriage?

Finally, little is known about the impact of severe illness and different antimicrobial strategies on the commensal and symbiotic anaerobes of the gastrointestinal tract. SDD was designed to have a limited impact on anaerobes, whereas many broad-spectrum systemic antibiotic regimens used to treat "nosocomial" infections are lethal to many anaerobic species.

References

1. Sarginson RE, Taylor N, Reilly N et al (2004) Infection in prolonged pediatric critical illness: a prospective four-year study based on knowledge of the carrier state. Crit Care Med 32:839–847
2. Gastmeier P (2007) Evidence – based infection control in the ICU (except catheters). Curr Opin Crit Care 13:557–562
3. Jardine M, Galvez I, Taylor N, Thorburn K et al (2007) Abnormal (resistant) flora in children with cerebral palsy requiring intensive care. Arch Dis Child 92(S1):A24
4. Bischoff WE, Wallis ML, Tucker BK et al (2006) "Gesundheit" sneezing, common colds, allergies, and Staphylococcus aureus dispersion. J Infect Dis 194(8):1119–1126
5. Thorburn K, Kerr S, Taylor N, van Saene HKF (2004) RSV outbreak in a paediatric intensive care unit. J Hosp Infect 57:194–201
6. Baxby D, van Saene HKF, Stoutenbeek CP, Zandstra DF (1996) Selective decontamination of the digestive tract: 13 years on, what it is and what it is not. Intensive Care Med 22:699–706
7. van Saene HKF, Petros AJ, Ramsay G, Baxby D (2003) All great truths are iconoclastic: selective decontamination of the digestive tract moves from heresy to level 1 truth. Intensive Care Med 29:677–690
8. Liberati A, D'Amico R, Pifferi S, Torri V, Brzzi L (2004) Antibiotic prophylaxis to reduce respiratory tract infections and mortality in adults receiving intensive care. Cochrane Database Syst Rev CD 00 00 22

9. Silvestri L, van Saene HKF, Milanese M, Gregori D, Gullo A (2007) Selective decontamination of the digestive tract reduces bacterial bloodstream infections and mortality in critically ill patients. Systematic review of randomized controlled trials. J Hosp Infect 65:187–203

10. Silvestri L, van Saene HKF, Casarin A et al (2008) Impact of selective decontamination of the digestive tract on carriage and infection due to Gram-negative and Gram-positive bacteria: a systematic review of randomised controlled trials. Anaesth Intensive Care 36:324–338

11. Silvestri L, van Saene HKF, Milanese M et al (2005) Impact of selective decontamination of the digestive tract on fungal carriage and infection: systematic review of randomized controlled trials. Intensive Care Med 31:898–910

12. Silvestri L, van Saene HKF (2008) Survival benefit of the full regimen of selective decontamination of the digestive tract (SDD). J Crit Care (in press)

13. Arnow PM, Carandang GC, Zabner R et al (1996) Randomised controlled trial of selective bowel decontamination for prevention of infections following liver transplantation. Clin Infect Dis 22:997–1003

14. Hellinger WC, Yao JD, Alvarez S et al (2002) A randomised, prospective, double-blind evaluation of selective bowel decontamination in liver transplantation. Transplantation 73:1904–1909

15. Hammond JMJ, Potgieter PD, Saunders GL, Forder AA (1992) Double-blind study of selective decontamination of the digestive tract in intensive care. Lancet 340:5–9

16. Silvestri L, van Saene HKF (2006) Selective decontamination of the digestive tract does not increase resistance in critically ill patients: evidence from randomised controlled trials. Crit Care Med 34:2027–2030

17. de Jonge E, Schultz M, Spanjaard L et al (2003) Effects of selective decontamination of the digestive tract on mortality and acquisition of resistant bacteria in intensive care: a randomised controlled trial. Lancet 363:1011–1016

18. Barret JP, Jeschke MG, Herndon DN (2001) Selective decontamination of the digestive tract in severely burned pediatric patients. Burns 27:439–445

19. Ruza F, Alvarado F, Herruzo R et al (1998) Prevention of nosocomial infection in a PICU through the use of selective digestive decontamination. Eur J Epidemiol 14:719–727

20. Smith SD, Jackson RJ, Hannakan CJ et al (1993) Selective decontamination in pediatric liver transplants. A randomized prospective study. Transplantation 55:1306–1309

21. Zobel G, Kuttnig M, Grubbauer HM et al (1991) Reduction of colonization and infection rate during pediatric intensive care by selective decontamination of the digestive tract. Crit Care Med 19:1242–1246

22. Abecasis F, Kerr S, Sarginson RE et al (2007) Comment on: emergence of multidrug-resistant Gram-negative bacteria during selective decontamination of the digestive tract on an intensive care unit. J Antimicrob Chemother 60:445

23. Gastinne H, Wolff M, de la Tour F et al (1992) A controlled trial in intensive care units of selective decontamination of the digestive tract with nonabsorbable antibiotics. N Engl J Med 326:594–599

24. Ferrer M, Torres A, Gonzalez J et al (1994) Utility of selective decontamination in mechanically ventilated patients. Ann Intern Med 120:389–395

25. Wiener J, Itokazu G, Nathan C et al (1995) A randomised, double-blind, placebo-controlled trial of selective digestive decontamination in a medical-surgical intensive care unit. Clin Infect Dis 20:861–867

26. Lingnau W, Berger J, Javorsky F et al (1997) Selective intestinal decontamination in multiple trauma patients: prospective, controlled trial. J Trauma 42:687–694

27. Verwaest C, Verhhaegen J, Ferdinande P et al (1997) Randomized, controlled trial of selective digestive decontamination in 600 mechanically ventilated patients in a multi-disciplinary intensive care unit. Crit Care Med 25:63–71

28. de la Cal MA, Cerda E, Garcia-Hierro P et al (2005) Survival benefit in critically ill burned patients receiving selective decontamination of the digestive tract. Ann Surg 241:424–430

29. Thorburn K, Taylor N, Saladi SM et al (2006) Use of surveillance cultures and enteral van-comycin to control methicillin-resistant *Staphylococcus aureus* in a paediatric intensive care unit. Clin Microbiol Infect 12:35–42
30. Silvestri L, van Saene HKF, Milanese M et al (2004) Prevention of MRSA pneumonia by oral vancomycin decontamination: a randomized trial. Eur Respir J 23:921–926
31. Viviani M, van Saene HKF, Dezzoni R et al (2005) Control of imported methicillin-resist-ant *Staphylococcus aureus* (MRSA) in mechanically ventilated patients: a dose-response study of enteral vancomycin to reduce absolute carriage and infection. Anaesth Intensive Care 33:361–372
32. de la Cal MA, Cerda E, van Saene HKF et al (2004) Effectiveness and safety of enteral van-comycin to control endemicity of methicillin-resistant *Staphylococcus aureus* in a medical/surgical intensive care unit. J Hosp Infect 56:175–183
33. Cerdá E, Abella A, de la Cal MA et al (2007) Enteral vancomycin controls methicillin-resist-ant *Staphylococcus aureus* endemicity in an intensive care burn unit: a 9-year prospective study. Ann Surg 245:397–407
34. Bergmans DCJJ, Bonten MJM, Gaillard CA et al (2001) Prevention of ventilator associated pneumonia by oral decontamination. Am J Respir Crit Care Med 164:382–388
35. Gaussorgues Ph, Salard F, Sirodot M et al (1991) Nosocomial bacteremia in patients under mechanical ventilation and receiving beta-inotropic drugs: efficacy of digestive decontami-nation. Rean Soins Intens Med Urg 7:169–174
36. Korinek AM, Laisne MJ, Nicolas MH et al (1993) Selective decontamination of the diges-tive tract in neurosurgical intensive care unit patients: a double-blind, randomized, placebo-controlled study. Crit Care Med 21:1466–1473
37. Krueger WA, Lenhart FP, Neeser G et al (2002) Influence of combined intravenous and top-ical antibiotic prophylaxis on the incidence of infections, organ dysfunctions and mortality in critically ill surgical patients. Am J Respir Crit Care Med 166:1029–1037
38. Pugin J, Auckenthaler R, Lew DP, Suter PM (1991) Oropharyngeal decontamination decreases incidence of ventilator-associated pneumonia. JAMA 265:2704–2710
39. Schardey HM, Joosten U, Fiuke U et al (1997) The prevention of anastomotic leakage after total gastrectomy with local decontamination. Ann Surg 225:172–180
40. Morar P, Singh V, Makura Z et al (2002) Differing pathways of lower airway colonization and infection according to mode of ventilation (endotracheal vs tracheotomy). Arch Otolaryngol Head Neck Surg 128:1061–1066
41. Huskins WC (2007) Interventions to prevent transmission of antimicrobial-resistant bacteria in the intensive care unit. Curr Opin Crit Care 13:572–577
42. Brun-Buisson C, Legrand P, Rauss A et al (1989) Intestinal decontamination for control of nosocomial multi-resistant Gram-negative bacilli. Ann Intern Med 110:873–881
43. van Saene HK, Taylor N, Damjanovic V, Sarginson RE (2008) Microbial gut overgrowth guarantees increased spontaneous mutation leading to polyclonality and antibiotic resistance in the critically ill. Curr Drug Target 9:419-21
44. Verma N, Clarke RW, Bolton-Maggs PH, van Saene HK (2007) Gut overgrowth of van-comycin-resistant enterococci (VRE) results in linezolid-resisant mutation in a child with severe congenital neutropenia: a case report. J Pediatr Hematol Oncol 29:557–560

Chapter 18

Pediatric Palliative Care in the Intensive Care Unit

Stephen Liben

Introduction

Despite the advances in pediatric intensive care technology and the uncontested desire to have every child survive into adulthood, the fact remains that some children die and, in wealthier countries, many do so in the setting of an intensive care unit (ICU). Should all deaths in the pediatric ICU (PICU) be seen as failures and all children who survive, irrespective of the degree of suffering and debilitated outcome, be seen as successes?

The success of intensive care is not, therefore, to be measured only by the statistics of survival, as though each death were a medical failure. It is to be measured by the quality of lives preserved or restored; and by the quality of the dying of those in whose interest it is to die; and by the quality of human relationships involved in each death [1].

Mortality rates in PICUs vary depending on the patient population (e.g. referral centers managing children after complex cardiac surgery have higher mortality rates, and 4–7% is a range often quoted [2, 3]. Another way of looking at mortality rates is to estimate that in a PICU with 800 admissions per year and an average 5% mortality rate that there will be more than three deaths per month or almost one for every week of the year. Most of the children who die in the PICU are less than 4 years old and most die while still sedated and ventilated. In North American PICUs the most common mode of death is after active withdrawal of "life-sustaining treatment" (LST) such as removing a ventilator or following decisions to not attempt cardiopulmonary resuscitation [4]. The frequency of removal of LST may be lower in South America and Europe. However, taking into consideration the possibility of "untruthful records" the rate may be more similar to North American estimates [5].

A statement by the European Association for Palliative Care recently published suggests standards for pediatric palliative care in Europe [6]. Using the World Health Organization's (WHO) inclusive and comprehensive definition of

M. Astuto (ed), *Basics*, Anesthesia, Intensive Care and Pain in Neonates and Children. ISBN 978-88-470-0654-6 © Springer-Verlag Italia 2009

pediatric palliative care, the standards call for a broad range of measures, and include core standards that although admirable in their scope remain far from the current reality of care delivered to the majority of very ill children in most countries. What follows in this brief chapter is an outline of how these principles of good palliative care can be applied to the pediatric intensive care setting that do not require a major shift from current practice, but rather reflect a first small step in how to improve the care of children who die and their bereaved families.

Integrating Pediatric Palliative Care and Intensive Care

Given that the PICU is the place where many children die, it makes sense that a core skill set of a PICU physician would include many of those of a specialist pediatric palliative care physician. What is needed is not a retraining of the PICU physician, but rather a reemphasis and reexploration of what options are available for care at the end of life in the PICU. What is missing in many clinical settings is the range of personnel required to meet the many and varied needs of the dying child and the family. Meeting the WHO definition "palliative care for children is the active total care of the child's body, mind and spirit, and also involves giving support to the family" requires the active participation of a dedicated team that may include disciplines such as social worker, pastoral services, music and child life therapy, and psychology, in addition to those of a physician and nurse skilled in end of life care of children. Knowing how to communicate (mostly meaning how to *actively listen*), appreciating the meaning of illness and suffering, and assessing and treating pain and other symptoms are some of the clinical competencies required of a PICU physician for effective end of life care.

A previously well 2-year-old boy, Dino, is admitted to the PICU postoperatively after evacuation of a large epidural hematoma subsequent to a severe head trauma. Massive brain swelling is noted in the operating room and the prognosis for survival is poor. The child returns to the PICU intubated, hyperventilated and in a barbiturate coma. Both parents and grandparents are present and there is a 15-year-old sister, Maria, who is waiting at home.

Pain and Symptom Management

With many critically ill neonates and children it is unclear, both to family members and to professional care-givers, when the child is in pain. Parents and staff meeting to discuss how to assess the child's expression of pain in different ways can help in the preparation of a care plan that both respects professional expertise on pain assessment and acknowledges that parents have unique insights into their own children [7]. Many children in the ICU receive continuous infusions of sedatives and analgesics that were started either postoperatively or at the initiation of mechanical ventilation. Some children are placed on continuous or regular intermittent doses of neuromuscular blockers that result in muscle relaxation and paralysis of skeletal muscle without any analgesic or sedative effects. Children on neuromuscular blocking drugs cannot move or breathe unaided. In most circumstances it is possible and desirable to interrupt the use of regular neuromuscular blockers in order to assess the level of comfort and sedation of the child [8].

In situations where the child has undergone an acute neurological event it may be difficult for both parents and staff to appreciate the level of neurological function in the presence of high doses of sedatives/analgesics. In these circumstances carefully reducing the degree of sedation may allow better evaluation of the level of consciousness and amount of pain the child may be experiencing. There is no indication or rationale for increasing sedatives just because the child "has suffered enough". Rather the point of sedative/analgesic administration is to respond to pain by first assessing its cause and intensity and then to selectively apply pain management principles as would be done for any child in pain whether the child is "palliative" or not.

Nonpharmacological pain management techniques can be adapted for use in the ICU. Massage therapy, music therapy, and for older children who are conscious art therapy, and even zoo therapy may sometimes be possible in certain circumstances. Less complex and at no cost but perhaps the most powerful way to help both child and parent is to not only allow but encourage parents to hold their critically ill child in their arms even whilst the child remains connected to a ventilator and many infusion pumps. For parents of ill newborns this may be their only chance to hold their child in their arms, and may be a powerful experience that would not have happened without the encouragement of the ICU staff.

While still attached to the ventilator Dino is held in his mother's arms while in a rocking chair. The lights are dimmed and his favorite music is played.

Communication with Children and Families

The majority of children who die in the ICU do not have the ability to communicate verbally because they were either preverbal due to their young age or nonverbal because of their preexisting medical condition. For verbal children in the ICU communication is still very limited either because of the illness itself or the life-support technology. These limitations restrict these ill children's opportunity to talk about their illness and ability to communicate their fears, wishes, dreams, hopes and desires about their life in general and about their possible death in particular.

Maintaining hope is a cornerstone of pediatric palliative care and is a common and challenging task for children, parents, and professionals. The difficult question is sometimes asked directly—"How can we maintain hope in the face of our child's death?" —or indirectly in other ways: "What do we do now?" "How can we go on?" "What is the point of anything?" These questions speak to the need to maintain hope and the struggle to find meaning in the tragic loss that is the death of a child. In the face of such questions (which may be unspoken), the role and challenge for the pediatric palliative care professional are to assist in reframing what hope can be when cure is no longer possible. For example, it can be comforting to know that other families have found a way to maintain hope by shifting from hope for cure to hope for a meaningful life or hope for a peaceful death. A starting point for the health-care professional is to recognize his or her own need to maintain hope and find meaning in the work that he or she does. "Hoping" is understood to be distinct from "wishing". Hope is the understanding that things will somehow be all right, no matter what the outcome. Wishing may be another way to deny reality and is the insistence that, despite the facts, the outcome will somehow "magically" be different. Practical approaches to maintaining hope are to:

1. Accept that, at times, loss of hope may be part of the process
2. Be an active listener as families may find their own way to meaning
3. Facilitate the process that leads to a shift from hoping for cure, to hoping for quality of life, to hoping that death will be as comfortable as possible.

Parents may wish health-care professionals to talk to their extended family, especially grandparents or the parents' brothers or sisters. One study that looked at the relative value parents placed amongst different people involved in decision-making for their children in the PICU (staff versus extended family) found that it was the staff that the family found the most helpful and supportive around difficult decisions such as removing life-supporting therapy [9]. Parents stated that the people who "knew what was really going on" were PICU staff, and they placed a high level of trust in professional care-givers when making decisions for their child even though they had known the professionals for only a short period of time.

After 3 days of hemodynamic instability Dino has stabilized from the cardiovascular perspective and is being weaned off barbiturates. His family has been present at all times and has had many discussions with the hospital chaplain, psychologist, PICU physician and primary care nurse. While being hopeful for a "miracle" the family has been told it is possible that despite all interventions Dino may not survive and that if he dose survive that he will likely have significant brain damage. Dino loved certain lullaby songs and they are being played to him on a recording made by his sister for him to listen to in his room in the PICU. His mother reads a favorite book of Dino's out loud to him while he remains unresponsive on the ventilator. The family continues to pray for him.

The Unit of Care is the Child and Family

Having a supportive team that is available to focus on the psychological, emotional and spiritual issues that children with life-threatening illness and their families face is an essential component of palliative care. It should be a basic principle of intensive care that the emotional, psychological and spiritual needs of children and families in crisis need to be addressed on a regular (as opposed to an as-required) basis. Seen in this light the presence of trained personnel to support the mind and soul of both the child and their family becomes an essential component of intensive care.

While it is important to provide supportive care to family members who are confronted with the possible death of their child, parents also emphasize the importance of the physical environment on their well being and ability to adapt and cope with what is for most of them the most traumatic experience of their lives. Physical facilities for parents such as showers, family rooms for overnight accommodation and kitchenettes, together with an open visiting policy, help to make the point that parents are not "visitors" but are rather the key people with the most at stake in their child's illness. For parents who are confronted by the possible death of their child the ICU environment can at first be a confusing place. The multiple rotating caregivers, lack of privacy, and total disruption of daily life routine coupled with a busy bright physical environment make for a disorienting experience. It can be helpful to have preprepared written materials for parents that explain the structure, hierarchy, and options available to them. Another useful resource for families is access to books and videos and web sites that are relevant to their own situation.

Siblings can be helped to cope with their brother's or sister's death by being given the opportunity to help with their care in a supervised manner. ICUs can facilitate this by having visiting policies that encourage parents to bring siblings for short visits. For example, a young sibling may be provided with crayons and paper to make a drawing for their sick brother or sister. Older siblings may choose to prepare a favorite recording to be played for their ill sibling. Child life specialists (play specialists) can be especially helpful in creating the space for siblings to be involved and to assist them express and come to terms with their sibling's illness or possible death.

Once the barbiturates and sedatives have worn off it becomes clear that Dino has only minimal brain function with preservation of a few brainstem reflexes. He has some gasping respirations but not enough to sustain him off the ventilator. It is possible that he may progress to brain death or may remain in a severely brain-damaged condition. He makes facial grimacing when suctioned in his endotracheal tube and appears to be calmer when gently massaged.

Decision Making

One challenge in pediatric palliative care is to help parents make decisions that respect what is in the best interests of their child versus those decisions that may help to alleviate only their own legitimate suffering. When it is difficult to separate the nonverbal child's suffering from that of the parents, it can be helpful to reframe the situation by asking parents to try to interpret what their child may be "telling" them in actions as opposed to in words. Some parents come to interpret repeated life-threatening episodes as meaning that their child is "ready to go" and may find some solace in knowing that they have found a way to "listen" to the nonverbal messages their child is sending.

Palliative care places a high value on care of the whole person that recognizes the importance of body, mind, and soul. Traditionally most ICUs have been developed to focus on care of the body with varying degrees of emphasis placed on other aspects of the child as a whole person. When cure is no longer possible and the child is likely to die, a shift in goals can be helpful for the child and their family as well as for health-care professionals. Whole-person care is one means to reestablish hope and meaning in the child's care. While most ICU professionals are adept at reducing pain caused by bodily symptoms, they may have less training in addressing the suffering that results from unresolved existential, psychological, emotional, and spiritual issues. Palliative whole-person care emphasizes the ability to heal even when cure is no longer possible. While dying "healed" may be an unrealistic goal for many children in the ICU, there is still much to be gained by addressing issues related to the child and family's emotional and spiritual needs. The beginning of addressing these needs begins with an assessment of the child and family as whole persons. In practice this evaluation of the whole person means asking questions not necessarily traditionally addressed in pediatric critical care such as:

- What is the most important thing in your life right now?
- What is happening in the ICU that is stopping you from making the most of the time you have with your child right now?
- Are there important celebrations that you would consider having on the ICU very soon, even before the "real" date? (e.g. birthdays, Christmas, etc.)

Establishing the child and family's priorities, what really matters to them right now, is often a catalyst for ICU staff to align their care giving in ways that help meet the most urgent needs of the child and family. For example, some families focus on trying to ensure that their ill child survives in order to be present at important milestone holidays. It can be suggested to such families that they consider celebrating an important holiday or birthday now, instead of waiting for the correct calendar date. Should the child survive until the "real" date then families are often more than happy to celebrate the occasion again. This approach of doing whatever the family feels is important to them now, instead of later, can help to relieve pressure.

Setting Goals

Acknowledging that a child is terminally ill is especially difficult in an intensive care environment. An advantage of doing so is that all diagnostic tests and therapies are redirected towards a new common goal: to increase the comfort and quality of life of the child (as opposed to the usual goal of striving to maintain life). For example, a child who suffered an anoxic insult with subsequent seizures will clearly be more comfortable not seizing and therefore the use of anticonvulsants is indicated even if the child is terminally ill, but should the same child develop pneumonia the question of the use of antibiotics is less clear and requires thoughtful and sensitive discussion about benefits and burdens of therapy. However, one should avoid an order for "no tests" or "do not escalate" placed in the chart but rather do everything possible to ensure maximum comfort and quality of life for the child. Seen in this light a palliative care philosophy is congruent with good medical care and is based on a positive attitude of doing as much as possible to meet agreed goals that serve to make the most of the life of the terminally ill child.

Dino becomes completely apneic over the next week and a diagnosis of brain death is made. The parents are told that Dino's brain has died and that it cannot recover.

As the Time of Death Approaches

There are children who die in the ICU with little prior warning for parents. Examples are neonates born at term but who unexpectedly die from birth complications, sepsis or have congenital heart or other congenital abnormalities; older children may die following severe trauma or sepsis. Another group are children with known conditions that were thought to be stable. For these children there may be little or no time available to plan for how death will occur, and palliative care may have more to offer the family survivors after the child has died. In one review of circumstances surrounding end of life in a PICU, it was found that decisions to forgo LST required one or two meetings before consensus was reached [4]. For the many children who die in the ICU after a decision to withdraw LSTs it is often possible to guide families as to what to expect and to offer options for different ways that the end of life can happen.

As the time of withdrawal of LSTs approaches the family may appreciate being transferred to a private room. For some families it is important that the extended family get to say goodbye and to hold the child in their arms before extubation. For other families it may be important to have very few people present in the room at the time of withdrawal of LSTs. Some ICUs take pictures of the child and family, make footprints of infants, or cut a lock of hair to keep as physical memories. Some families are keen for the child to go home or to a hospice on ventilator support with removal of the ventilator occurring once the child is at home or hospice [10]. However, there are considerable logistic and staffing implications in achieving this, and the proportion of children transferred out of intensive care units to the community is small.

Many parents find it both hard and at the same time comforting to have their child in their arms before and while the tracheal tube is being removed. Some mothers have commented that they were present for the entry of their child into the world and they want to be present when their child leaves. The discussion as to what would be the best environment to die is not an easy one for all involved and yet decisions made from this discussion may remain important memories for all those involved for years to come. What is important is to discuss with the family what may be most meaningful to them and not to assume what is best for them. Once the decision has been made to withdraw mechanical ventilatory support the child and family should be guided through how the process will unfold. It is important to be sure that family, as well as ICU staff, understand that the child is not having care withdrawn, but is instead having a treatment removed that no longer has more benefits than burdens. For children on full ventilator support it is important to establish a plan for the control of dyspnea and secretions upon withdrawal of the ventilator [11].

After the Death

Once the child has died families should be allowed to stay with their child in the room until they are ready to leave. Prior to bathing/washing the body ICU staff can remove sutures holding catheters in place and medical devices can be removed. Some parents appreciate being offered the opportunity to clean and bathe the body with staff.

A discussion should take place concerning the possible benefits of an autopsy, which will usually have been considered before death. In some situations an autopsy is mandated by law, otherwise the fact that autopsy examination often reveals additional information needs to be highlighted. Adverse publicity about autopsies regarding the removal and storage of tissue samples and organs has resulted in a marked decline in the autopsy acceptance rate. In the UK, detailed consent has to be obtained including a description of the procedure and specific agreement obtained about the storage and disposal of tissues and organs and their use for research. Although some parents feel that their child has "suffered enough" and instinctively want to decline an autopsy, it should be explained that having as complete information as possible is often helpful to best understand the cause of their child's death and that this information may be important for them and their family in the future. This is especially important when the cause of death is uncertain, even though at the time of death parents may not appreciate just how much not "having an answer" may preoccupy them in the future. An autopsy is the only opportunity to settle the question of "what really happened". It should be explained that an autopsy does not affect the face and that when clothed the child's appearance will be unaffected. Parents should be given some time to reflect on the benefits for them and their family of an autopsy before making their decision. Physicians asking for an autopsy should recognize that it is something that may help bring some closure to a family and is in the family's best interest. If there is any question of a genetically transmitted disease the results of the autopsy may affect the health of future siblings and generations. For these reasons, even if parents initially reject an autopsy because they feel their child has suffered enough, time should be taken to explain again the potential benefits.

Most institutions have a forum for the team to review morbidities and mortalities that happened in the unit. These reviews are often oriented around medical issues pertaining to pathology and symptom control and lessons for the future. They also offer the opportunity to look at the psychological impact of deaths on the families and the health-care professionals. They also allow staff not on duty at the time of the child's death to be brought up to date and understand the full circumstances surrounding the death and to ask questions and consider unresolved issues.

After a child dies there are a number of ways to commemorate the child. Staff may write messages for the family in a card that can be sent to the family in the following weeks. This also gives staff that were absent at the time of death the opportunity to offer their condolences to the family. Staff may also wish to create a "communication book" for the PICU in which those who were present at the time of the death can write down what happened as well as their thoughts and feelings about the child. All who knew the child or family can contribute. There may be a memorial book in the PICU, chapel or elsewhere in the hospital, and families may wish to co-design a commemorative page in the book. Offering parents different options on how to commemorate their child who died in the PICU can also help avoid the creation of a large "memorial wall of plaques" in the PICU that parents of other temporarily hospitalized children may find uncomfortable.

The family needs to be informed of the many different forms of bereavement support available from the hospital or in the community. In addition, all relevant health professionals in the hospital and community need to be informed of the child's death.

Families are usually appreciative of staff being present at the child's funeral. Additionally some units hold memorial services for children who have recently died. Staff and family attendance and participation can help them cope with the child's death, and is an opportunity for staff who were unable to say goodbye to the family after the child's death to also find some closure [12].

The senior physician may see the family a few weeks after the child's death. This meeting provides an opportunity to review events in the PICU and address any unanswered questions about their child's care. Some parents may appreciate telling the "story" one more time to the doctor who was involved with their child's life at such a vulnerable time, and allows misconceptions to be addressed. If an autopsy was performed this will need to be reviewed together with an explanation of the significance of its findings. It also allows the physician to review how the family is coping with their bereavement and if additional assistance might be beneficial [13].

Many families welcome bereavement follow-up from a health-care professional who knew the family in the PICU. Providing family counseling requires both training and ongoing support for those who participate in the often-difficult phone calls and meetings with the bereaved family in the subsequent year or two. Important times to make contact with the family include the child's birthday, anniversary of the death, and important religious and other holiday periods.

Acknowledgements
Specified excerpts from "Integrating Pediatric Palliative Care into the PICU" by Liben S. in "Oxford Handbook of ICU and Palliative Care", edited by Rocker G. et al. (2009), Oxford University Press, with permission, and from "Pediatric Palliative Care" by Liben S. (Chapter 10, Section 2, pp.431-440) in "Palliative Care Core Skills and Clinical Competencies", edited by Emanuel L., Librach L. (2007), Saunders Elsevier, with permission.

References

1. Dunstan GR (1985) Hard questions in intensive care. A moralist answers questions put to him at a meeting of the Intensive Care Society, Autumn, 1984. Anaesthesia 40:479–482
2. Arias Y, Taylor DS, Marcin JP (2004) Association between evening admissions and higher mortality rates in the pediatric intensive care unit. Pediatrics 113:e530–e534
3. Field MJ, Behrman RE (eds) (2003) when children die: improving palliative and end-of-life care for children and their families. Chapter 2. Committee on Palliative and End-of-Life Care for Children and Their Families, Institute of Medicine. The National Academies Press, Washington DC
4. Garros D, Rosychuk RJ, Cox P (2003) Circumstances surrounding end of life in a pediatric intensive care unit. Pediatrics 112:e371–e379
5. Garros D (2003) A "good" death in pediatric ICU: is it possible?. J Pediatr (Rio J) 79 [Suppl 2]:S243–S254
6. European Association for Palliative Care (2007) IMPaCCT: standards for paediatric palliative care in Europe. Steering Committee of the EAPC task force on palliative care for children and adolescents. Eur J Palliative Care 14:109–114
7. Contro N, Larson J, Scofield S, et al (2002) Family perspectives on the quality of pediatric palliative care. Arch Pediatr Adolesc Med 156:14–19
8. Hawryluck LA, Harvey WR, Lemieux-Charles L, Singer PA (2002) Consensus guidelines on analgesia and sedation in dying intensive care unit patients. BMC Med Ethics 3:E3
9. Meyer EC, Burns JP, Griffith JL, Truog RD (2002) Parental perspectives on end-of-life care in the pediatric intensive care unit. Crit Care Med 30:226–231
10. Craig F, Goldman A (2003) Home management of the dying NICU patient. Semin Neonatol 8:177–183
11. von Gunten C, Weissman DE (2003) Ventilator withdrawal protocol. J Palliat Med 6:773–776
12. Macdonald ME, Liben S, Carnevale FA, et al (2005) Parental perspectives on hospital staff acts of kindness and commemoration after a child's death. Pediatrics 116:884–890
13. Macnab AJ, Northway T, Ryall K, et al (2003) Death and bereavement in a paediatric intensive care unit: parental perceptions of staff support. Paediatr Child Health 8:357–362

Chapter 19

Chronic Pain Management: Organization, Techniques and Guidelines

Joëlle Desparmet

Introduction

Chronic pain is a significant problem in the pediatric population. It is estimated that it affects 15% to 20% of children at some point in their life. Abdominal pain, recurrent chest pain, complex regional pain syndromes (CRPS), musculoskeletal pain and diffuse widespread pain are just a few examples of chronic pain in children. Chronic pain is defined as pain persisting beyond a period of time in which an initial injury would be expected to heal, usually but not necessarily 3 to 6 months. A good example is severe pain occurring a few weeks after a fracture. This could be CRPS type I (previously known as reflex sympathetic dystrophy, or RSD) where the fracture is clinically healed but the patient suffers from intense burning pain in the limb. Chronic pain sometimes occurs in the absence of an identifiable injury or causal event as is the case in myofascial pain and fibromyalgia [1]. Chronic pain can also occur during life-long diseases such as sickle cell anemia, diabetes or juvenile arthritis, to name but a few.

Chronic pain has social, emotional, psychological [2, 3], mental and spiritual repercussions for the child. Marni Jackson, the author of *Pain, the fifth vital sign* compared chronic pain to the toxic spill of oil by a tanker at sea, "which spreads far beyond the original site". The child decreases or ceases school attendance, withdraws from his friends and social activities and feels peers and family do not understand him. Some children show their despair to the point of having clinical depression or suicidal ideation. Chronic pain also often has an impact on the family and the disruption to everyone's life is sometimes dramatic. The child's life, and often his family's, is on hold until the pain goes away at a crucial time of physical, social, intellectual and spiritual development.

The pain's primary impact on the child is a reduction in physical activity. This in turn will increase the degree of pain. There are three hallmarks of the degree of impact of chronic pain on a child's life: impairment, disability and handicap. *Impairment* refers to the original primary pain complaint with the vicious cycle of pain–inactivity–more pain–more inactivity. An example of impairment is diffuse widespread pain. This soon leads to *disability*. The child

M. Astuto (ed), *Basics*, Anesthesia, Intensive Care and Pain in Neonates and Children.
ISBN 978-88-470-0654-6 © Springer-Verlag Italia 2009

is unable to function physically in an age-appropriate way due to the pain. A previously active child stops participating in sports at school or playing with his friends, refuses to attend school because of pain and may end up sitting on a couch in front of a television set or a computer game all day. He becomes physically and emotionally isolated from his peers from family members. With time the psychological and mental consequences of this disability results in a *handicap*. The child is unable to function normally in his usual environment be it at school, with his friends, in his family setting and in life in general. The child may have major sleep disturbances that will further prevent him for having normal daily activities due to fatigue. He/she may have feelings of hopelessness or despair and may withdraw totally. Because a child is a developing human being, chronic pain can further prevent him from reaching normal developmental stages and thus keep him from reaching his full potential.

This description of the impact of pain on a child's life demonstrates the absolute necessity for the management of pain in children to be multidisciplinary and to address the physical, emotional, familial and social aspects of pain. Early and vigorous treatment is warranted to prevent a simple impairment from evolving into a disability or a handicap. In the case of a child with chronic pain, the principal goal of pain management is return to normal function rather than an absolute resolution of the pain. A child may return to school with residual pain but the normalization of function will lead to the further progressive reduction of pain.

Organization

The recommendations of the International Association for the Study of Pain (IASP) [4] and the American Society of Anesthesiologists (ASA) [5] concerning chronic pain clinic programs stipulate that they must be multidisciplinary, have a core team with at least one physician, and have access to other health-care professionals such as a psychologist, psychiatrist, physiotherapist and various other consultants. Many pediatric chronic pain clinics have a structure in which patients meet with different specialists on the same day in order to have a comprehensive initial evaluation [6, 7]. At the Montreal Children's Hospital, we use a simultaneous interview technique (SIT) [8] by which all members of the team see the patient together in the clinic. Between clinic visits, the patients attend therapy sessions in the Physiotherapy and Psychology Departments, and the team discusses the progress of all the patients weekly. Our core team consists of a physician, a physiotherapist, a psychologist and a nurse practitioner who provides counseling for the family and coordinates care.

Unlike an adult, a child relies on his parents to make decisions about his care; nevertheless, every effort should be made to involve him as much as possible. Additionally, for a child, the most influential life models are his parents and their beliefs about pain and their personal stress are major factors in how he will "live" his pain. This is why the whole family must be part of the treatment team and must be listened to, assisted, and involved in the care of their child. It takes a convinced parent to convince a child to continue long treatments.

Children and adolescents are not small adults. They have specific pain syndromes, so that the management of chronic pain in children differs from that in adults. Specific training in pediatric chronic pain is recommended. It is important when setting up a chronic pain clinic to secure a large enough room for patients, families and all members of the team. Trainees should be able to follow the interviews in an adjacent room with a one-way mirror. One should also have a facility in which to do blocks. Children are usually sedated or anesthetized for these blocks and access to a fully equipped operating room or equivalent is mandatory. Some blocks are done with the help of fluoroscopic imaging, and this should be available.

Techniques

Assessment

The management of chronic pain in children starts with a thorough assessment, which must include the history and characteristics of the pain, previous treatments and laboratory tests and their results as well as previous medical and surgical history. This initial assessment must also explore the impact of the pain on the child's life, specifically with regard to sleep disturbances, school attendance and socialization with friends, and the impact on the entire family. The family situation and possible stresses that can influence the pain should be determined, so that they can later be addressed by the psychologist and social workers if needed. The child's affect and interaction with team members and with his family during the interview are important clues to the impact of the pain on the child.

Finally, great care should be given to the discovery of beliefs pertaining to pain of the child and his family. Constraining beliefs are those that hinder progress. An example would be the belief that because the neighbor's best friend's child had the same pain, "my child will have this all his life too". A facilitating belief is one that helps progress for instance, "I know that all the tests are normal, so I will surely get better". This is an important step in the assessment because, in order to progress, one must create a context for changing beliefs by establishing trust and by challenging, altering and modifying constraining beliefs while identifying, affirming and solidifying facilitating beliefs. In our clinic, this initial assessment lasts one hour.

The physical examination should be general first and then more targeted to the painful area. It evaluates the pain and its impact on overall function including general condition, gait, posture, range of movement, and strength. It then concentrates on the particular area or areas of pain by careful and methodical visual examination and palpation and a measure of pain at rest and during mobilization. A neurological examination should be included to determine the impact on neuromuscular function and the main neurological systems.

Diagnosis

The diagnosis of the chronic pain syndrome is based on the results of the interview and the examination. It is essential to explain in easily understandable
terms the diagnosis, and what prognosis can be expected. Often the child and the
family have consulted many specialists before arriving at the pain clinic. They
may have misunderstood or misinterpreted what they were told during an often
too-brief visit in an overcrowded clinic. Sometimes, having found no obvious
cause of the pain, the physician expressed doubt as to the very existence of the
pain. It is when giving feedback to the patient and his family about his condition
that trust can be established and no effort should be spared to answer all questions, no matter how insignificant.

In children and adolescents the most common types of chronic pain are musculoskeletal pain secondary to trauma, an inflammatory process or a tumor,
headaches and migraines, recurrent abdominal pain, CRPS, pain of sickle cell
disease, neuropathic pain secondary to chemotherapy or a neurological disease,
and phantom limb pain. McGrath et al. [9] found that the majority of children
followed in their chronic pain clinic had either limb pain (4–33%) or abdominal
pain (6–15%) or nonmigraine headaches (6–29%), or a combination of these
pain problems. The different pain syndromes seen in our clinic in during 2006
are shown in Table 19.1. Figure 19.1 shows the steady progression of the number of patients referred to our clinic. It demonstrates the increase in trust in the
multidisciplinary approach to the management of chronic pain in the pediatric
population and the need for it.

Table 19.1 Pain syndromes treated in our clinic in 2006

Syndrome	Percent of total cases
Headache	20
Recurrent abdominal pain	15
Widespread diffuse pain (WDP)	30
Musculoskeletal pain	10
Complex regional pain syndrome	5
Chronic cancer pain and postchemotherapy pain	4
Neuropathic pain	10
Phantom limb pain	1
Post trauma pain	1
Disease-related pain	4

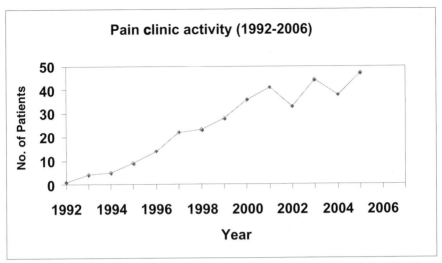

Fig. 19.1 Increase in the number of new patients per year referred to the Chronic Pain Clinic

CRPS

CRPS type 1 was previously known as RSD or Sudeck's atrophy. A lower extremity is more frequently involved in children, and girls are more often affected than boys [10–12]. There are physical signs of neuropathic involvement (burning pain, allodynia, hyperesthesia, numbness) and signs of autonomic dysfunction (swelling, sweating, mottling, temperature and skin color changes). The initial cause of the pain cannot be attributed to a specific nerve lesion and the distribution of the pain is in a sock or glove pattern. Sympathetic involvement is not consistently found but may be a contributing factor in the persistence of the clinical signs [13]. The syndrome typically evolves in three phases. During the acute phase, the limb is warm and red and the pain is nonspecific. The second, or dystrophic, phase the limb changes color from one day to another, alternating between red and hot to mottled or blue and cold, and the pain is burning. During the final, or atrophic, phase the limb remains cold and mottled, the pain is intense and there is dystonia and motor weakness. During this late stage there is also hyperhidrosis and trophic changes (nails and hair). However, these stages are not always distinguishable from one another, and the child may present with muscle atrophy and motor weakness at the first visit to the pain clinic if the syndrome was not previously recognized. After an original improvement, a few recurrent episodes can occur, but the prognosis is better in children than adults and total resolution is expected.

The diagnosis is generally based on clinical findings and additional investigations such as radiographic imaging are rarely contributory.

Treatment modalities include intense physiotherapy, short prescriptions analgesics such as nonsteroidal anti-inflammatory drugs or minor opioids longer-term medications for neuropathic pain such as tricyclic antidepressants and anticonvulsants. Transcutaneous electrical stimulation (TENS) can help reduce the pain in some cases [12]. If the pain is too severe to perform efficient physiotherapy, an intravenous, peripheral or central block is done [14, 15].

CRPS type II, also known as causalgia, results from the injury of a specific nerve or plexus. The clinical signs and treatment approach are similar to those of CRPS type I, but the prognosis is often dependent on the gravity of the nerve lesion. CRPS type III, or myofascial pain, also known as fibromyalgia, is more diffuse and less specific in children. Instead of the classical 18 trigger points, palpation reveals diffuse pain. Children report having "pain all over". The children also often complain of fatigue and sleep disturbance. Injection of lidocaine as well as "dry" needling without the local anesthetic into the trigger points have been suggested, but the relief of pain is temporary and the injections often need to be repeated. Children rarely accept multiple injections, and physiotherapy, anticonvulsants and cognitive behavioral therapy often lead to complete remission within a few weeks [16–24].

Headaches

Headaches are a frequent complaint in children referred to a chronic pain clinic. The majority of headaches in children and adolescents are benign. However, the most common causes of headaches seen in an emergency room are infections, migraine, tension and intracranial abnormalities [25, 26].

Migraine is characterized by episodic headaches separated by pain-free intervals. The prevalence of headaches is between 3% and 50% depending on age. The International Headache Society requires certain criteria for the diagnosis of migraine. Headaches should last 4 to 72 hours, and have two of the following characteristics: unilateral, pulsating, moderate to severe intensity, worsened by activity and be accompanied by nausea and/or vomiting, photophobia and/or sonophobia. There should be at least five attacks that fulfill these criteria and there should be no underlying organic disease.

In 70% of patients, there is a family history of migraine and a personal history of motion sickness. Certain foods can trigger attacks, and anxiety, stress and fatigue are often factors. Tension headaches are most frequently seen after puberty. They differ from migraine in that they are diffuse and symmetrically distributed, have a gradual onset and nausea and vomiting are usually absent. School or family-related stress is a common feature. Psychological issues should ⁀ine if psychological intervention is indicated.

ain

↑ (RAP) is defined as three or more bouts of abdominal eriod severe enough to interfere with a child's normal activity. RAP will be experienced by 10–15% of children at some point. Functional abdominal pain is by far the most common cause of RAP. The cause of RAP is controversial and it is thought that it could be akin to CRPS type I of the intestinal tract or visceral hypersensitivity. Onset often occurs between 5 and 19 years of age. Most episodes last less than an hour and the pain is diffuse and non-specific. Stress may be a factor and the child may have difficulty falling asleep due to the pain. Nausea, vomiting, pallor or flushing and palpitations may be associated with the pain. An organic cause to the pain should be ruled out. Reassurance and explanations about the possibility of having abdominal pain without an underlying disease is essential. Psychological interventions are often necessary to improve sleep and decrease stress. Sometimes a short pharmacological treatment with a low-dose antidepressant or an anticonvulsant will prove beneficial [27].

Treatment

A multimodal approach often is more effective than a single sequential treatment approach. Medications, physiotherapy and psychological interventions are prescribed simultaneously as appropriate. Either one of these interventions alone will rarely give results. Education of the patient and the family about the pain, its mechanism and its impact is a major step as it leads to reassurance, trust and compliance.

Medications

Pharmacological treatment is given systemically or regionally. The oral route is recommended rather than the intramuscular route whenever possible. Opioid and nonopioid analgesics can be given for short periods (doses are shown Table 19.2). They should be given only while waiting for the antidepressants or anticonvulsants to take effect. They should be given in conjunction with acetaminophen and/or an NSAID for a synergistic effect.

There are very few studies on the use of antidepressants for pain relief in children although they are commonly used. Antidepressants block the reuptake of noradrenaline and serotonin and block sodium channels. Tricyclic antidepressants inhibit serotonin and norepinephrine reuptake. Selective serotonin reuptake inhibitors (SSRI) are not commonly prescribed in children. Low-dose antidepressants of the tricyclic family are recommended rather than SSRIs due to the latter's side effect profile. Amitriptyline (Elavil) is given if there are sleep disturbances as it has a strong sedative effect. If there are no problems with sleep or if the child becomes too somnolent during the day with amitriptyline, nortriptyline is the preferred antidepressant. For both drugs, one should start with a low dose of 10 mg given at bedtime for 5 to 10 days to see how the patient tolerates the drug. This can be increased to 20 mg at bedtime as needed. Side effects include dry mouth and somnolence.

Table 19.2 Doses of commonly used opioids in chronic pain in children

Drug	Equipotent dose	Dosage
Morphine	1	10–60 mg orally every 4 h
MS Contin		15–100 mg orally
Hydrocodone	1/30–1/8	5–10 mg orally every 4–6 h
Hydromorphone	7	2–4 mg orally every 4–6 h
Codeine	1/30–1/8	0.5 mg/kg orally every 4 h
Methadone	1–3	0.05–0.1 mg/kg orally every 3–4 h
Tramadol	1/8	50–100 mg orally every 4–6 h (max 400 mg/day)

Anticonvulsants bind to calcium channels in the dorsal horn decreasing excitatory neurotransmitters (glutamate, substance P). Anticonvulsants such as gabapentin (Neurontin) and pregabalin (Lyrica) are commonly used for neuropathic pain. Metoclopramide (Tegretol) is indicated in neurogenic pain such as that seen in neurofibromatosis and topiramate (Topomax) in migraine headaches. The most frequent but transient side effects are dizziness, fatigue, tremors, constipation and diarrhea. The side effects can be avoided by starting at a low dose and increasing slowly every 5 to 8 days to effect or side effects. Doses are shown in Table 19.3.

In CRPS type I, mobilization of the affected limb is an essential part of the treatment. If it is impossible to mobilize the affected limb due to the intense pain, a block is done both to enable physiotherapy and to provide a sympathetic block. This can be done as either a central block or a peripheral venous (Bier) block. An algorithm for the treatment of CRPS is presented in Figure 19.2 [28].

Table 19.3 Doses of antidepressants and anticonvulsants for chronic pain

Drug	Dosage
Amitriptyline/nortriptyline	Initial dose: 0.1 mg/kg orally at bedtime Titrate up to 0.50–2 mg/kg every 3–4 weeks by 10-mg increments
Gabapentin	Initial dose: 100 mg orally three times daily Titrate up to 300 mg three times daily in increments of 100 mg three times daily every 5–7 days. Then increase to 800 mg three times daily as needed every 4–6 weeks
Pregabalin	Initial dose: 50 mg orally Increase to 150–300 mg/day as needed
Carbamazepine	Initial dose: 50 mg orally twice daily Titrate up to 100–300 mg twice daily as needed

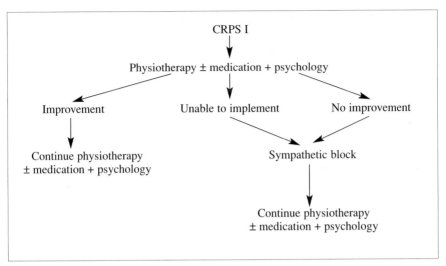

Fig. 19.2 Algorithm for the treatment of CRPS I

Blocks

Central blocks are useful in CRPS type I of the lower extremity, the most frequent site in children. Sympathetic involvement is not consistently found but may be a contributory factor in the persistence of the clinical signs.

Lumbar epidural blocks are the most frequent central blocks used. They can be done as an outpatient procedure under sedation (intravenous midazolam 0.1–0.2 mg/kg) or general anesthesia (nitrous oxide in oxygen with or without sevoflurane, for example) in very anxious children. In any case, the blocks should be done in an operating room, or equivalent, with all safety precautions pertaining to a general anesthetic. The person performing the block should have an assistant who will perform the anesthesia.

The epidural space is accessed at the appropriate vertebral interspace (L3-4 or L4-5). A mixture of equal volumes (0.3–0.5 ml/kg) of lidocaine 1% for quick onset and bupivacaine 0.25% (for long duration) can be used to diagnose and treat CRPS type I of the lower extremity. Temperature monitors are placed on each foot to measure the change in temperature of the affected versus the nonaffected foot. The affected foot is usually colder by 2–4°C than the unaffected foot and the temperatures rise in both feet and equalize within 15–30 minutes. The efficacy of the block is ascertained by the presence of motor and sensory blocks. Passive progressive and controlled manipulation of the foot commences in the postanesthesia care unit (PACU) as soon as tolerated by the patient. When the motor block wears off, the patient is asked to actively mobilize the foot if possible. In severe cases, the child is hospitalized and an epidural catheter is placed for a continuous infusion of a low concentration of local anesthetic (0.05–0.1% bupivacaine or 0.3–0.5% lidocaine) over 4–7 days. This will allow the physiotherapist to provide intense daily passive and active exercises.

Intravenous regional blocks (Bier blocks) have been proposed for the treatment of CRPS types I and II. The use of a number of medications such as guanethidine is described in the literature [29]. Clonidine, ketorolac and bretylium have been studied in adults, but not in children [30–32].

Sympathetic Blocks

Stellate ganglion block is used for the management of CRPS of the upper extremity. The block is most often done under sedation or general anesthesia in children who are under 10 years of age or who are uncooperative.

In the neck, the sympathetic trunks are anterior and lateral to the vertebral column, beginning at the level of C1. These trunks are associated with three cervical sympathetic ganglia: superior, middle and inferior. The inferior cervical ganglion fuses with the first thoracic ganglion to form the stellate ganglion. The stellate ganglion supplies sympathetic innervation to the upper extremity. This star-shaped (*stella*, a star) ganglion lies anterior to the transverse process of C7 just superior to the neck of the first rib on each side and posterior to the origin of the vertebral artery. Injection of 0.2 ml/kg of 0.25% bupivacaine (up to 14 ml) at the site of the stellate ganglion results in a sympathetic block of the ipsilateral upper limb [33].

The block usually results in Horner's syndrome (myosis, ptosis and nasal congestion) due to sympathetic nerve interruption to the head. Because the recurrent laryngeal nerve can also be blocked due to the diffusion of local anesthetic solution, bilateral stellate ganglion blockade is not recommended. Other complications include blockade of the phrenic nerve, partial blockade of the brachial plexus if the needle is too posterior, respiratory insufficiency (following intraspinal injection) or convulsions (following intravascular injection), as well as pneumothorax.

For lumbar sympathetic block, the child is asleep and the procedure is done under fluoroscopy. The lumbar sympathetic ganglia are situated anterior and medial to the lateral border of the second and third lumbar vertebral bodies. Correct needle placement is confirmed by injection of radiocontrast solution which shows the spread of the solution in front of the vertebral bodies. A bolus of 0.4–0.5 mg/kg of 0.1–0.25% bupivacaine is injected in small increments resulting in a rise in skin temperature, and vasodilation in the ipsilateral limb [34].

Physiotherapy

The physiotherapist acts as a coach and trains the patient back to a normal level of function. Rehabilitation and general conditioning rather than pain relief are the goal. Indeed, when a child start moving again, sometimes after months of inactivity, pain increases just as it would in an athlete who has not trained in a while. Certain techniques such as laser and ultrasound are used to decrease swelling. Hot and cold contrast baths and whirlpool baths desensitize the limbs. A TENS may help as well.

Patients with CRPS types I and II in our clinic benefit from intense physiotherapy, a program developed to provide physiotherapy three to four times a week rather than the standard once a week session used for other conditions. Some centers hospitalize the children for two to three weeks and provide daily physiotherapy, psychological support and family counseling.

Psychological Interventions

Because pain has an impact on a patient's emotional status and emotions such as stress, sadness and fear may change the level of pain and hinder progress, psychological interventions are as important as medications and mobilization in decreasing the pain. Self-hypnosis, relaxation, and stress management techniques all help the patient cope with pain. Sleep disturbances are a constant finding in patients who have chronic pain and changing sleep patterns is essential. Biofeedback, a technique in which the patient trains himself to relax a set of muscles through visualization on a monitor, has been shown to exceed medication in efficacy for the treatment of headaches in children. Dealing with school absenteeism and school avoidance, frequent aspects of prolonged pain, is often necessary. A progressive return to school is implemented as the pain decrease.

Conclusion

Chronic pain has long been unrecognized and undertreated in children. Classically, children were seen by different specialists separately and proper management was delayed or denied because these specialists could not find an organic cause to their pain. Multidisciplinary centers specializing in pediatric chronic pain are increasing in number and provide the best hope for these often misunderstood patients.

Chronic pain affects the whole person and a multidisciplinary approach to its treatment gives the best results. This approach targets the physical, emotional and social aspects of pain. Lack of information leads to fear, and fear increases the pain. Information and reassurance are key. Immobility is the worst enemy of a patient in pain and a comprehensive physiotherapy program is an important part of the treatment.

References

1. Sherry DD, McGuire T, Mellins E et al (1991) Psychosomatic musculoskeletal pain in childhood: clinical and psychological analyses of 100 children. Pediatrics 88:1093–1099

2. Sherry DD, Wallace CA, Kelley C et al (1999) Short- and long-term outcomes of children with complex regional pain syndrome type I treated with exercise therapy. Clin J Pain 15:218–223

3. International Association for the Study of Pain (1990) Desirable characteristics for pain treatment facilities. IASP, Seattle, WA

4. American Society of Anesthesiologists (1997) Practice guidelines for chronic pain management: a report by the American Society of Anesthesiologists Task Force on Pain Management, Chronic Pain Section. Anesthesiology 86:995–1004

5. Berde C, Sethna NF, Masek B et al (1989) Pediatric pain clinics: recommendations for their development. Pediatrician 16:94–102

6. Berde CB, Soloniuk J (2003) Multidisciplinary programs for management of acute and chronic pain in children. In: Schechter N, Berde CB, Yaster M (eds) Pain in infants, children and adolescents, 2nd edn. Lippincott Williams & Wilkins, Philadelphia, pp 472–486

7. Desparmet JF, Aquan-Assee J, Bradley K et al (2000) L'entrevue simultanée dans un centre de douleur chronique pédiatrique. Doul Analg 1:15–19

8. McGrath PA (1999) Chronic pain in children. In: Crombie IK, Croft PR, Linton SJ, LeResche L, Von Korff M (eds) Epidemiology of pain. IASP Press, Seattle, pp 81–101

9. McGrath PA, Ruskin D (2007) Caring for children with chronic pain: ethical considerations. Pediatr Anesth 17:505–508

10. Berde CB, Lebel A (2005) Complex regional pain syndromes in children and adolescents. Anesthesiology 102:252–255

11. Finniss DG, Murphy PM, Brooker C et al (2006) Complex regional pain syndrome in children and adolescents. Eur J Pain 10:767–770

12. Lee BH, Scharff L, Sethna NF et al (2002) Physical therapy and cognitive-behavioural treatment for complex regional pain syndromes. J Pediatr 141:135–140

13. Anthony KK, Schanberg LE (2005) Pediatric pain syndromes and management of pain in children and adolescents with rheumatic disease. Pediatr Clin North Am 52:611–639

14. Wilder RP (1995) Reflex sympathetic dystrophy in children and adolescents: differences from adults. In: Janig W, Stanton-Hicks M (eds) Reflex sympathetic dystrophy: a reappraisal, vol 6. IASP Press, Seattle, pp 67–77

15. Dadure C, Motais F, Ricard C et al (2005) Continuous peripheral nerve blocks at home for treatment of recurrent complex regional pain syndrome I in children. Anesthesiology 102:387–391

16. Reid GJ, McGrath PJ, Lang BA (2005) Parent-child interactions among children with juvenile fibromyalgia, arthritis, and healthy controls. Pain 113:201–210

17. Conte PM, Walco GA, Kimura Y (2003) Temperament and stress response in children with juvenile primary fibromyalgia syndrome. Arthritis Rheum 48:2923–2930

18. Imbierowicz K, Egle UT (2003) Childhood adversities in patients with fibromyalgia and somatoform pain disorder. Eur J Pain 7:113–119

19. Brown GT, Delisle R, Gagnon N et al (2001) Juvenile fibromyalgia syndrome: proposed management using a cognitive-behavioural approach. Phys Occup Ther Pediatr 21:19–36

20. Gedalia A, Garcia CO, Molina JF et al (2000) Fibromyalgia syndrome: experience in a pediatric rheumatology clinic. Clin Exp Rheumatol 18:415–419

21. Breau LM, McGrath PJ, Ju LH (1999) Review of juvenile primary fibromyalgia and chronic fatigue syndrome. J Dev Behav Pediatr 20:278–288

22. Mikkelsson M (1999) One-year outcome of preadolescents with fibromyalgia. J Rheumatol 26:674–682

23. Clark P, Burgos-Vargas R, Medina-Palma C et al (1998) Prevalence of fibromyalgia in children: a clinical study of Mexican children. J Rheumatol 25:2009–2014

24. Siegel DM, Janeway D, Baum J (1998) Fibromyalgia syndrome in children and adolescents: clinical features at presentation and status at follow-up. Pediatrics 101(3 Pt 1):377–382

25. Lewis DW (2001) Headache in the pediatric emergency department. Semin Pediatr Neurol 8:46–51

26. Burton LG, Quinn B, Pratt JL et al (1997) Headache etiology in a pediatric emergency department. Pediatr Emerg Care 13:1–4 .

27. Di Lorenzo C, Youssef NN, Sigurdson L et al (2001) Visceral hyperalgesia in children with functional abdominal pain. J Pediatr 139:838–843
28. Wilder RT, Berde CB, Woholan M et al (1992) Reflex sympathetic dystrophy in children. Clinical characteristics and follow-up in seventy patients. J Bone Joint Surg Am 74:910–919
29. Rosenblatt R, Pepitone-Rockwell F, McKillop MJ (1979) Continuous axillary analgesia for traumatic hand injury. Anesthesiology 51:565–566
30. Maneksha FR, Mirza H, Poppers PJ (2000) Complex regional pain syndrome (CRPS) with resistance to local anesthetic block: a case report. J Clin Anesth 12:67–71
31. Jadad AR, Carroll D, Glynn CJ et al (1995) Intravenous regional sympathetic blockade for pain relief in reflex sympathetic dystrophy: a systematic review and a randomized, double-blind crossover study. J Pain Symptom Manage 10:13–20
32. Kaplan R, Claudio M, Kepes E et al (1996) Intravenous guanethidine in patients with reflex sympathetic dystrophy. Acta Anaesthesiol Scand 40:1216–1222
33. Lunn R, Sethna N, Berde C et al (1989) Stellate ganglion blockade in infants and children. Anesthesiology 71:A1023
34. Wilder RT (2002) Regional anesthetic techniques for chronic pain management in children. In: Schecter NL, Berde CB, Yaster M (eds) Pain in infants, children, and adolescents, 2nd edn. Lippincott Williams & Wilkins, Baltimore, pp 396–416

Subject Index

Acetaminophen 23, 178, 179, 247
Acute pain 173, 182
Acute Pain Service 173, 177, 181-183
Adrenal gland 151, 156
Adrenal insufficiency in children 156
Adrenergic receptors 5, 180
Airway
    difficult pediatric airway 33-35, 41-43,
      46
    management 31, 32, 42, 72, 188, 192,
      210
Alertness/sedation scale 103
Allergies 76
Amnesia 89, 102, 105
Anesthesia
    a.-related adverse events 71
    level of a., 103
    outside the operating room 185
    regional a. 105, 113, 116, 117, 120, 121,
      123, 130, 144, 181
Anticonvulsants 189, 237, 246-248
Antidepressant 247
Antidiuretic hormone 143, 153
Antifibrinolytics 168
Anxiety 9, 12-15, 86-88, 105, 189, 208, 210,
    246
Aprotinin 168
Ascending arousal system 102, 104
Asthma and bronchial hyperreactivity 75

Bispectral index 107
Bloodstream infection 61, 62
Blood substitutes 139
Blood transfusion 138, 139
Bupivacaine 25, 116-120, 125-128, 181,
    249, 250

Carriage 64, 138, 216-218, 225-228
Central venous catheter 49, 50, 53, 57
Cerebral state index 108
Child
    difficult child 11, 15
Clonidine 25, 116, 117, 119, 120, 121, 127,
    180, 182, 190, 250
Clowns 14, 86
Complications 7, 31, 33, 34, 46, 51-54, 57,
    77, 80, 91, 93, 96, 116, 117, 123, 125, 127,
    130, 141, 151, 158, 162, 166, 173, 178,
    186, 189, 198-202, 237, 250
    infections 200
Consciousness 76, 102, 105-109, 187, 233
Corticosteroid replacement in the pediatric
    intensive care unit 157
Cricothyrotomy 36, 199
Critical care 8, 138, 158, 236

Depth monitoring of anesthesia 104
Diabetes 77, 78, 174, 241
Diagnosis of acute adrenal insufficiency 157
Distraction 14
Drug
    formulations 23
    licensed drugs 19, 20
    off-label drugs 19, 20, 22, 23, 25
    unlicensed drugs 25

Electrocardiogram 101, 104-109, 166, 167
EMLA 93, 175
End-of-life care 232
Enteral antimicrobials 54
Entropy 107
Environment 12, 15, 73, 85-89, 102, 142,
    166, 203, 207-209, 223, 235, 238, 242

Epidural analgesia 116, 117
Exogenous 61, 63, 64, 1155, 215, 218, 219, 222-226

Family 11, 13, 15, 16, 72, 73, 77, 85-87, 197, 207-210, 232, 234-239, 241-244, 246, 247, 251
Fasting 6, 77-80, 135, 136, 144, 189, 190
Fentanyl 25, 88, 120, 164, 165, 179, 181, 190
Fluid balance 144, 146, 168
Food and Drug Administration 20, 107, 108
Functional residual capacity 4, 77

Glomerular filtration 6
Glucose 6, 54, 78, 126, 140, 141, 144, 146, 152

Headaches 244, 246, 248, 251
Heart murmurs 76
Hygiene 54, 63, 64, 215, 217, 223, 225, 226
Hyoid bone 31, 35, 197
Hypnosis 14, 88, 89, 105, 107, 191, 251
Hyponatremia 143-145, 155, 156
Hypothalamic adrenal axis 151

Iliohypogastric nerve block 117, 130
Ilioinguinal and iliohypogastric nerve block 115-117, 130
Immature respiratory control 4
Induction 13-15, 33, 41, 42, 44, 79, 85-97, 108, 136, 144, 164, 190
Infection mortality 224
Inpatient procedures 79
Intensive care 22-24, 43, 46, 49, 51, 61, 62, 66, 109, 110, 135, 138, 142, 154, 156-158, 168-170, 174, 205, 206, 209, 215, 224, 231, 23, 235-237, 240
Intravenous cannula 89-91, 93, 96
Intravenous induction 41, 87, 90, 93, 95, 97, 190

Ketamine 42, 88, 89, 94, 120, 121, 164, 165, 173, 180, 182, 190

Levobupivacaine 116, 119, 125, 126, 128
Licensing process 19, 20
Long-term steroid treatment 78
Lumbar blocks 118

Macroglossia, crycoid cartilage 3
Meta-analysis 33, 65, 157
Midazolam 14, 88, 89, 92, 94, 120, 121, 165, 190, 249
Monitoring 23, 39, 49, 73, 85, 90, 91, 93, 95, 101, 102, 106, 107, 109, 113, 118, 127, 144, 146, 161, 165, 166, 171, 182, 186, 207, 208
Multidisciplinary approach 11, 244, 251

Narcotrend 108
Near infrared spectroscopy 166
Negative intrathoracic pressure 4
Neonates 3-8, 21, 33, 55, 90, 105, 113-120, 126-128, 130, 139, 154, 157, 158, 162, 169, 174-176, 178, 205, 210, 215, 232, 237
Neurological diseases 77
Neuromonitoring 166, 167, 170
Nitric oxide 165
NSAIDs 173, 179, 180

Obesity 77, 78, 179
Off-patent medicines 20
Off-site sedation 185
Opioids 102, 117, 173, 178-182, 190, 245, 248

Pain 7, 11, 12, 15, 79, 80, 89, 90, 93, 95, 105, 113, 116, 117, 119, 143, 153, 173-183, 189, 232, 233, 236, 241-251
Palliative care 231-237, 240
Paravenous infusion 95
Parenteral antimicrobials 64
Parental presence 13, 14, 87, 88, 93, 191
Pediatric
    airways 3
    anesthesiologist 16, 90, 95
    care 12
    critical illness 151, 157, 158
    drug formulation 23-25
    intensive care 22, 24, 51, 66, 110, 135, 138, 154, 156-158, 174, 205, 206, 215, 231, 232
    intensive care unit 66, 135, 215, 217-219, 222, 224, 227, 231, 232, 234, 237, 239
    pain scale 177
    palliative care 231, 235

sedation 188
Tracheotomy Teams 209
Percutaneous tracheotomy 199
Perioperative information 12
Peripheral nerve blocks 115, 130
Pharmacological premedication 14, 88
Physical restraint 16
Plasma expanders 138, 141
Postoperative apnea 4, 80
Post-tracheotomy stenosis 198
Premedication 13, 14,85-89, 93, 180
Preoperative evaluation 71, 72, 79, 161
Preoperative period 11
Primary endogenous 63, 64, 215, 218, 222, 224, 225
Propofol 25, 42, 43, 93-96, 106, 107, 109, 164, 190
Pulmonary hypertension 34, 76, 162, 165

Rapid Response Systems 209
Rapid sequence induction 91, 96, 136
Recurrent abdominal pain 244, 246
Regional anesthesia 105, 113, 116, 117, 120, 121, 123, 130, 144, 181
Regional blocks 117, 181, 250
Resistance 4, 37, 50, 90, 121, 122, 143, 152, 154, 164, 165, 226, 227
Respiratory muscles 4, 32
Risk group 209, 210
Ropivacaine 116, 117, 119, 120, 125, 126, 128, 181
Routine laboratory testing 81

Secondary endogenous 64, 215, 218, 222-224, 226
Sedation 42, 43, 101-103, 105, 108-110, 120, 121, 142, 180-182, 185-192, 223, 249, 250
Selective digestive decontamination 54
Sevoflurane 42, 43, 81, 89-92, 164, 180, 190, 249
Single-breath vital capacity technique 92
Speaking valve 204, 205
Starling response 5, 6
Steroids treatment in pediatric ICU 157
Stress dose of steroids in children 155
Subgroup analysis 209, 210
Suggestion 14, 87, 89
Surgery 6, 7, 12, 14, 15, 34, 39, 41, 43, 71-73, 75, 76, 78-80, 85, 88, 90, 96, 115, 117, 119, 122, 123, 125, 130, 138, 140-142, 144, 153-156, 161, 162, 165, 166, 168, 170, 173-176, 178, 180, 185, 204, 217, 224, 225, 228, 231
Surveillance cultures 63, 64, 216-219, 224
Sympathetic blocks 250

Thoracic block 115, 118, 122
Tidal volume 4, 92
Tracheal incision 198
Tracheostomy 200, 202-205, 209, 226
Tracheotomy 44, 197-210
Transacral block 118, 122, 123
Transcranial Doppler 166
Troposmia 89
Tubular function 6

Ultrasonography 55, 56, 130
Upper respiratory tract infections 74, 75

Ventilator support 197, 237, 238
Ventricular assist device 169

Printed in October 2008